COGNITIVE THERAPY WITH
CHILDREN AND ADOLESCENTS

COGNITIVE THERAPY WITH CHILDREN AND ADOLESCENTS

A Casebook for Clinical Practice

SECOND EDITION

Edited by
MARK A. REINECKE
FRANK M. DATTILIO
ARTHUR FREEMAN

Foreword by Aaron T. Beck

THE GUILFORD PRESS
New York   London

©2003 The Guilford Press
A Division of Guilford Publications, Inc.
72 Spring Street, New York, NY 10012
www.guilford.com

Printed in the United States of America

This book is printed on acid-free paper.

Last digit is print number: 9 8 7 6 5 4 3 2 1

Library of Congress Cataloging-in-Publication Data

Cognitive therapy with children and adolescents : a casebook for
clinical practice / edited by Mark A. Reinecke, Frank M. Dattilio, Arthur
Freeman.— 2nd ed.
      p. cm.
Includes bibliographical references and index.
   ISBN 1-57230-853-2
  1. Cognitive therapy for children. 2. Cognitive therapy for
teenagers. 3. Cognitive therapy for children—Case studies. 4.
Cognitive therapy for teenagers—Case studies. I. Reinecke, Mark A.
II. Dattilio, Frank M. III. Freeman, Arthur M.
RJ505.C63 C65 2003
618.92'89142—dc21

                                              2002015671

About the Editors

Mark A. Reinecke, PhD, ABPP, ACT, is Associate Professor and Chief of the Division of Psychology at Northwestern University's Feinberg School of Medicine. He is a Distinguished Fellow and former president of the Academy of Cognitive Therapy, and is a diplomate of the American Board of Professional Psychology. Dr. Reinecke's research and clinical interests include childhood depression and suicide, cognitive and social vulnerability for depression, and cognitive mediation of adjustment to chronic illness.

Frank M. Dattilio, PhD, ABPP, ACT, is Clinical Associate Professor in the Department of Psychiatry at Harvard University Medical School; Clinical Associate in Psychiatry at the Center for Cognitive Therapy, University of Pennsylvania School of Medicine; and Clinical Director of the Center for Integrative Psychotherapy in Allentown, Pennsylvania. Dr. Dattilio is a Fellow of the Academy of Cognitive Therapy and the American Board of Professional Psychology. His research and clinical interests include marital and family therapy, crisis management, and cognitive-behavioral treatment of anxiety disorders.

Arthur Freeman, EdD, ABPP, ACT, is Professor and Chair of the Department of Psychology at the Philadelphia College of Osteopathic Medicine. He has been the president of the Association for Advancement of Behavior Therapy and is a Fellow of the Academy of Cognitive Therapy and the American Board of Professional Psychology. Dr. Freeman's research and clinical interests include marital and family therapy, and cognitive-behavioral treatment of depression, anxiety, and personality disorders.

Contributors

Anne Marie Albano, PhD, is Assistant Professor of Psychiatry at the New York University School of Medicine, where she is on the faculty of the NYU Child Study Center. Dr. Albano completed her doctorate in clinical psychology at the University of Mississippi and is a Fellow of the Academy of Cognitive Therapy. Her clinical and research interests center on anxiety and mood disorders among children.

Arthur D. Anastopoulos, PhD, is Professor of Psychology at the University of North Carolina at Greensboro. He received his doctorate in clinical psychology from Purdue University. Dr. Anastopoulos's clinical and research interests center on the assessment and treatment of attention-deficit/hyperactivity disorder among children, adolescents, and adults.

Arnold E. Andersen, MD, is Professor of Psychiatry at the University of Iowa College of Medicine. He received his medical degree from Cornell University, and is a diplomate of the American Board of Psychiatry and Neurology. His clinical interests center on developing integrative treatment strategies for eating disorders. The author of over 200 publications, his research focuses on medical complications, cultural factors, gender differences, neurological and neuropsychological concomitants, and vulnerability for eating disorders.

Dean W. Beebe, PhD, is Assistant Professor of Clinical Pediatrics at Children's Hospital Medical Center in Cincinnati, Ohio. He received his doctorate in clinical psychology from Loyola University Chicago. Dr. Beebe completed an internship in clinical psychology at the University of Chicago, and a postdoctoral fellowship in pediatric neuropsychology at Children's Hospital Medical Center.

Wayne A. Bowers, PhD, is Professor of Psychiatry at the University of Iowa College of Medicine. He completed his doctorate at the University of Iowa. Dr. Bowers is a Fellow of the Academy of Cognitive Therapy and a diplomate in behavioral psychology of the American Board of Professional Psychology. His clinical and research interests center on cognitive-behavioral therapy for eating disorders.

Kathy L. Bradley-Klug, PhD, is Assistant Professor of School Psychology at the University of South Florida. She completed her doctorate in school psychology at Lehigh University. Her clinical and research interests center on remediation of academic skills deficits.

Rebecca Burwell is a graduate student in clinical child psychology at the University of Denver. She completed her master's degree in social and developmental psychology at Cambridge University.

John F. Curry, PhD, is Assistant Professor of Psychiatry and Behavioral Sciences at Duke University. He received his doctorate in clinical psychology from Catholic University of America, and is a diplomate of the American Board of Professional Psychology and a Fellow of the American Psychological Association. His clinical and research interests center on adolescent depression and substance abuse.

Frank M. Dattilio, PhD (see "About the Editors").

Esther Deblinger, PhD, is Associate Professor of Clinical Psychiatry and Clinical Director of the Center for Children's Support at the University of Medicine and Dentistry of New Jersey. She received her doctorate from the State University of New York at Stony Brook. Her clinical and research interests center on the treatment of traumatized and abused children.

David L. DuBois, PhD, is Associate Professor of Community Health Sciences at the University of Illinois at Chicago. He received his doctorate in clinical–community psychology from the University of Illinois and completed an internship in clinical child psychology at the University of Chicago. Dr. DuBois's research interests include risk and resilience among children and adolescents and the role of the self system in adaptation.

Norman B. Epstein, PhD, is Professor of Family Studies at the University of Maryland. He received his doctorate from UCLA and is a Fellow of the Academy of Cognitive Therapy and the American Psychological Association. Dr. Epstein is widely published, and his clinical and research interests center on the assessment and treatment of couples and family problems.

Kay Evans, RN, MA, is a clinical nursing specialist at the University of Iowa Hospitals and Clinics. She completed both her undergraduate and graduate degrees at the University of Iowa. Her clinical interests center on the treatment of patients with eating disorders.

Robert D. Felner, PhD, is a Professor and Director of the School of Education at the University of Rhode Island. He received his doctorate in clinical psychology from the University of Rochester. Dr. Felner has published extensively in the fields of child clinical and community psychology, particularly in the area of prevention initiatives for children and families at risk.

Edna B. Foa, PhD, is Professor of Clinical Psychology and Psychiatry and Director of the Center for the Treatment and Study of Anxiety at the University of Pennsylvania. She received her doctorate in clinical psychology and personality from the University of Missouri and has devoted her academic career to studying the psychopathology and treatment of anxiety disorders. Dr. Foa has been the chair of the Treatment Guidelines Task Force of the International Society for Traumatic Stress Studies and of the DSM-IV Subcommittee for OCD, and is co-chair of the DSM-IV Subcommittee for PTSD. She is the author of over 250 articles and book chapters, and has received numerous awards.

Martin E. Franklin, PhD, is Assistant Professor of Psychiatry at the Center for the Treatment and Study of Anxiety at the University of Pennsylvania School of Medicine. He received his doctorate from Rhode Island University. Dr. Franklin's clinical and research interests center on cognitive-behavioral therapy for obsessive–compulsive disorder, trichotillomania, and social anxiety.

Arthur Freeman, PhD (see "About the Editors").

Lisa M. Gerrard is a graduate student in clinical psychology at the University of North Carolina at Greensboro.

Susan Harter, PhD, is Professor of Psychology and Head of the Developmental Psychology Program at the University of Denver. She received her doctorate from Yale University. Her research centers on the causes, correlates, and consequences of self-esteem among youth.

Anne Hope Heflin, PhD, is Associate Professor at the American School of Professional Psychology, Argosy University, in Washington, DC. She received her doctorate from the University of North Carolina at Chapel Hill. Her clinical and research interests center on children's response to trauma and sexual abuse.

Susan M. Knell, PhD, completed her doctorate at Case Western Reserve University, where she is an Adjunct Assistant Professor of Psychology. She also serves as a staff psychologist in the employee assistance program at Progressive Insurance. Dr. Knell's clinical and research interests center on child psychopathology, play therapy, and cognitive-behavioral therapy with preschool children.

Daniel LeGrange, PhD, is Assistant Professor of Psychiatry at the University of Chicago School of Medicine. He completed his doctorate in psychology at the University of London and postdoctoral fellowships at the Institute of Psychiatry of the University of London and Stanford University Medical School. He is a Fellow of the Academy of Eating Disorders and currently holds an NIMH career development award. Dr. LeGrange's clinical and research interests center on interpersonal, cognitive-behavioral, and family-based treatments of eating disorders.

John E. Lochman, PhD, is Saxon Professor of Psychology at the University of Alabama. He received his doctorate in clinical psychology from the University of Connecticut and is a Fellow of the American Psychological Association. His research interests center on the development and treatment of aggressive and antisocial behavior among youth.

Erika M. Lockerd is a graduate student at the University of Missouri at Columbia.

Cristy Lopez, PhD, is a postdoctoral fellow at the Preventive Intervention Research Center of Arizona State University.

John S. March, MD, MPH, is Professor and Chief of the Division of Child and Adolescent Psychiatry at Duke University Medical School. His clinical and research interests center on anxiety and mood disorders among youth and on clinical trials in pediatric psychiatry. Major accomplishments include successfully rolling his sea kayak.

David F. O'Connell, PhD, is a consulting psychologist with the Caron Foundation. His clinical interests center on cognitive-behavioral therapy for substance abuse.

Dustin A. Pardini is a graduate student in clinical psychology at the University of Alabama.

Gilbert R. Parra is a graduate student at the University of Missouri at Columbia.

Henry O. Patterson, PhD, is Assistant Professor of Psychology and Co-coordinator of the Applied Psychology Program at the Pennsylvania State University–Berks Lehigh Valley Campus. He received his doctorate from Temple University. Dr. Patterson's clinical and research interests center on group dynamics, organizational culture, and leadership.

Mark A. Reinecke, PhD (see "About the Editors").

Andrea Rigby is a graduate student in clinical psychology at the Philadelphia College of Osteopathic Medicine. She holds a master's degree in clinical psychology from Millersville University and a master's degree in education from the Pennsylvania State University.

Susan Risi, PhD, is Assistant Professor in the College of Education at the University of New Mexico. She received her doctorate in clinical psychology from Florida State University and completed a 3-year research fellowship at the University of Chicago. Her clinical and research interests center on autism and severe developmental disabilities.

Christine D. Ruma, MSW, is Coordinator of the Sexual Abuse Treatment Team and Clinical Supervisor at the Child Guidance Center of Greater Cleveland. She specializes in individual, group, and family treatment of children who have been sexually abused.

Moira Rynn, MD, is Medical Director of the Mood and Anxiety Disorders Section at the Hospital of the University of Pennsylvania. Her clinical and research interests center on medications for the treatment of mood and anxiety disorders across the lifespan.

Stephen E. Schlesinger, PhD, serves on the faculty of the Department of Psychiatry and Behavioral Sciences at Northwestern University's Feinberg School of Medicine. He completed his doctorate in clinical psychology at the State University of New York at Stony Brook. His clinical and research interests center on cognitive-behavioral therapy for substance abuse, anxiety, and relationship problems.

Edward S. Shapiro, PhD, is Iacocca Professor of Education and School Psychology at Lehigh University. He received his doctorate from the University of Pittsburgh and is the former editor of *School Psychology Review*. The author of eight books and over 80 articles, his research interests center on assessment and intervention of academic skills problems.

Stephen Shirk, PhD, is Director of the Child Study Center at the University of Denver. He received his doctorate in clinical psychology from the New School for Social Research and completed his internship at the Judge Baker Children's Center and the Children's Hospital in Boston. His research interests center on interpersonal processes in child psychotherapy and child psychopathology.

Foreword

It is quite pleasing to me any time a text on cognitive therapy appears in a second edition. This is particularly important as it signifies that cognitive therapy has continued to grow and be well accepted among mental health professionals throughout the world.

I also am honored that three of my former students are contributing to the continually growing literature on child and adolescent treatment. Drs. Reinecke, Dattilio, and Freeman are all former students of mine through the Center of Cognitive Therapy and the University of Pennsylvania in Philadelphia. Dr. Reinecke, now at Northwestern University's Feinberg School of Medicine, where he is Chief of the Division of Psychology, has proven himself to be an excellent researcher as well as an active practitioner in the field of child and adolescent psychology. Dr. Dattilio worked with me for years at the University of Pennsylvania School of Medicine and also, on occasion, at the Beck Institute in our extramural training program. Dr. Dattilio has many years of experience working with children and adolescents and is known throughout the world for his work in cognitive therapy with couples and families. Dr. Freeman, who served with me as senior staff member at the University of Pennsylvania for 15 years, now continues to train cognitive therapists in Philadelphia and worldwide. He is noted for his clear presentation style, as well as his many fine publications in the field.

During my career, I often have found children and adolescents quite receptive to cognitive therapy, due to its clear and structured approach and to the fact that this age group can be so resilient and impressionable. Cognitive therapy has achieved one of the highest rates of success with children and adolescents according to the outcome data. This success is clearly reflected in the course of this text, which is well supported by the literature.

The various chapters appear right on target, addressing the most critical areas of treatment. Unfortunately, our youth have only become more challenging to work with in recent times, and, therefore, effective treatments are now more critical than ever. Drs. Reinecke, Dattilio, and Freeman, in my opinion, have once again embarked on an ambitious undertaking in assembling a fine composition of important cases in the treatment of children and adolescents. The manner in which the text is organized, with its clear writing style and illuminating case material, allows the reader to sit in on master clinicians at work and obtain a good feel for how the art of cognitive therapy is applied with challenging cases.

This book is destined to become a major reference for students, clinicians, and researchers for years to come. I am confident that its importance will increase over time, as the interest and popularity of cognitive therapy continue to grow.

AARON T. BECK, MD
University Professor of Psychiatry
University of Pennsylvania School of Medicine
The Beck Institute, Philadelphia

Acknowledgments

One might think that compiling a second edition of a text should be easier than the first since there is a fairly solid framework to work from, as well as plenty of opportunities and experiences to reflect on. The fact of the matter is, however, that often a second edition of a text is more difficult than the first, particularly when the first edition was done so well. We have found that the first edition of this text has been a hard act to follow, and our attempts to produce an improved product have certainly required special efforts. Thus, our efforts would not have been possible without the help and support of many. Among the most essential, of course, is our expert typist and coordinator, Ms. Carol Jaskolka, who has been very patient in coordinating numerous texts and helping us with all of the infinite details. In addition, we would like to extend our gratitude to the fine staff of The Guilford Press, particularly our Editor-in-Chief, Seymour Weingarten, whose direction, patience, and guidance have always proven to be an effective ingredient in helping us produce a top-notch reference.

Finally, we thank our spouses and families for their patience with our absences and short attention spans during the preparation of this volume.

MARK A. REINECKE
FRANK M. DATTILIO
ARTHUR FREEMAN

Contents

COGNITIVE THERAPY WITH CHILDREN AND ADOLESCENTS

1

What Makes for an Effective Treatment?

MARK A. REINECKE
FRANK M. DATTILIO
ARTHUR FREEMAN

This volume provides an overview of recent advances in cognitive-behavioral treatments of behavioral and emotional difficulties experienced by youth. Even a cursory review of recent book titles and issues of journals in the fields of child psychiatry and clinical child psychology indicates that cognitive-behavioral approaches have generated considerable clinical and empirical attention over the past several years (Carr, 2000; Friedberg & McClure, 2002; Graham, 1998; Hibbs & Jensen, 1996; Kendall, 2000). Cognitive-behavioral therapy has been successfully applied to a wide range of clinical problems experienced by youth, including depression, anxiety, anger and aggression, eating disorders, learning problems, and autism. Given the breadth of this literature, and the speed with which it has advanced, this seemed an opportune time to review recent empirical, conceptual, and clinical work on cognitive-behavioral psychotherapy with children and adolescents and to describe how these approaches might be used in practice.

Epidemiological research indicates that a significant percentage of youth experience disabling behavioral and emotional difficulties. Although estimates vary depending on the nature of the sample and the methodologies employed, prevalence studies suggest that between 15 and 22% of youth will experience significant adaptive difficulties at some time (Costello, 1989; McCracken, 1992). Unfortunately, the majority of these individuals do not receive effective treatment. This is of particular concern insofar as longitudinal studies indicate that behavioral and emotional difficulties

1

among youth are often recurrent, and can be associated with a significantly increased risk of psychopathology during adulthood (Robins & Rutter, 1990). With these concerns in mind, it becomes important to develop efficient, cost-effective treatments, and to make them available to children and families. It also becomes important to understand factors associated with vulnerability for psychopathology so that effective prevention programs can be developed and implemented.

COGNITIVE-BEHAVIORAL THERAPY WITH YOUTH

Morris and Kratochwill (1991) observed that the child mental health literature is relatively young, and can be traced only to the early 20th century. The use of psychotherapy for treating children and adolescents dates to Freud's (1905/1953) treatment of Dora, an 18-year-old girl suffering from low spirits, headaches, nervous coughing, and social withdrawal. This case is of interest in that Freud's concern was not with Dora's developmental status or the social context in which her concerns arose. Rather, he was interested in elaborating upon his dynamic drive/structure model and in understanding the ways in which this may be expressed through dream content. The importance of adopting a developmental perspective for understanding and treating youth was not recognized until a number of years later. Developmentally and socially focused psychoanalysts during the 1920s and 1930s (including Anna Freud, Harry Stack Sullivan, and Melanie Klein) and those who viewed psychopathology as related to a lack of self-esteem (such as Sandor Rado, Otto Fenichel, and Edward Bibring) anticipated many of the issues confronting cognitive therapy today. The mental hygiene movement and the establishment of child guidance centers during the 1920s contributed to an increased concern for children's emotional development and an awareness of their mental health needs. Although child guidance programs provided clinical services to children and their families, they were not developed with the goal of supporting empirical research into the development of psychopathology or its treatment. The recognition of the value of adopting an objective, empirical approach for assessing, conceptualizing, and treating childhood emotional disorders did not begin to emerge until more recently. Cognitive-behavioral therapy deserves praise, then, for its concern with factors that place individuals at risk for developing behavioral and emotional problems, for its attention to the role of the family and social environment in the development and maintenance of these difficulties, for its attention to tacit beliefs about the self and how these may influence behavioral and emotional adjustment, and for its emphasis on empirically testing models of psychopathology and the effectiveness of interventions derived from them.

Cognitive therapy is founded upon the assumption that behavior is adaptive and that there is an interaction between an individual's thoughts, feelings, and behaviors (Dobson & Dozois, 2001; Freeman & Reinecke, 1995). A major emphasis in cognitive-behavioral therapy with youth is on understanding the development of an individual's behavioral repertoire and the accompanying cognitive and perceptual processes. Cognitions are viewed as an organized set of beliefs, attitudes, memories and expectations, along with a set of strategies for using this body of knowledge in an adaptive manner. As Kendall and Dobson (1993) note, "Cognition is not a singular or unitary concept, but is rather a general term that refers to a complex system" (p. 9). Cognitions refer to one's current thoughts or self-statements, as well as perceptions, memories, appraisals, attributions, tacit beliefs or schemas, attitudes, goals, standards, values, expectations, and images. It can be useful to attend to each of these variables when conceptualizing and treating behavioral and emotional difficulties among youth. The term "cognition" refers not only to cognitive "contents," but also to the ways information is represented in memory and the mediational or control processes by which the information is processed or used.

Cognitions, as such, may be viewed as a set of complex skills (Weimer, 1977) that incorporate problem-solving or coping strategies, communication and linguistically based knowledge, interpersonal skills, and affect regulation capacities. This notion, that cognitions and cognitive processes may be viewed as skills, is conceptually important. It allows us to understand the development and use of these processes and capacities as we would other capacities acquired during childhood (Fogel, 1993; Vygotsky, 1962). It provides a point of contact between the cognitive therapy and developmental psychology literatures. From this perspective, all cognitive development (including the development of maladaptive beliefs and processes) occurs in a social context. It is impossible, then, to draw a line between the cognitive and the social. Cognitive contents and processes are acquired, maintained, and function in social contexts. They are modeled and reinforced by parents and others in the child's community, and serve an adaptive function in organizing and regulating the child's responses to stressful life events. This perspective is consistent with the clinical observation that it can be quite difficult, in practice, to conceptualize and treat clinical problems experienced by children and adolescents without attending to their home environment and peer group. One rarely anticipates that children or adolescents would demonstrate substantially similar behavioral or emotional reactions if there were significant changes in their home environment or social network.

One of the fundamental assumptions of cognitive-behavioral therapy is that cognitions influence emotions and behavior. Children and adolescents, like adults, are believed to respond to cognitive representations of events, rather than to the events themselves. This is an important assumption in that it designates cognitive change as a prerequisite to behavioral and emotional improvement. This is not to say, however, that cognitive factors are necessary or sufficient causes of psychopathology. No single factor appears to "cause" psychopathology in childhood. Rather, research suggests that behavior and adaptation are multiply determined (Rutter, 1989), and that a number of factors interact in contributing to the emergence of behavioral and emotional problems. Biological, genetic, social, cognitive, and environmental factors reciprocally influence one another in placing children at risk for developing behavioral and emotional problems. In a similar manner, there appears to be a range of interpersonal, cognitive and social factors that serve a protective function and ameliorate these risks. As a consequence, some children, when exposed to stressful life events, experience only mild distress, whereas others experience relatively severe adjustment problems. The concept of multifinality, borrowed from the field of developmental psychopathology, captures this notion. Put simply, it refers to the fact that children born with similar conditions, or who are exposed to similar experiences, may demonstrate markedly different outcomes later in life. Our goal is to identify factors that may account for these different outcomes. Our challenge, as clinicians and researchers, is to attempt to understand the ways in which cognitive, biological, and environmental factors interact over time in mediating the emergence of psychopathology during childhood. This task is complicated by the fact that different factors appear to be more or less important at different stages of development, and that specific etiological factors may differ from one form of psychopathology to another. Although we are not suggesting that cognitive factors "cause" psychopathology among youth, strong evidence suggests that there are cognitive and behavioral differences between children who manifest difficulties in adaptation and those who do not (Kendall & MacDonald, 1993). It is these cognitive and behavioral factors that become the focus of our clinical interventions.

Emotional and behavioral responses to events in one's day-to-day life are a influenced by how these events are perceived, the recollection of similar events in the past, attributions that are made about the causes of the event, and the ways in which the events affect one's self-perceptions and the pursuit of one's goals. These cognitive processes are believed to be influenced, in turn, by underlying beliefs that individuals maintain about themselves, the world, and their future. These tacit beliefs or schemas are actively constructed over the course of development, and might be thought of as "lenses" or "templates" guiding the perception, processing, recollection, interpretation, and analysis of incoming information. When children's behavioral or emotional responses to an event are maladaptive—that is, they are inappropriate given the nature or severity of the event or significantly impair the child's social or academic adjustment—it is presumed that they may lack more appropriate cognitive or behavioral skills, or that their beliefs (cognitive contents) or problem-solving capacities (cognitive processes) are in some way disturbed. The latter difficulties may reflect cognitive deficiencies or distortions (Kendall, 2000). "Cognitive deficiencies" refer to the lack of effective cognitive processing, as might be demonstrated by an inattentive child who approaches problems in an impulsive, nonreflective manner. "Cognitive distortions," in turn, refer to beliefs and attitudes founded on irrational or "distorted" logic, as might be manifested by a depressed teenager who systematically minimizes his or her abilities, and who selectively dismisses or overlooks support provided by others. With this in mind, cognitive-behavioral therapists endeavor to assist children and adolescents by facilitating the acquisition of new cognitive and behavioral skills, and by providing children with experiences that will facilitate cognitive change.

COGNITIVE-BEHAVIORAL THERAPY IN PRACTICE

Therapy most often begins with a careful assessment of factors contributing to the child's behavioral and emotional difficulties. This typically involves collection of objective and subjective reports from the child, caregivers, and school officials. When possible, it is desirable to augment these data with direct behavioral observation. Assessments are made not only of the child's mood and behavior, but also of the full range of cognitive, social, and environmental factors that may underlie and maintain his or her distress. An outline of this assessment strategy is presented in Table 1.1.

This assessment is followed by the introduction of interventions

TABLE 1.1. Cognitive-Behavioral Assessment Strategy

Source	Domain	Respondent
Objective measures	Emotion	Child
Subjective report	Behavior	Caregiver(s)
Behavioral observation	Social adjustment	Teacher(s)
	Academic adjustment	Clinician
	Environmental stressors/supports	

	Cognition
	    Automatic thoughts
	    Schemas
	    Problem solving
	    Self-concept
	    Attributions
	    Expectations
	    Goals, standards, and values
	    Memories
	    Cognitive distortions/bias	

designed to increase behavioral competence, as well as techniques designed to correct maladaptive beliefs or cognitions. As in the practice of cognitive-behavioral therapy with adults, cognitive-behavioral therapy with children is (1) active, (2) structured, (3) problem-oriented, (4) collaborative, and (5) strategic. It is based upon a cognitive-behavioral formulation of factors maintaining the individual's difficulties. An outline of a standard course of cognitive-behavioral therapy is presented in Table 1.2.

Ellis (1962) and Beck (1976) are often credited with introducing the concept of "cognitive restructuring" to the clinical literature. This term refers to the use of Socratic questioning or rational disputation to modify maladaptive or "distorted" thoughts. This approach was subsequently refined (Kendall & Hollon, 1979; Meichenbaum, 1977), and then applied to the treatment of depression and anxiety experienced by children and adolescents. Other cognitive interventions include exercises in social perspective taking, rational problem solving, guided imagery, relaxation training,

---

TABLE 1.2. Outline of Standard Course of Cognitive-Behavioral Therapy

1. Therapist elicits information regarding the development of specific symptoms, as well as situational determinants and temporal course. Objective and subjective data are collected (preferably from multiple informants) regarding the nature of the presenting problem.

2. A goal list is developed with the child and the parents or other caregiver. Cognitive-behavioral formulation and treatment recommendations are shared with the child and his or her parents.

3. Underlying beliefs, attitudes, assumptions, expectations, attributions, goals, and self-statements or automatic thoughts are identified. Patients learn to monitor negative or maladaptive thoughts and emotions. Attempts at self-monitoring are rewarded.

4. Specific behavioral and interpersonal skills deficits are identified.

5. Medical, social, and environmental factors maintaining the symptoms are identified. The latter may include stressful life events (both major and minor, short-term and chronic) or the modeling and reinforcement of the symptoms by others in the child's life.

6. Cognitive and behavioral interventions are selected and introduced based upon the specific needs of the child.

7. Homework is assigned. The patient practices the cognitive or behavioral skills during the session. Attempts are made to ensure that the interventions are clearly understood, that the child is motivated to attempt the assignment, and that they expect the intervention to be helpful. Factors that may interfere with the successful completion of the homework assignment are identified and addressed.

8. Effectiveness of the intervention is evaluated through objective ratings, behavioral observations, and subjective reports.

9. Relapse prevention interventions are introduced. Follow-up or booster sessions are scheduled.

and the use of adaptive self-statements. These interventions (and others) may be introduced based on the specific needs of the child. Cognitive-behavioral interventions have also been developed to remediate cognitive deficiencies. These take the form of techniques introduced to facilitate the development of reflective thought, effective problem solving, and self-regulation.

As noted, virtually all of these interventions—including cognitive restructuring, enhancement of self-control skills, and social problem-solving techniques—were initially developed for treating emotional disorders among adults and are based on rationalist models of human adaptation (Mahoney & Nezworski, 1985). These techniques must be adapted for use with children and adolescents in that children often lack the social, linguistic, and cognitive sophistication to benefit from these techniques if they are introduced in an unmodified form. School-age children, for example, are often unable to discriminate and label emotional states or to readily identify their thoughts and concerns. Young children appear, as well, to be less able than adults to recall emotions apart from the environmental events that generated them. The use of rational disputation and Dysfunctional Thought Records (DTRs)—staples of cognitive-behavioral therapy with older adolescents and adults—are, as a consequence, not feasible with this population. With this in mind, we must simplify our interventions such that they are commensurate with the abilities of our patients, or assist children in developing the requisite skills so that they may benefit from these techniques.

Cognitive-behavioral therapy with children and adolescents requires more, however, than the modification of techniques developed for use with adults for this younger population. Rather, it requires that we recast cognitive-behavioral theories of psychopathology and psychotherapy in developmental terms.

THE IMPORTANCE OF MAINTAINING A DEVELOPMENTAL PERSPECTIVE

Rationally based models of psychotherapy have been criticized as being insensitive to developmental issues and tasks faced by children and adolescents. Moreover, it has been suggested that they do not attend to the self-organizing, constructive processes of child development (Mahoney & Nezworski, 1985). These criticisms are, in some ways, reasonable. Tacit beliefs regarding the reliability of relationships ("working models" in the attachment literature), personal security, and the stability of the family, for example, are of critical importance to school-age children, but are rarely explored in the cognitive therapy literature. Moreover, these factors are rarely incorporated into cognitive-behavioral conceptualizations of childhood emotional disorders. In a similar manner, the developmental tasks of adolescence—the establishment of an adult identity, developing a sense of autonomy from one's family, developing vocational goals, and stabilization of self-concept—have not received a great deal of attention from cognitive-behavioral researchers or clinicians. It is worth noting, however, that relationships between early attachment, adult attachment style, and interpersonal schemas have received an increasing amount of attention since we prepared the first edition of this book (Ingram, Miranda, & Segal, 1998; Randolph & Dykman, 1998; Reinecke & Rogers, 2001; Roberts, Gotlib, & Kassel, 1996; Whisman & McGarvey, 1995). It is worth acknowledging, as well, that recently developed approaches for treating depressed adults (Gotlib & Hammen, 1992) and youth (Curry & Reinecke, Chapter 5, this volume) explicitly attend to attachment security and its relationship to mood and adjustment.

There are a number of reasons why it may be important to adopt a developmental perspective when developing cognitive-behavioral models for treatment of youth. Childhood and adolescence are characterized by dramatic changes in social, cognitive, behavioral, affective, and physical abilities. Competencies developed in each of these domains serve as the foundation for effective functioning as an adult. Not surprisingly, failures in the development of these skills and competencies can place the child at risk for later behavioral and emotional problems. Childhood and adolescence can be viewed, then, as critical periods for the acquisition of adaptive skills and as a period when an individual's developmental trajectory can more readily be influenced.

Second, changes in cognitive, social, and affective competencies during childhood and adolescence influence the nature and frequency of behavioral, emotional, and social problems experienced. Important changes have been observed, for example, in the rates, symptom patterns, gender distribution, and course of behavioral and emotional difficulties over the course of development. Developmental changes also influence the ways in which we think about the adaptiveness (or maladaptiveness) of certain forms of behavior. Various fears (e.g., the dark, being left by a parent), for example, are relatively common during early childhood (and are seen as normal), but may be indicative of clinically significant anxiety at a later age. Similarly, heightened sensitivity to social rejection is relatively common among adolescents, and may serve an adaptive developmental function during this period. It may, however, be indicative of a clinically significant difficulty at another age. Any comprehensive model of child psychopathology must account for these developmental differences.

Third, it is important to attend to transactional relationships between cognitive and socioenvironmental risk and protective factors (Reinecke & DuBois, 2001). As we have noted, human behavior is multiply determined. Although something of a truism, this simple concept is often overlooked in the development of treatment strategies for children. A range of biological, social, cognitive, and environmental factors are associated with risk for psychopathology during childhood and adolescence (Cicchetti & Cohen, 1995; Lenzenweger & Haugaard, 1996). Any comprehensive treatment cognitive-behavioral model must, as a consequence, attend to the full range of factors associated with vulnerability for psychopathology among youth and to the ways in which these factors interact over time.

With this in mind, adaptation during childhood and adolescence, and the acquisition of skills necessary for effective functioning as an adult, can best be viewed from a developmental-systems perspective (Mash & Dozois, 2003; Rutter, 1986). This viewpoint offers a useful paradigm for understanding risk for psychopathology within a broader framework of normative developmental processes (Cicchetti & Schneider-Rosen, 1986; Garber, Braafladt, & Zeman, 1991; Holmbeck et al., 2000). Emotional and behavioral development are influenced by a range of factors that cut across multiple systems that are both internal and external to the child (Mash & Dozois, 2003). Moreover, children develop in a number of contexts. Their behavioral and emotional adaptation, as well as the acquisition of affective, cognitive, social, and vocational skills, are influenced by their family, peers, school, and community. A developmental-systems perspective can be useful in allowing for an integrative and systematic understanding of the effects of individual-level characteristics of the child or adolescent and those that are socially or environmentally based (Reinecke & DuBois, 2001). Whereas an emphasis has been placed during recent years on understanding factors associated with cognitive vulnerability for psychopathology (Ingram et al., 1998; Ingram & Price, 2001), a developmental-systems perspective also directs attention toward factors that promote healthy functioning. Comprehensive cognitive-behavioral models should attend to moderator variables that serve to insulate or protect individuals from developing behavioral and emotional problems (Anthony & Cohler, 1987; Cicchetti & Garmezy, 1993; Compas, Hinden, & Gerhardt, 1995). These variables—referred to by such terms as invulnerability, resilience, competence, and protective factors—may play a particularly important role in the development of prevention programs.

In sum, a developmental psychopathology perspective allows us to address a number of important issues and observations that have not been addressed in the cognitive-behavioral treatment literature. Moreover, it highlights the importance of examining multiple interacting risk and protective factors during specific stages of life, as well as the manner in which they may be manifest in both internal and external sources of risk and resilience.

Insofar as emotional adaptation during childhood and adolescence is influenced by a range of social, environmental, biological, and cognitive factors, our understanding of psychopathology and treatment will be advanced if we attend to the ways in which these factors interact over time. As cognitive, social, behavioral, and affective skill acquisition occurs in a developmental context, an emphasis should be placed on understanding normative development and the ways in which deviations from normal developmental processes influence adjustment.

Although robust evidence suggests that cognitive-behavioral interventions can be effective for treating affective and anxiety disorders among adults (including clinical depression, obsessive–compulsive disorder, panic, generalized anxiety disorder, and social anxiety), it is necessary to modify both our models and techniques before these approaches can be applied with youth. How can we know whether our models and interventions are "developmentally appropriate"? A few simple questions provide the answer:

- Does the model or intervention attend to age-related differences in the cognitive, behavioral, social, or emotional competencies of the child or adolescent?
- Does the model or intervention attend to the contexts in which the child or adolescent is functioning?
- Could the study be conducted with adults using the same design and measures? Could the same intervention be used with adults without modification?
- Does the model or intervention attend to vulnerability or protective factors?
- Are the constructs, variables, and measures used in the study relevant to understanding child development?

Research in developmental psychopathology provides a range of tools and constructs for understanding emotional and behavioral difficulties experienced by youth. These concepts—including developmental trajectories, multifinality, developmental tasks, and resilience—can provide useful insights into vulnerability for psychopathology among youth and may allow for the development of more effective treatments. This paradigm directs us, for example, to attend to the timing of stressful life events, the impact of multiple, concurrent traumatic events, and the long-term effects of stressful life events on adjustment. Similarly, it guides us to attend to the developmental needs and tasks of the child or adolescent (e.g., development of affect regulation skills, affiliation with peer group, autonomy from parents), the resources available in the family or environment to address these needs, and the ways in which these affect the child's mood and adjustment. Finally, it encourages us to consider the ways in which cognitive and socioenvironmental factors interact over time in contributing to risk for psychopathology. This perspective is not far removed, then, from contemporary cognitive diathesis–stress models of psychopathology (Clark & Beck, 1999; Gotlib & Hammen, 1992). Although important advances have been made during recent years in understanding cognitive vulnerability for psychopathology (Ingram & Price, 2001; Reinecke & Clark, 2003), the field of cognitive-behavioral therapy has not fully incorporated the broad range of developmental psychopathology findings and principles into its techniques and models.

Cognitive therapy is based on the assumption that behavioral and emotional difficulties stem from the activation of maladaptive beliefs, from the use of biased information-processing strategies, or from a lack of effective behavioral skills. Clinical work with children and adolescents requires that we attend to how these cognitive contents and processes develop, the social contexts in which they function, and their implications for functioning later in life. It is possible, from a developmental perspective, to view behavioral and emotional difficulties experienced by youth as stemming, at least in part, from failures in the management of normative developmental tasks, or from breakdowns in the development of essential competencies (including affect regulation, rational problem solving, and social skills).

FUTURE DIRECTIONS

Cognitive-behavioral therapy with children and adolescents has developed rapidly during the past 10–15 years. The models are compelling, and many of the interventions derived from these approaches have received empirical support. Our understanding of vulnerability for psychopathology, processes of change, treatment effectiveness, and prevention of psychopathology are growing quickly, and will be facilitated by an ever-closer integration of findings and approaches from the cognitive-behavioral therapy, developmental psychology, and developmental psychopathology literatures.

In order to address developmentally oriented questions, developmentally oriented research designs must be used. We would suggest that future research with children and adolescents should, whenever possible and appropriate, use longitudinal (rather than cross-sectional) designs. In this way developmental trajectories (for both clinical and nonclinical populations) can be followed such that causal relationships between cognitive, social, environmental, and biological variables can be better understood. Second, research designs should attend to both risk and resilience factors, and to the contexts in which development occurs. Particular attention should be given to identifying moderator and mediator variables, and to using statistical techniques that are appropriate for delineating their relationships with outcome variables. Third, it will be useful to examine adaptation at developmentally important transition points (e.g., puberty, transition to early adolescence, transition from adolescence to early adulthood), and the ways in which cognitive-behavioral psychotherapy influences psychosocial adjustment at these times. Finally, we would suggest using a broader range of outcome variables in studies of therapeutic outcome and process. Relatively few studies, for example, have examined the development of schemas among children and adolescents, the stability of tacit beliefs over time and how they are influenced by the beliefs and attitudes of parents and peers, their relationships to broader indices of adaptation (most studies focus solely on their relationship to measures of mood, such as the Beck Depression Inventory), or their implications for adjustment during adulthood. Follow-up studies are critically important, not only to document the stability of therapeutic gains, but also to clarify the effects of our interventions on broader indicators of social and emotional functioning.

The Effectiveness of Cognitive-Behavioral Psychotherapy with Youth

Research completed over the past 20 years on the effectiveness of cognitive-behavioral treatments for behavioral and emotional difficulties among youth has been substantial and, for the most part, positive. Although the volume of this literature is modest in comparison with work completed on the treatment of adult disorders, it is nonetheless impressive and a number of tentative conclusions can be drawn. First, cognitive-behavioral interventions appear to do some good, at least for some problems and under some conditions. Controlled outcome studies suggest that cognitive-behavioral therapy is superior to no-treatment and to placebo controls for treating a range of affective, anxiety, and behavioral disorders among youth. The effect sizes observed in these studies are comparable to those observed in outcome research with adults, and gains often are maintained over time (Reinecke, Ryan, & DuBois, 1998; Weisz & Weiss, 1993). It is worth acknowledging, however, that the number of controlled outcome studies completed is relatively small, most have employed nonclinical samples, few have included viable alternative forms of treatment as a control, and few have examined the stability of treatment gains for more than a few weeks or months. Moreover, specific interventions may be more effective at different ages, and few dismantling studies have been completed examining which components of the treatment protocols are most closely associated with clinical improvement. Second, cognitively based interventions may be effective, at least in the short term, for preventing some forms of affective, anxiety, and behavioral disorders. Finally, cognitive-behavioral interventions appear to be effective in alleviating both internalizing and externalizing difficulties. A caveat is in order here, as well, in that cognitive-behavioral therapy does not appear to be indicated as a primary form of treatment for attention-deficit/hyperactivity disorder. It may, however, serve as a useful adjunct for other interventions.

What are the characteristics of effective forms of psychotherapy with youth? It is difficult, based upon a review of the empirical literature, to draw firm conclusions. Empirically supported forms of psychotherapy appear, however, to share a number of characteristics. They tend, for example, to be active and problem-focused, rather than nondirective and primarily supportive in nature. Second, they tend to emphasize the development of a parsimonious treatment rationale and to share this with the patient and his or her family. This serves at least three purposes: It provides a shared vocabulary for the therapist and the family to understand the child's difficulties; it allows for the development of specific treatment recommendations; and, as a consequence, it leads the child and caregivers to feel understood and provides them with a sense of hope. This is not a minor contribution insofar as the family often views the child's difficulties as inexplicable and feels powerless to rectify them. Third, effective treatments encourage action. They assist the child to develop specific adaptive skills, and support the child's caregivers and school officials in their efforts to alleviate stressors in the child's life, provide reliable and consistent support, and reinforce the child's adaptive efforts. Effective forms of psychotherapy also tend, as a group, to encourage the child (or parents) to monitor moods and behavior and to modify these efforts on the basis of feedback about which techniques have been most useful. Empirically supported treatment programs tend to include a psychoeducational component, and attempt to develop specific cognitive and behavioral skills. They tend, as well, to attend to the family or community context in which the child is developing. Finally, effective psychosocial interventions typically attend to the generalizability of treatment gains and take steps to prevent recurrence or relapse.

As the astute reader will note, many of these characteristics also describe other, noncognitive, forms of empirically supported psychotherapy (such as Interpersonal Psychotherapy; Mufson, Moreau, Weissman, & Klerman, 1993). We mention this as the processes of therapeutic change in psychotherapy with youth are not well understood. Alternative forms of psychotherapy may, in practice, be similar. Moreover, there may be multiple pathways to change. The mechanisms of change in short-term psychodynamic psychotherapy, for example, may differ from those in cognitive-behavioral therapy. Pathways to change in alternative forms of psychotherapy may or may not be similar. Finally, it is worth noting that controversies exist regarding the relative importance of nonspecific (e.g., trusting therapeutic rapport, warmth, genuineness) and theory-specific technical factors for therapeutic improvement, and the impact of patient, therapist, family, and community variables on short- and long-term outcome.

Looking Forward

This volume includes chapters addressing several of these issues and concerns. Anastopoulos and Gerrard (Chapter 2), for example, directly address the fact that there is limited evidence for the efficacy of cognitive-behavioral therapy as a primary treatment of attention-deficit/hyperactivity disorder. They propose that it may be necessary to reconceptualize this disorder, and direct our attention to understanding factors associated with failures in the development of inhibitory controls among youth. Along similar lines, Curry and Reinecke (Chapter 5) propose a "modularized" treatment approach for adolescent depression based upon findings in the cognitive therapy and developmental psychopathology literatures. They propose that interventions can be tailored to the needs of individual patients based upon an understanding of specific cognitive and behavioral deficits maintaining their dysphoria. They suggest that attention should be paid to attachment style and the development of affect regulation skills, and have incorporated intervention strategies to address these issues into their program.

Several of our contributors borrow from the adult psychotherapy literature in developing treatment programs for children and adolescents. Bowers, Evans, LeGrange, and Andersen (Chapter 10), for example, describe how empirically supported treatment protocols developed by Fairburn for treating eating disorders among adults may be adapted for work with adolescents. They explicitly attend to developmental differences that may influence the nature and course of treatment. Albano (Chapter 6) proposes an innovative, integrated cognitive-behavioral program for treating social anxiety among youth, what has been referred to as the "neglected anxiety disorder," and Heflin and Deblinger (Chapter 9) describe the ways in which cognitive and behavioral principles can inform the treatment of posttraumatic stress disorder among youth.

Programmatic research plays a particularly important role in the development of cognitive-behavioral models and treatment programs. Extended and intensive lines of investigation allow models to be put to the test and facilitate the refinement of clinical techniques. Programmatic research into the psychopathology of externalizing behavior problems and anxiety serve as the basis for treatment programs for oppositional defiant disorder (Pardini & Lochman, Chapter 3) and obsessive–compulsive disorder (Franklin, Rynn, Foa, & March, Chapter 7).

This volume also includes several chapters applying cognitive-behavioral therapy to "nontraditional" problems. Patterson and O'Connell (Chapter 4), for example, describe a cognitive-behavioral approach for understanding and treating chemical dependence among adolescents, Bradley-Klug and Shapiro (Chapter 11) describe procedures for assisting youth with academic problems or learning disabilities, and Beebe and Risi (Chapter 14) propose that cognitive-behavioral principles can be used in developing treatment programs for high functioning autistic youth. Freeman and Rigby (Chapter 16) address a highly controversial issue—the diagnosis and treatment of personality disorders among youth. They suggest that developmental precursors of personality disorders can be identified among children and adolescents, and that cognitive-behavioral interventions may be useful in addressing these potentially serious clinical problems. These are challenging clinical concerns, and press the bounds of cognitive-behavioral practice with youth.

Several of our contributors attempt to redefine cognitive-behavioral models of psychopathology. Shirk, Burwell, and Harter (Chapter 8), for example, discuss the relationship of self-concept to psychopathology among youth, and outline how insights from research on self-esteem can inform and enhance cognitive-behavioral therapy. This is particularly important given the fact that self-concept is typically viewed as a dependent variable in cognitive-behavioral research, and the central importance of the self-schema in cognitive models of vulnerability to psychopathology. Along similar lines, DuBois (Chapter 15) elaborates upon his quadripartite model of social competence and describes how it may be applied in treating children and adolescents. These approaches are noteworthy in that they draw heavily on work in developmental psychology and developmental psychopathology, and attend to factors associated with resilience and positive adaptation among youth.

Finally, several of our contributors have developed treatment programs that touch upon and invigorate older lines of clinical practice. Epstein and Schlesinger (Chapter 12), for example, provide a comprehensive, systematic, and scholarly discussion of the ways that cognitive-behavioral approaches can be applied in family therapy; and Knell and Ruma (Chapter 13) discuss how traditional play therapy techniques can be incorporated into effective cognitive-behavioral treatment programs for school-age children.

CONCLUSION

Cognitive-behavioral therapy with children and adolescents is promising in that it explicitly recognizes the importance of cognitive, behavioral, affective, and social factors in the etiology and maintenance of behavioral and emotional disorders. It is consistent with contemporary integrationist and constructivist models of behavior change, and maintains the objective, empirical focus that is the hallmark of cognitive therapy with adults. Cognitive-behavioral therapy with children and adolescents is fundamentally similar, both in theory and in practice, to cognitive therapy with adults. It challenges these models, however, by requiring us to carefully attend to the interpersonal contexts in which children's beliefs, attitudes, competencies, and skills develop, as well as developmental factors associated with behavioral and emotional change and adaptation.

REFERENCES

Anthony, E., & Cohler, B. (Eds.). (1987). *The invulnerable child.* New York: Guilford Press.

Beck, A. (1976). *Cognitive therapy and the emotional disorders.* New York: New American Library.

Carr, A. (Ed.). (2000). *What works with children and adolescents? A critical review of psychological interventions with children, adolescents and their families.* London: Routledge.

Cicchetti, D., & Cohen, D. (1995). *Developmental psychopathology: Vol. 2. Risk, disorder and adaptation.* New York: Wiley.

Cicchetti, D., & Garmezy, N. (1993). Prospects and promises in the study of resilience. *Development and Psychopathology, 5,* 497–502.

Cicchetti, D., & Schneider-Rosen, K. (1986). An organizational approach to childhood depression. In M. Rutter, C. Izard, & P. Read (Eds.), *Depression in young people: Developmental and clinical perspectives* (pp. 71–134). New York: Guilford Press.

Clark, D., & Beck, A. (1999). *Scientific foundations of cognitive theory and therapy of depression.* New York: Wiley.

Compas, B. E., Hinden, B. R., & Gerhardt, C. A. (1995). Adolescent development: Pathways and processes of risk and resilience. *Annual Review of Psychology, 46,* 265–293.

Costello, E. (1989). Developments in child psychiatric epidemiology. *Journal of the American Academy of Child and Adolescent Psychiatry, 28,* 836–841.

Dobson, K., & Dozois, D. (2001). Historical and philosophical bases of the cognitive-behavioral therapies. In K. Dobson (Ed.), *Handbook of cognitive-behavioral therapies* (2nd ed., pp. 3–39). New York: Guilford Press.

Ellis, A. (1962). *Reason and emotion in psychotherapy.* New York: Lyle Stuart.

Fogel, A. (1993). *Developing through relationships: Origins of communication, self, and culture.* Chicago: University of Chicago Press.

Freeman, A., & Reinecke, M. (1995). Cognitive therapy. In A. Gurman & S. Messer (Eds.), *Essential psychotherapies: Theory and practice* (pp. 182–225). New York: Guilford Press.

Freud, S. (1953). A case of hysteria. In J. Strachey (Ed. and Trans.), *The standard edition of the complete psychological works of Sigmund Freud* (Vol. 7, pp. 1–122). London: Hogarth Press. (Original work published 1905)

Friedberg, R., & McClure, J. (2002). *Clinical practice of cognitive therapy with children and adolescents: The nuts and bolts.* New York: Guilford Press.

Garber, J., Braafladt, N., & Zeman, J. (1991). Affect regulation in depressed and nondepressed children and young adolescents. *Development and Psychopathology, 7,* 93–115.

Gotlib, I., & Hammen, C. (1992). *Psychological aspects of depression: Toward a cognitive-interpersonal integration.* New York: Wiley.

Graham, P. (Ed.). (1998). *Cognitive-behaviour therapy for children and families.* Cambridge, UK: Cambridge University Press.

Hibbs, E., & Jensen, P. (Eds.). (1996). *Psychosocial treatments for child and adolescent disorders: Empirically based strategies for clinical practice.* Washington, DC: American Psychological Association.

Holmbeck, G., Colder, C., Shapera, W., Westhoven, V., Kenealy, L., & Updegrove, A. (2000). Working with adolescents: Guides from developmental psychology. In P. Kendall (Ed.), *Child and adolescent therapy: Cognitive-behavioral procedures* (2nd ed., pp. 334–385). New York: Guilford Press.

Ingram, R., Miranda, J., & Segal, Z. (1998). *Cognitive vulnerability to depression.* New York: Guilford Press.

Ingram, R., & Price, J. (Eds.). (2001). *Vulnerability to psychopathology: Risk across the lifespan.* New York: Guilford Press.

Kendall, P. (Ed.). (2000). *Child and adolescent therapy: Cognitive-behavioral procedures* (2nd ed.). New York: Guilford Press.

Kendall, P., & Dobson, K. (1993). On the nature of cognition and its role in psychopathology. In K. Dobson & P. Kendall (Eds.), *Psychopathology and cognition* (pp. 3–17). San Diego: Academic Press.

Kendall, P., & Hollon, S. (1979). Cognitive-behavioral interventions: Overview and current status. In P. Kendall & S. Hollon (Eds.), *Cognitive-behavioral interventions: Theory, research, and procedures* (pp. 1–9). New York: Academic Press.

Kendall, P., & MacDonald, J. (1993). Cognition in the psychopathology of youth and implications for treatment. In K. Dobson & P. Kendall (Eds.), *Psychopathology and cognition* (pp. 387–427). San Diego: Academic Press.

Lenzenweger, M., & Haugaard, J. (Eds.). (1996). *Frontiers of developmental psychopathology.* New York: Oxford University Press.

Mahoney, M., & Nezworski, M. (1985). Cognitive-behavioral approaches to children's problems. *Journal of Abnormal Child Psychology, 13*(3), 467–476.

Mash, E. J., & Dozois, D. J. A. (2003). Child psychopathology: A developmental–systems perspective. In E. J. Mash & R. A. Barkley (Eds.), *Child psychopathology* (2nd ed., pp. 3–71). New York: Guilford Press.

McCracken, J. (1992). The epidemiology of child and adolescent mood disorders. *Child and Adolescent Psychiatric Clinics of North America, 1,* 53–72.

Meichenbaum, D. (1977). *Cognitive-behavior modification: An integrative approach.* New York: Plenum Press.

Morris, R., & Kratochwill, T. (1991). Introductory comments. In T. Kratochwill & R., Morris (Eds.), *The practice of child therapy* (2nd ed., pp. 3–5). New York: Pergamon Press.

Mufson, L., Moreau, D., Weissman, M., & Klerman, G. (1993). *Interpersonal psychotherapy for depressed adolescents.* New York: Guilford Press.

Randolph, J., & Dykman, B. (1998). Perceptions of parenting and depression-proneness in the offspring: Dysfunctional attitudes as a mediating mechanism. *Cognitive Therapy and Research, 22,* 377–400.

Reinecke, M., & Clark, D. (Eds.). (2003). *Cognitive therapy across the lifespan.* Cambridge, UK: Cambridge University Press.

Reinecke, M., & DuBois, D. (2001). Socio-environmental and cognitive risk and resources: Relations to mood and suicidality among inpatient adolescents. *Journal of Cognitive Psychotherapy, 15,* 195–222.

Reinecke, M., & Rogers, G. (2001). Dysfunctional attitudes and attachment style among clinically depressed adults. *Behavioural and Cognitive Psychotherapy, 29,* 129–141.

Reinecke, M., Ryan, N., & DuBois, D. (1998). Cognitive-behavioral therapy of depression and depressive symptoms during adolescence: A review and meta-analysis. *Journal of the American Academy of Child and Adolescent Psychiatry,* 37(1), 26–34.

Roberts, J., Gotlib, I., & Kassel, J. (1996). Adult attachment security and symptoms of depression: The mediating roles of dysfunctional attitudes and low self-esteem. *Journal of Personality and Social Psychology, 70,* 310–320.

Robins, L., & Rutter, M. (Eds.). (1990). *Straight and devious pathways from childhood to adulthood.* Cambridge, UK: Cambridge University Press.

Rutter, M. (1986). The developmental psychopathology of depression: Issues and perspectives. In M. Rutter, C. Izard, & P. Read (Eds.), *Depression in young people: Developmental and clinical perspectives* (pp. 3–30). New York: Guilford Press.

Rutter, M. (1989). Pathways from childhood to adult life. *Journal of Child Psychology and Psychiatry, 30,* 23–51.

Vygotsky, L. (1992). *Thought and language.* Cambridge, MA: Massachusetts Institute of Technology Press.

Weimer, W. (1977). A conceptual framework for cognitive psychology: Motor theories of mind. In R. Shaw & J. Bransford (Eds.), *Perceiving, acting and knowing* (pp. 267–311). Hillsdale, NJ: Erlbaum.

Weisz, J., & Weiss, B. (1993). *Effects of psychotherapy with children and adolescents.* Newbury Park, CA: Sage.

Whisman, M., & McGarvey, A. (1995). Attachment, depressotypic cognitions, and dysphoria. *Cognitive Therapy and Research, 19,* 633–650.

2

Facilitating Understanding and Management of Attention-Deficit/Hyperactivity Disorder

ARTHUR D. ANASTOPOULOS
LISA M. GERRARD

A fundamental premise of standard models of cognitive therapy (Beck, 1976; J. Beck, 1995) is that faulty thinking—that is, maladaptive or negativistic thought patterns—contributes to the development and maintenance of many psychological problems. For disorders whose defining features include patterns of faulty thinking (e.g., depression, anxiety), cognitive therapy has an impressive track record, with many years of research and clinical practice supporting its use (Dobson, 1989; Harrington, Campbell, Shoebridge, & Whittaker, 1998; Solomon & Haaga, in press). Unfortunately, this same type of success has not been evident in the treatment of attention-deficit/hyperactivity disorder (AD/HD). To many in the field, this limitation in the effectiveness of cognitive therapy as it applies to AD/HD comes as no great surprise, because it is assumed that faulty cognitions do not play a prominent role in the etiology of this disorder. Assuming this to be true, does this mean that cognitive therapy has no place in the clinical management of children and adolescents with AD/HD? The short answer to this question is no, but such a response requires qualification.

The intent of this chapter is to provide such clarification, beginning with a brief overview of what is now known about AD/HD. Against this background, a case example is then presented to illustrate the various ways in which cognitive-behavioral therapy strategies can be employed with this population.

CLINICAL PRESENTATION

Primary Symptoms and Diagnostic Criteria

AD/HD is a chronic and pervasive condition characterized by developmentally deviant levels of inattention, impulsivity, and/or hyperactivity. Clinical descriptions of children with AD/HD frequently include difficulties sustaining attention to task, not following through on instructions, being easily distracted, fidgeting, talking excessively, and interrupting others.

The diagnostic criteria for AD/HD appear in the fourth edition of the *Diagnostic and Statistical Manual of Mental Disorders* (DSM-IV; American Psychiatric Association, 1994). To receive a diagnosis of AD/HD, an individual must first display a high enough frequency of its primary symptoms. In keeping with the results of factor analytic studies, DSM-IV presents these primary symptoms in two lists: one pertaining to inattention symptoms (e.g., often fails to give close attention to details, often does not seem to listen when spoken to directly, often has difficulty organizing tasks), the other related to hyperactivity–impulsivity concerns (e.g., often leaves seat, often on the go, often blurts out answers, often has difficulty awaiting turn). To meet the frequency requirement, DSM-IV stipulates that at least six of nine inattention symptoms and/or six of nine hyperactive–impulsive symptoms must be present. If so, there must also be evidence that these symptoms occur in two or more settings and that they are associated with some degree of functional impairment in an individual's daily life. Moreover, these symptoms must be developmentally deviant, have a duration of 6 months, arise prior to 7 years, and not be due to other medical and mental health conditions that better account for their existence.

According to these guidelines, *all* AD/HD diagnoses must now be accompanied by one of several possible subtyping distinctions. What distinguishes one major subtype from another is whether or not the criteria for one or both of the primary symptom lists are met. For example, if six or more symptoms from both lists are present, and if all other AD/HD criteria are met, AD/HD, combined type (Code 314.01), is the appropriate diagnosis. When there are six or more inattention symptoms, but less than six hyperactivity–impulsivity symptoms present, and all other AD/HD criteria are met, a diagnosis of AD/HD, predominantly inattentive type (314.00), is in order. The other possible scenario that might unfold is when there are six or more hyperactivity–impulsivity symptoms, but less than six inattention symptoms present. Assuming that all other AD/HD criteria are met, the proper diagnosis for this situation is AD/HD, predominantly hyperactive–impulsive type (314.01).

Many individuals incorrectly regard the predominantly inattentive and the predominantly hyperactive–impulsive classifications as pure or exclusive subtyping categories. In view of this possibility, clinicians and researchers must bear in mind that both subtyping categories can include symptoms that go beyond what is suggested in their labeling. Thus, children with the predominantly inattentive type can have subclinical hyperactive–impulsive features that require therapeutic attention. Conversely, the same is also true for children with the predominantly hyperactive–impulsive classification.

Situational Variability

AD/HD is not an all-or-none phenomenon, either always present or never present. Rather, it is a condition whose primary symptoms fluctuate in response to situational demands (Zentall, 1985). One of the most important factors determining this variation is the degree to which children with AD/HD are interested in what they are doing. AD/HD symptoms are much more likely to occur in situations that are highly repetitive, boring, or familiar, versus those that are novel or stimulating (Barkley, 1977). Another determinant of situational variation is the amount of imposed structure. In many free play or low-demand settings, where children with AD/HD have the freedom to do as they please, their behavior is often indistinguishable from that of normal children (Luk, 1985). Significant AD/HD problems may arise, however, when others place demands on them or set rules for their behavior. Presumably due to increased demands for behavioral self-regulation, group settings are far more problematic for children with AD/HD than would be the case in one-to-one situations. There is also an increased likelihood for AD/HD symptoms to arise in situations where feedback is dispensed infrequently or on a delayed basis (Douglas, 1983).

   In view of this tendency for AD/HD symptoms to vary in response to situational factors, it should come as no surprise that children with AD/HD often display inconsistency in their task performance, both in terms of productivity and accuracy (Douglas, 1972). Such variability may be evident with respect to their in-class performance, test scores (e.g., getting a grade of 90 one day, 60 the next), completion of homework, or chores at home. Although it may be argued that all children display a certain amount of variability in their daily activities, it is clear from clinical experience and research that children with AD/HD exhibit this to a much greater degree. Thus, instead of reflecting "laziness" as some might infer from their behavior, the inconsistent performance of children with AD/HD may represent yet another manifestation of this disorder.

PREVALENCE

The overall prevalence of AD/HD among children—that is, the sum total of all subtyping categories—is 3–5% (American Psychiatric Association, 1994). Community-based estimates of the prevalence have ranged from 7.5% to 21.6% for both parent- and teacher-generated samples (DuPaul et al.,

1998; Gaub & Carlson, 1997). That these would be higher than the 3–5% prevalence described in DSM-IV is not surprising, given the fact that community rates were derived primarily on the basis of the AD/HD symptom frequency requirement alone. Such figures likely include many children for whom AD/HD would not be diagnosed, due to the fact that they would not meet all the other DSM-IV criteria.

DEVELOPMENTAL COURSE

Most individuals with AD/HD begin to display their symptoms in early childhood, with hyperactive–impulsive difficulties typically preceding inattention. Although symptoms typically appear at 3 to 4 years, they can also become apparent during infancy or upon school entrance. Upon reaching late childhood and early adolescence, many children with AD/HD begin to display fewer hyperactive–impulsive symptoms. Some may also show a reduction in their overall level of inattention, but to a much lesser degree. This change in symptom presentation may help to explain why only 50–80% of the children identified as AD/HD will continue to meet full diagnostic criteria for this condition as adolescents (Barkley, Fischer, Edelbrock, & Smallish, 1990). Although only 30% of adolescents with ADHD continue to meet diagnostic criteria for this condition as adults (Gittelman, Mannuzza, Shenker, & Bonagura, 1985; Mannuzza, Klein, Bessler, Malloy, & LaPadula, 1993), as many as 50% will continue to exhibit subclinical levels of these symptoms, which interfere with daily functioning (Weiss & Hechtman, 1993). The overall frequency of AD/HD symptoms seems to decline gradually across adulthood (Murphy & Barkley, 1996b). Unlike what has been observed for children and adolescents, such declines are evident for both hyperactive–impulsive and inattention symptoms.

PSYCHOSOCIAL IMPACT

Having AD/HD places individuals at risk for a multitude of psychosocial difficulties across the life span. The exact nature of these complications is determined in large part by a consideration of what is considered typical or normal at any given stage of development. Preschoolers with AD/HD place enormous caretaking demands on their parents (Shelton et al., 1998) and frequently display aggressive behavior when interacting with siblings or peers (Campbell, 1990). Difficulties acquiring academic readiness skills may be evident as well, but these tend to be of less clinical concern than the family or peer problems that preschoolers present. As children with AD/HD move into the elementary school years, academic problems take on increasing importance (DuPaul & Stoner, 1994). Together with their ongoing family (Johnston, 1996) and peer relationship problems (Lahey, Carlson, & Frick, 1997), such school-based difficulties set the stage for the development of low self-esteem and other emotional concerns (August, Realmuto, MacDonald, Nugent, & Crosby, 1996). Similar problems persist into adolescence, but on a much more intense level. New problems may develop as well (e.g., traffic violations, experimentation with alcohol and drugs), stemming from the increased demands for independence, self-regulation, and self-control that teenagers with AD/HD face (Barkley, Anastopoulos, Guevremont, & Fletcher, 1992; Klein & Mannuzza, 1991). AD/HD can also make the transition into adulthood difficult. Noteworthy in this regard are the obstacles that AD/HD imposes on adults in their efforts to establish and maintain a family or career (Murphy & Barkley, 1996a).

COMORBIDITY

In addition to being affected by its primary symptoms, individuals with AD/HD are at increased risk for having secondary or comorbid diagnoses. Preschoolers and children with AD/HD frequently display oppositional defiant disorder (ODD; Jensen, Martin, & Cantwell, 1997). Among adolescents with AD/HD, conduct disorder (CD) is quite common (Barkley, Anastopoulos, Guevremont, & Fletcher, 1991). When AD/HD is accompanied by ODD or CD, there is also an increased risk for depression and anxiety disorders to be present (August et al., 1996). Antisocial personality disorder, major depression, and substance abuse are just a few of the many comorbid problems that may be found among adults with AD/HD (Klein & Mannuzza, 1991). In combination with AD/HD, such comorbid conditions increase the severity of an individual's overall impairment, thereby making the prognosis for such individuals less favorable.

ETIOLOGY

Biological Accounts

Several lines of evidence point toward the involvement of biological factors in the etiology of AD/HD. In particular, research has suggested that abnormalities in brain chemistry (Arnsten Steere, & Hunt, 1996), brain structure (Castellanos et al., 1996), and brain function (Zametkin et al., 1990) may play a role. Multiple pathways presumably lead to these abnormalities. Among these, genetic mechanisms (Levy, Hay, McStephen, Wood, & Waldman, 1997) and certain pregnancy complications, such as excessive maternal consumption of alcohol and/or nicotine (Streissguth, Bookstein,

Sampson, & Barr, 1995), very likely account for the largest percentage of children who have AD/HD. For some children, AD/HD may be acquired after birth, resulting from head injury, elevated lead levels, or other biological complications.

Psychosocial Conceptualizations

Although some environmental theories have been proposed to explain AD/HD (Block, 1977; Jacobvitz & Sroufe, 1987), there is little empirical justification for claiming that poor parenting, chaotic home environments, or poverty *cause* AD/HD. The results of twin studies indicate that less than 5% of the variance in AD/HD symptomatology can be accounted for by environmental factors (Levy et al., 1997). When AD/HD is found among children who come from such family circumstances, one might reasonably speculate that the parents of such children may themselves be individuals with childhood and adult histories of AD/HD. If so, this would help to explain why their homes might be so chaotic and, at the same time, provide support for a genetic explanation for the child's AD/HD condition. Under this same scenario, the resulting chaos in the home might then be viewed as a factor exacerbating, rather than causing, the child's inborn AD/HD condition.

Psychological Conceptualizations

Building on what is now known about the biology of AD/HD, recent theories have taken on a distinctive neuropsychological flavor, emphasizing the impulsivity features of this disorder. Quay (1997), for example, proposed that AD/HD stems from an impairment in a neurologically based behavioral inhibition system. In an extensive elaboration of this same theme, Barkley (1998) has contended that a deficit in behavioral inhibition leads to impairment in four areas of executive functioning—working memory, emotion regulation, internalization of language, and reconstitution. Such deficits in executive functioning lead directly to the various academic, behavioral, and social deficits observed within AD/HD populations.

Cognitive Models

Cognitive models of AD/HD and its associated features have periodically appeared in the literature over the past 30 years. Most of these models were inspired by the seminal work of Meichenbaum and Goodman (1971), who observed significant reductions in impulsivity among children participating in their cognitive self-instructional training (CSIT) program. Borrowing from the Russian psychologists Vygotsky and Luria, Meichenbaum and

Goodman (1971) developed a theoretically driven treatment program that assumed that the behavioral difficulties of impulsive children stemmed from deficiencies in the acquisition and use of verbal mediation skills. Mimicking the developmental progression that presumably led to the verbal control of behavior, CSIT begins with an adult verbally coaching the child through the steps necessary to complete a task. Next, the adult encourages the child to use overt language to guide his or her own behavior. Thereafter, the child whispers self-instructions to guide behavior. In the final step of the program, the child "thinks" through the self-instructions necessary to guide him- or herself through an assigned task. In this way, CSIT achieves two important therapeutic goals that parallel normal development, namely, shifting control of the child's behavior from other to self, and shifting control of the child's behavior from overt to covert (internalized) language.

The success of Meichenbaum and Goodman's (1971) study and the theoretical appeal of their treatment approach spawned a tremendous amount of interest in the use of CSIT and related treatments that emphasized verbal self-regulation training (Bornstein & Quevillon, 1976; Kendall & Braswell, 1985). Included among these were various self-monitoring, self-reinforcement, and self-instructional techniques. Much of the appeal for their clinical application stemmed from their apparent focus on some of the primary deficits of AD/HD, including impulsivity, poor organizational skills, and difficulties with rules and instructions. Also contributing to their popularity was their presumed potential for enhancing treatment generalization, above and beyond that achieved through more traditional contingency management programs.

Research on self-monitoring has shown that it can improve on-task behavior and academic productivity in some children with AD/HD (Shapiro & Cole, 1994). The combination of self-monitoring and self-reinforcement can also lead to improvements in on-task behavior and academic accuracy (Hinshaw, Henker, & Whalen, 1984), as well as in peer relations (Hinshaw, 2000). Behavioral improvements have also been reported for aggressive AD/HD children who received a combination of self-control and anger management training (Miranda & Presentacion, 2000). As for self-instructional training, the picture is less clear, with many studies (Abikoff & Gittelman, 1985) failing to replicate earlier reported successes (Bornstein & Quevillon, 1976; Meichenbaum & Goodman, 1971).

Overall, CSIT and other verbal self-regulation treatment approaches began with much promise but have received modest empirical support at best. Although they can be helpful for *some* children with AD/HD (Kendall, 2000), such verbal training techniques often do not produce the kinds of behavioral improvements that would be considered therapeutically meaningful. Thus, there is little justification for routinely including them in treatment plans for children with AD/HD.

COGNITIVE MODELS IN A DIFFERENT LIGHT

Given their theoretical appeal, why haven't these cognitive models of AD/HD received the kind of strong empirical support so many expected? Part of the answer to this question may come from a consideration of recent conceptualizations of AD/HD. As noted earlier, Barkley (1998) has postulated that a deficit in the behavioral inhibition center of the brain interferes with the development and subsequent performance of four major executive functions, which in turn leads to the clinical presentation of AD/HD. As conceptualized by Barkley, an underaroused cortical inhibition center makes it difficult for individuals with AD/HD to (1) stop before initiating a response, (2) stop a response that has already been initiated, and/or (3) block out mental interference. This failure to inhibit interferes with the development and subsequent functioning of an individual's nonverbal working memory, internalization of speech, self-regulation of affect, and capacity for reconstitution. Of particular relevance for the present discussion is the executive function that Barkley (1998) terms "internalization of speech." This executive function is nothing more than the same verbal self-regulation process that captured the attention and interest of Meichenbaum and Goodman (1971) and others (Bornstein & Quevillon, 1976; Kendall & Braswell, 1985). What makes Barkley's reference to this process different is where he places it in his model. Rather than being the starting point for AD/HD, verbal self-regulation deficits are thought to play a mediating role, linking deficits in behavioral inhibition to the expression of AD/HD. More to the point, if an individual cannot block out mental interference, he or she will not be able to utilize internal language to guide behavior, at least not effectively. Thus, for internal speech and the other executive functions to be maximally effective, the cortical inhibition center must be functioning normally. Presumably, such is not the case for individuals with AD/HD.

With this in mind it becomes easier to understand why CSIT and other verbal self-control training programs do not work particularly well as a treatment for reducing primary AD/HD symptoms. To the extent that they address an executive function (i.e., internalization of speech) and not the core deficit (i.e., behavioral inhibition) that precedes it, the likelihood for success is slim. Stated another way, verbal self-regulation training is too far downstream in the process that leads to AD/HD. To be successful, therefore, the focus of treatment needs to be more upstream, targeting the behavioral inhibition deficit, which is the presumed starting point of the process leading to AD/HD.

OPPORTUNITIES FOR USING COGNITIVE INTERVENTIONS

In light of Barkley's (1998) conceptualization of AD/HD and the absence of strong empirical support, CSIT and other types of verbal self-regulation training programs do not appear to be well suited for addressing AD/HD, at least in terms of reducing its primary symptoms. This need not mean, however, that there is no room for cognitive interventions in the clinical management of AD/HD. Based upon a consideration of how AD/HD presents itself clinically, there are numerous ways in which cognitive therapy strategies can be employed both in the assessment and treatment of individuals who have this condition. Such opportunities are discussed in the context of the following case illustration.

CASE EXAMPLE

Background Information

At the time clinical services were sought, Jason D., a Caucasian male, was 9.5 years old and enrolled in a regular fourth-grade classroom. He was initially referred for services by his parents who, along with his teachers, were concerned about his long-standing home and school difficulties, including excessive fidgeting, difficulties following through on assigned tasks, and not working up to his potential.

Jason's developmental history was unremarkable. He had been in good health throughout his lifetime. He had not taken any prescription medications for behavior management purposes nor for any other reason. He and his two younger half-siblings lived with their parents in a home where the family had resided for more than a year. Jason maintained typical relations with his siblings, neither of whom had any major medical, behavioral, or learning problems. Mr. and Mrs. D. had been together for nearly 7 years but were married for only the past 3 years. Their relationship was generally stable, with no history of major marital difficulties. No recent psychosocial stressors had occurred. Although there was no extended family history of AD/HD, several maternal relatives had displayed conduct problems and antisocial behavior, as well as learning disorders.

Throughout his schooling Jason had been performing at grade level to somewhat below grade level in all facets of his academic work. Moreover, the quality and quantity of his work was highly variable from day to day. Both his parents and his teachers believed that his academic achievement was well below his intellectual potential. Amplifying on this point, Jason's current teacher, Mrs. S., had recently remarked:

> "Jason is a child with great potential! He appears to be very bright, has much general knowledge, a wonderful oral vocabulary, and seems to absorb a lot even if I think he is not listening. *But* he will not produce unless an adult is standing right next to him. When left on his own after work is thoroughly explained, nothing gets done. It is difficult to evaluate where he stands as far his grade level because many times work is incomplete or hurried at the last minute. I have no doubt, however, that

Jason could easily produce above grade level in all areas if he applied himself."

Despite such long-standing concerns, Jason had never undergone school-based testing or received psychological testing. He carried no prior diagnoses and had never received any ongoing psychotherapy or special education assistance.

Assessment Process

Prior to embarking on a course of treatment, Jason underwent a formal psychological evaluation. In particular, a comprehensive multimethod assessment was performed (Anastopoulos & Shelton, 2001), so as to capture the situational variability of Jason's AD/HD, as well as its comorbid features and impact on home, school, and social functioning. This included not only the traditional methods of parent and child interviews, but also standardized child behavior rating scales, parent self-report measures pertaining to personal and family functioning, clinic-based psychological testing, and a review of prior medical and school records.

Like many parents, Mr. and Mrs. D. were initially confused by their level of involvement in the assessment process. "After all," they reasoned, "if you're trying to find out whether our child has AD/HD, why are you spending so much time interviewing us and having us fill out questionnaires. . . . Why aren't you spending more time testing our child?" Left unanswered, such matters might have caused them to feel threatened or to question the competence of the evaluating clinician. This in turn might have interfered with their acceptance of diagnostic feedback, as well as their willingness to implement subsequent treatment recommendations. The rationale for this assessment approach was therefore explained. In particular, Mr. and Mrs. D. were told that directly testing Jason involved relatively novel and interesting psychological test materials that are administered under closely supervised, high feedback, one-to-one conditions. Such circumstances decrease the likelihood that AD/HD symptoms would surface. For this reason, the most accurate sampling of Jason's behavior stemmed from their input and from that of his teacher, based on their observations of Jason in situational contexts that are more likely to elicit AD/HD symptomatology. This explanation alleviated their initial concerns.

Diagnostic Conceptualization

An abbreviated summary of Jason's multimethod assessment results appears in Tables 2.1 and 2.2. The Diagnostic Interview Schedule for Children (DISC), ADHD Rating Scale–IV, and Behavioral Assessment System for Children (BASC) findings provided strong evidence that Jason met DSM-IV criteria for a diagnosis of attention-deficit/hyperactivity disorder, combined type (314.01). In addition, it was quite clear from the DISC and BASC that he met DSM-IV criteria for a secondary diagnosis of oppositional defiant disorder (313.81). Together, these conditions very likely were responsible for his diminished academic productivity on the Academic Performance Rating Scale (APRS), the significant gap between his predicted Wechsler Intelligence Scale for Children—Third Edition (WISC-III) and actual Wechsler Individual Achievement Test (WIAT) levels of educational achievement, and the elevated parenting stress reported by his parents on the Parenting Stress Index—Short Form (PSI-SF). No other major diagnostic concerns emerged from this evaluation. However, there was evidence (BASC) to suggest that depression concerns might be emerging. Moreover, the possibility of a visual–motor deficit (Coding subtest of the WISC-III) was raised. In addition to these child concerns, there was reason to believe that Mrs. D. might be having adult AD/HD difficulties, as well as mild depressive symptoms and other types of psychological distress as indicated by the Symptom Checklist 90—Revised (SCL-90-R).

TABLE 2.1. Abbreviated Summary of Significant Multimethod Assessment Findings Obtained from Mother and Teacher

	Mother	Teacher
Diagnostic Interview Schedule for Children (DISC)	Positive for AD/HD, ODD	n/a
ADHD Rating Scale–IV		
Inattention	24	17
Hyperactive–Impulsive	26	24
Behavior Assessment System for Children (BASC)		
Hyperactivity	83	74
Aggression	72	67
Depression	67	68
Attention problems	71	57
Academic Performance Rating Scale (APRS)		
Academic success	n/a	27
Productivity	n/a	26
Parenting Stress Index—Short Form (PSI-SF)		
Total stress	97	n/a
Symptom Checklist 90—Revised (SCL-90-R)		
General severity	63	n/a
Adult AD/HD Rating Scale		
Total severity	29	n/a

TABLE 2.2. Abbreviated Summary of Significant Multimethod Assessment Findings Obtained from Jason

Wechsler Intelligence Scale for Children—Third Edition (WISC-III)	
Verbal IQ	129
Performance IQ	123
Full Scale IQ	129
Verbal Comprehension Index	136
Perceptual Organization Index	133
Freedom from Distractibility Index	98
Processing Speed	86
Picture Completion	17
Information	16
Coding	5
Similarities	16
Picture Arrangement	9
Arithmetic	10
Block Design	19
Vocabulary	15
Object Assembly	17
Comprehension	18
Symbol Search	9
Digit Span	9

Wechsler Individual Achievement Test (WIAT)	
Reading Standard Score	91
Math Standard Score	96
Spelling Standard Score	93

Feedback Session

During a subsequent feedback session, Mrs. D. respectfully challenged the conclusion that Jason displayed the combined type of AD/HD. While acknowledging that Jason had problems paying attention, she firmly believed that "he was not hyperactive." Implicit in this response is the faulty belief that motor restlessness has to be extreme before it can be labeled hyperactivity. Moreover, she appeared to assume that hyperactivity could only be expressed through physical actions. To help correct these misperceptions and thereby facilitate parental acceptance of the diagnosis and subsequent treatment recommendations, Mrs. D. was first told that hyperactivity can be displayed both motorically and vocally. Also pointed out was that while most people think of hyperactivity in its extreme form (e.g., "bouncing off the walls"), it can also present itself in less severe forms, such as "fidgeting when seated," or "talking excessively." With this explanation in mind, Mrs. D.'s understanding of Jason's lifelong history of being a "motor-mouth" and having difficulties sitting still in church suddenly made far more sense to her.

Another complication that arose during the feedback session was Mr. D.'s resistance to accepting any diagnosis at all. As he stated, *"If he really does have AD/HD, then why can he pay attention to his video games . . . and why don't I have problems managing him?"* At the root of this difference of parental opinion is dichotomous, all-or-none thinking—that is, if he has AD/HD, it should always be evident. Cognitive restructuring techniques were then used to point out the all-or-none nature of this thinking. Also provided at this time was a more realistic view of how AD/HD symptoms vary in accordance with situational demands. Although initially skeptical, Mr. D. was generally receptive to these restructuring efforts, thereby making it possible for him to see this matter more in accordance with his wife.

As the feedback session progressed, both parents became more accepting of Jason's diagnostic status, at least with respect to his AD/HD. When news of his comorbid ODD was mentioned, yet another complication arose. Feeling like there must be something terribly wrong with their son, Mr. and Mrs. D. wondered out loud what they had done wrong to produce a child with so many problems. Some friends and relatives had gone so far as to tell them that they had erred. Hearing this additional diagnostic feedback served to confirm their worst fears—that they had indeed done something wrong and were bad parents, which increased their sense of guilt, frustration, and despair. To defuse the underlying overgeneralization in their thinking, it was pointed out that faulty parenting is *not* a cause of AD/HD. On the contrary, most of the current research points toward biological causes, including genetic transmission and prenatal complications. Emphasizing the biological nature of this disorder went a long way toward helping Mr. and Mrs. D. to see Jason's problems in a different light. Although this information did not eliminate their negative self-perception and feelings, it began the process of reframing their views of their contribution to his problems. This in turn set the stage for Mr. and Mrs. D. to let go of other maladaptive beliefs that they may have (e.g., "I must be a bad parent"), thereby reducing associated feelings of guilt and personal distress.

Treatment Plan

Given the multiple problems inherent in Jason's clinical presentation, it was quite clear that no one treatment could address all of his clinical management needs. Thus, a multimodal treatment plan, incorporating a combination of intervention strategies that recently has received empirical support (Jensen et al., 2001), was adopted. This included a trial of stimulant medication, classroom modifications, and home management strategies, as well as individual counseling for Mrs. D.

In view of the fact that Jason was also displaying mild symptoms of depression and anxiety, as well as peer relationship problems, Mr. and Mrs. D. were advised to monitor his status in these areas. Direct treatment of these problem areas was deferred, however, because there was reason to believe that these difficulties might be secondary manifestations of Jason's primary AD/HD and ODD symptoms. More specifically, it was assumed that as the preceding treatments brought his primary AD/HD and ODD symptoms under better control, concomitant improvements in his emotional and social functioning would likely ensue.

Given that Jason had been showing signs of a motor-based learning problem, further assessment of this matter was also recommended. Finally, to facilitate implementation of all of these recommendations, Mr. and Mrs. D. and Jason's teacher were strongly encouraged to increase their knowledge and understanding of AD/HD through various readings on the topic, as well as through videotaped presentations, websites, and local support groups.

Course of Treatment

To deal with Jason's AD/HD symptoms both at home and in school, a trial of stimulant medication was recommended. Although stimulant medications are an empirically supported treatment for AD/HD (Greenhill, 1998), Mr. and Mrs. D. were somewhat hesitant. Although they feared the unknown, as it were, they nonetheless agreed to give it a try. They were uncertain, however, as to how they would explain this to Jason. Recognizing their hesitancy about the matter, they asked for assistance in explaining this upcoming medication trial to Jason.

As Mr. and Mrs. D. had predicted, Jason was very apprehensive about taking medication. Much of this distress stemmed from negative comments about medication that he had heard from them in the past. Although they were now more ready to give this a try based on the new factual information they had acquired, Jason was much less willing to do so. To alleviate his concerns, visual imagery related to Jason's everyday life experience was used to reframe his view of medication. To create this mental picture, Jason was first asked: "Are you a fast runner?" Just about every child says yes, as did Jason. He was next asked, "What are the names of some kids that don't run as fast as you?" After offering "Jimmy," Jason was then told, "Let's suppose that you and Jimmy are about to run a race . . . but in this race, you have heavy weights attached to your ankles. . . . if that were to happen, who would win the race?" Jason acknowledged the obvious and admitted that Jimmy would. At this point he heard, "Having those weights on is a lot like having AD/HD. It keeps you from doing what you can do and know how to do. . . . What would happen if we took off those weights?" After he responded that he would run faster and win once again, the rationale for the medication trial was then offered, "Well, that's why we sometimes give special medication to children. . . . It helps remove some of the "weight" from you, and that makes it possible for you to do everything you're capable of doing." This type of visual imagery helped Jason see the benefits of medication while acknowledging its limitations. By highlighting that the medication would enable him to "be all that you can be," it reinforced the notion that therapeutic gains would in part be due to his own skills. This point is important as one wants to avoid having the child attribute any difficulties to not taking the medication, and similarly giving credit for all improvements to the medication. In short, the goal of this discussion was to help Jason understand the basics of medication in a developmentally appropriate fashion and to appraise the benefits of medication in a realistic and balanced way.

This goal was reached and the trial proceeded smoothly from start to finish. A 4-week, double-blind drug–placebo trial format was employed, comparing weekly administrations of low (5 mg), medium (10 mg), and high (15 mg) twice-daily doses of methylphenidate against a placebo condition. The outcome data from the trial demonstrated that Jason benefited from the medium and high stimulant doses in the absence of significant side effects. In cognitive therapy terms, such behavioral data served to disconfirm previously held fears and anxieties that Jason and his parents had. Thus, the family was most receptive to the idea of maintaining Jason on a long-term stimulant therapy regimen, under the close supervision of his pediatrician.

Parent training and classroom contingency management programs also stand as empirically supported treatments for AD/HD among youth (Pelham, Wheeler, & Chronis, 1998). Concurrent with Jason's medication trial, numerous school-based changes were introduced to create classroom conditions that would further reduce the impact of his AD/HD, thereby maximizing his academic performance. This included recommendations for, among other things, reducing his workloads, attaching an index card with classroom rules to his desk, using a high-interest curriculum, giving more immediate and frequent feedback throughout the day, and establishing a daily report card system. Although these recommendations were conceptually sound and empirically supported, Jason's teacher was reluctant to incorporate them. Why? As she explained, "If I change things for one child, then I'll have to change things for everyone else." By pointing out the overgeneralization in her statement, Mrs. S. was able to see Jason's situation in a different and more supportive light. Thus, she eventually agreed to implement the recommended modifications in order to create a classroom environment that, in combination with his stimulant medication regimen, ultimately facilitated Jason's school behavior and academic performance.

In order to deal with Jason's AD/HD and ODD problems in the home, which were identified by his parents as a priority for treatment, Mr. and Mrs. D. began receiving training in the use of specialized behavior management strategies tailored to the needs of children with AD/HD. This was accomplished in the context of a 9-week, clinic-based parent training program that was originally developed by Barkley (1987) and then later modified by his colleagues at the University of Massachusetts Medical Center (Anastopoulos & Barkley, 1990; Barkley, 1997).

Our goals during the first session were to acquaint Mr. and Mrs. D. with the mechanics of participating in the treatment program, to increase their knowledge of AD/HD, and to set appropriate expectations for therapeutic change. During the second session Mr. and Mrs. D. learned about a four-factor model for understanding parent–child conflict and gained knowledge of behavior management principles as they apply to children with AD/HD.

The main objective of Session 3 was to begin teaching them positive attending and ignoring skills in the context of special time. In particular, they were encouraged to "catch Jason being good" as often as possible, so as to see him in a different, more realistic, and more positive light. Doing so, of course, helped establish more positive parent–child relations.

During the next session Mr. and Mrs. D. learned how to extend positive attending skills to other situations, including times when Jason was displaying appropriate behavior that allowed Mr. and Mrs. D. to engage in activities without interruption. Like many other children with AD/HD, Jason often became disruptive when his parents were engaged in home activities, such as talking on the telephone, preparing dinner, or visiting with company. Why? Presumably because children with AD/HD have trouble waiting for things and delaying gratification, they frequently interrupt. After calling attention to the fact that most parents generally do not hesitate to stop an ongoing activity to address these disruptions, the following questions were posed: Should Mr. and Mrs. D. stop what they were doing to attend positively to Jason when he was engaged in independent play that was not disruptive? Like most parents, Mr. and Mrs. D. did not think so, citing a "let sleeping dogs lie" philosophy as their rationale. This assumption was first examined from a cognitive therapy perspective—as an example of jumping to conclusions (in this case, predicting a negative outcome). Mr. and Mrs. D. were then asked how certain they were that dispensing positive attention in this manner would be disruptive. They stated that they were pretty sure, but not 100%. While acknowledging that they might in fact be correct in their prediction, it was also pointed out that they may not be. Until their "sleeping dogs" philosophy was put to empirical test against an alternative hypothesis, it could neither be confirmed or disconfirmed. Additional justification for putting these competing assumptions to test was inferred from what was learned earlier in the review of general behavior management principles—namely, that when any behavior is ignored, this decreases its probability of occurring. This in turn increases the likelihood that various disruptive behaviors will develop inadvertently. If attended to positively, however, such independent play is much more likely to reappear in the future. With some degree of trepidation, Mr. and Mrs. D. put these competing hypotheses to test. As so often happens, they came back the following week with good news to report. Illustrative of their success, Mr. D. reported that he had actually read the newspaper uninterrupted for the first time in many years!

Establishing a reward-oriented home token system was the major focus of Session 5. The intent of such a system was to provide Jason with the external motivation he needed to complete parent-requested activities that may be of little intrinsic interest and that served to trigger his defiance. Mr. and Mrs. D.'s confidence and motivation, which had been increasing, began to waver at the start of this session. Like many parents, they believed that they had "already done something like this before and that it just doesn't work." These overgeneralizations were addressed by asking them to provide a detailed description of the techniques they had used. Against this background, the details of the current home token system were presented, emphasizing differences with their previous attempts. Although this information did not immediately convince Mr. and Mrs. D. that this new approach would work, they became more receptive to the idea that alternative approaches might exist. Consequently, they were willing to try the recommended home token system, which ultimately brought about major improvements in Jason's home behavior.

The primary purpose of Session 6 was to refine the home token system, including the addition of response-cost strategies for minor misbehavior. More specifically, Mr. and Mrs. D. were instructed to begin deducting poker chips for noncompliance with one or two requests. Similar penalties were introduced to address problematic behaviors, including physical aggression and talking back. Another punishment strategy was added during Session 7. Mr. and Mrs. D. learned how to use a version of time-out for dealing with more serious forms of noncompliance. As had been the case for the home token system, Mr. and Mrs. D. had unsuccessfully used a variation of the time-out strategy in the past. Their negative expectations were addressed via the same type of cognitive restructuring techniques that had been used to deal with their reluctance to using the home poker chip system.

Although Jason's behavior had improved, treatment effects rarely generalize to new settings without planning and effort. With this in mind, the purpose of Session 8 was to begin expanding Mr. and Mrs. D.'s use of the behavior management program to settings outside the home. Among the settings that were identified as problematic for Jason were department stores and restaurants. Modified versions of the strategies that had been used successfully at home were incorporated into this plan. In contrast their eagerness to use behavior management techniques at home, Mr. and Mrs. D. were much less enthusiastic about implementing these techniques in public. After all, they noted, "What will people think?" The fact that this reflected mind reading, a form of cognitive distortion, was highlighted as the basis for their reaching a negative conclusion. Alternative viewpoints as to what people might think, and the importance they were attaching to others' opinions as it pertained to Jason's welfare, were discussed. Addressing parental perceptions in this manner reduced their uneasiness, thereby increasing their motivation for trying such a new and challenging approach.

Session 9 served many purposes, including increasing Mr. and Mrs. D.'s knowledge of relevant school issues, discussing how to handle future problems that might arise, and preparing for termination by learning how to fade out the home-based behavior management program, among other issues. Given how well they had acquired the knowledge and skills of this program, Mr. and Mrs. D. agreed that termination from this phase of the multimodal treatment program was in order.

Although the contingency management system worked well for several weeks following termination, Jason began to display some resistance and his behavior began to deteriorate. This led Mr. and Mrs. D. to the erroneous conclusion that the program had not worked. During a follow-up telephone consultation, it was pointed out that this was not an unusual occurrence for children with AD/HD, given the fact that they are prone to become bored easily and that specific rewards may lose their salience over time. They were encouraged to make minor modifications in Jason's contingency management system, so as to increase its novelty, salience, and meaningfulness. It was hypothesized that doing so would increase his interest in the program. When put to test, this prediction was supported.

After several months, it was clear that the combination of stimulant medication therapy, parent training, and school-based modifications had brought about many improvements in Jason's psychosocial functioning, as noted in Table 2.3. Of additional importance is that Jason's parents reported feeling less stress and guilt in their roles as parents. Moreover, both parents indicated that they had learned to view and to accept Jason's AD/HD in a different light. This in turn reduced the disagreements they had over parenting issues. Equally important, Jason seemed to be happier and more involved in social activities with peers. Had an opposite outcome scenario unfolded – that is, had there been no concomitant improvements in his emotional and social functioning—it would then have been necessary to consider targeting these emotional and social areas more directly through the use of individual therapy and school-based social skills training, respectively.

Although not directly related to the management of Jason's AD/HD, one last finding from the multimethod assessment bears mentioning. Because there was evidence that Mrs. D. might be experiencing mild depression as well as adult AD/HD problems, this too needed to be addressed. Thus, a recommendation was made for her to undergo further evaluation and to begin receiving treatment as needed. To her credit she followed through on these recommendations. Through a combination of cognitive

TABLE 2.3. Abbreviated Summary of Psychosocial Changes Following Multimodal Treatment

	Mother		Teacher	
	Pre	Post	Pre	Post
ADHD Rating Scale–IV				
In/attention	24	22	17	10
Hyperactive–Impulsive	26	18	24	12
Behavior Assessment System for Children (BASC)				
Aggression	72	64	67	60
Depression	67	58	68	62
Academic Performance Rating Scale (APRS)				
Academic success	n/a	n/a	27	30
Productivity	n/a	n/a	26	32
Parenting Stress Index—Short Form (PSI-SF)				
Total stress	97	85	n/a	n/a
Symptom Checklist 90—Revised (SCL-90-R)				
General severity	63	55	n/a	n/a

therapy and stimulant medication, she was able to bring about improvements in her depression and AD/HD symptoms. This not only served to alleviate her personal distress but also allowed her to implement her newly acquired parent training techniques and other aspects of Jason's treatment plan more effectively.

CONCLUSIONS

Early applications of cognitive therapy with AD/HD populations emphasized the use of verbal self-regulation training. Such an approach was based on the assumption that verbal mediation deficits were central to understanding this disorder. Contrary to expectation, research findings have not provided strong support for using this type of treatment routinely in the clinical management of AD/HD. One possible explanation for the limited success of these cognitively based treatment strategies is that they do not target neurologically based deficits in behavioral inhibition, which presumably precede verbal self-regulation in the chain of events leading to the AD/HD.

Although verbal self-control training may not be well suited to addressing its primary symptoms, the manner in which AD/HD presents itself affords clinicians many opportunities for using restructuring, visual imagery, and other cognitive techniques. Such strategies can be used at many points in the clinical management of children and adolescents with AD/HD, including both the assessment and treatment phases.

The clinical examples described in this chapter should in no way be construed as exhaustive. On the contrary, there would seem to be no boundaries to the ways in which clinicians might employ cognitive therapy techniques in the assessment and treatment of children and adults with AD/HD. At present, few pertinent research findings are available to guide clinical practice. Therefore, there is a clear need within the field for specialists in AD/HD and cognitive-behavioral therapy to collaborate in developing assessment and treatment procedures that address the clinical needs of this population.

In the child domain, consideration could be given to developing assessment procedures that tap into parental assumptions about AD/HD as a disorder, including parental cognitions about its causes and beliefs about the efficacy of various treatments. Similar assessment devices might be developed for use with affected children and their teachers. Once developed, such measures might be used to examine the role cognitive variables play in predicting treatment outcome and in mediating previously reported treatment-induced changes in parenting functioning, such as decreased parenting stress following participation in cognitive-behavioral parent training programs (Anastopoulos, Shelton, DuPaul, & Guevremont, 1993). To the extent that parent and teacher cognitions interfere with the success of home and school-based interventions, it may also be useful for future researchers to begin examining how cognitive therapy, pitched systematically at these important adults in the child's life, can improve their implementation of and adherence to treatments that they deliver on behalf of the child.

These are but a few of the many possible directions that future research and clinical practice might take. Those who read this chapter, ideally, will be inspired to think of other ways in which cognitive therapy can be used when working with AD/HD populations.

REFERENCES

Abikoff, M., & Gittelman, R. (1985). Hyperactive children treated with stimulants: Is cognitive training a useful adjunct? *Archives of General Psychiatry, 42,* 953–961.

American Psychiatric Association. (1994). *Diagnostic and statistical manual of mental disorders* (4th ed.). Washington, DC: Author.

Anastopoulos, A. D., & Barkley, R. A. (1990). Counseling and training parents. In R. A. Barkley, *Attention-deficit hyperactivity disorder: A handbook for diagnosis and treatment* (pp. 397–431). New York: Guilford Press.

Anastopoulos, A. D., & Shelton, T. L. (2001). *Assessing attention-deficit/hyperactivity disorder.* New York: Kluwer Academic/Plenum.

Anastopoulos, A. D., Shelton, T. L., DuPaul, G. J., & Guevremont, D. C. (1993). Parent training for attention-deficit hyperactivity disorder: Its impact on parent functioning. *Journal of Abnormal Child Psychology, 21,* 581–596.

Arnsten, A. F. T., Steere, J. C., & Hunt, R. D. (1996). The contribution of alpha2 Noradrenergic mechanism to prefrontal cortical cognitive function. *Archives of General Psychiatry, 53*, 448–455.

August, G. J., Realmuto, G. M., MacDonald, A. W., Nugent, S. M., & Crosby, R. (1996). Prevalence of ADHD and comorbid disorders among elementary school children screened for disruptive behavior. *Journal of Abnormal Child Psychology, 24*, 571–595.

Barkley, R. A. (1977). The effects of methylphenidate on various measures of activity level and attention in hyperkinetic children. *Journal of Abnormal Child Psychology, 5*, 351–369.

Barkley, R. A. (1987). *Defiant children: A clinician's manual for parent training.* New York: Guilford Press.

Barkley, R. A. (1997). *Defiant children: A clinician's manual for assessment and parent training* (2nd ed.). New York: Guilford Press.

Barkley, R. A. (1998). *Attention-deficit hyperactivity disorder: A handbook for diagnosis and treatment* (2nd ed.). New York: Guilford Press.

Barkley, R. A., Anastopoulos, A. D., Guevremont, D. C., & Fletcher, K. E. (1991). Adolescents with attention deficit hyperactivity disorder: Patterns of behavioral adjustment, academic functioning, and treatment utilization. *Journal of the American Academy of Child and Adolescent Psychiatry, 30*, 752– 761.

Barkley, R. A., Anastopoulos, A. D., Guevremont, D. C., & Fletcher, K. E. (1992). Adolescents with attention deficit hyperactivity disorder: Mother–adolescent interactions, family beliefs and conflicts, and maternal psychopathology. *Journal of Abnormal Child Psychology, 20*, 263–288.

Barkley, R. A., Fischer, M., Edelbrock, C. S., & Smallish, L. (1990). The adolescent outcome of hyperactive children diagnosed by research criteria: I. An 8-year prospective follow-up study. *Journal of the American Academy of Child and Adolescent Psychiatry, 29*, 546–557.

Beck, A. T. (1976). *Cognitive therapy and the emotional disorders.* New York: New American Library.

Beck, J. (1995). *Cognitive therapy: Basics and beyond.* New York: Guilford Press.

Block, G. H. (1977). Hyperactivity: A cultural perspective. *Journal of Learning Disabilities, 110*, 236–240.

Bornstein, P. H., & Quevillon, R. P. (1976). The effects of a self-instructional package on overactive preschool boys. *Journal of Applied Behavior Analysis, 9*, 179– 188.

Campbell, S. B. (1990). *Behavior problems in preschool children: Clinical and developmental issues.* New York: Guilford Press.

Castellanos, F. X., Giedd, J. N., Marsh, W. L., Hamburger, S. D., Vaituzis, A. D., Dickstein, D. P., Sarfatti, S. E., Vauss, Y. C., Snell, J. W., Lange, N., Kaysen, D., Krain, A. L., Ritchhie, G. F., Rajapakse, J. C., & Rapoport, J. L. (1996). Quantitative brain magnetic resonance imaging in attention-deficit/hyperactivity disorder. *Archives of General Psychiatry, 53*, 607–616.

Dobson, K. S. (1989). A meta-analysis of the efficacy of cognitive therapy for depression. *Journal of Consulting and Clinical Psychology, 57*, 414–419.

Douglas, V. I. (1972). Stop, look, and listen: The problem of sustained attention and impulse control in hyperactive and normal children. *Canadian Journal of Behavioral Science, 4*, 259–282.

Douglas, V. I. (1983). Attention and cognitive problems. In M. Rutter (Ed.), *Developmental neuropsychiatry* (pp. 280–329). New York: Guilford Press.

DuPaul, G. J., Anastopoulos, A. D., Power, T. J., Reid, R., Ikeda, M. J., & McGoey, K. E. (1998). Parent ratings of attention-deficit/hyperactivity disorder symptoms: Factor structure and normative data. *Journal of Psychopathology and Behavioral Assessment, 20,* 83–102.

DuPaul, G. J., & Stoner, G. (1994). *ADHD in the schools: Assessment and intervention strategies.* New York: Guilford Press.

Gaub, M., & Carlson, C. (1997). Behavioral characteristics of DSM-IV AD/HD subtypes in a school-based population. *Journal of Abnormal Child Psychology, 25,* 103–111.

Gittelman, R., Mannuzza, S., Shenker, R., & Bonagura, N. (1985). Hyperactive boys almost grown up: I. Psychiatric status. *Archives of General Psychiatry, 42,* 937–947.

Greenhill, L. (1998). Childhood attention deficit hyperactivity disorder: Pharmacological treatments. In P. Nathan & J. Gorman (Eds.), *A guide to treatments that work* (pp. 42–64). New York: Oxford University Press.

Harrington, R., Campbell, F., Shoebridge, P., & Whittaker, J. (1998). Meta-analysis of CBT for depression in adolescents. *Journal of the American Academy of Child and Adolescent Psychiatry, 37,* 1005–1006.

Hinshaw, S. P. (2000). Attention-deficit/hyperactivity disorder: The search for viable treatments. In P. C. Kendall (Ed.), *Child and adolescent therapy: Cognitive-behavioral procedures* (pp. 88–128). New York: Guilford Press.

Hinshaw, S. P., Henker, B., & Whalen, C. K. (1984). Self-control in hyperactive boys in anger-inducing situations: Effects of cognitive-behavioral training and of methylphenidate. *Journal of Abnormal Child Psychology, 12,* 55–77.

Jacobvitz, D., & Sroufe, L. A. (1987). The early caregiver–child relationship and attention-deficit disorder with hyperactivity in kindergarten: A prospective study. *Child Development, 58,* 1488–1495.

Jensen, P. S., Hinshaw, S. P., Swanson, J. M., Greenhill, L. L., Conners, C. K., Arnold, L. E., Abikoff, H. B., Elliott, G., Hechtman, L., Hoza, B., March, J., Newcorn, J. H., Severe, J. B., Vitiello, B., Wells, K., & Wigal, T. (2001). Findings from the NIMH Multimodal Treatment Study of ADHD (MTA): Implications and applications for primary care providers. *Journal of Developmental and Behavioral Pediatrics, 22,* 60–73.

Jensen, P. S., Martin, D., & Cantwell, D. P. (1997). Comorbidity of ADHD: Implications for research, practice, and DSM-V. *Journal of the American Academy of Child and Adolescent Psychiatry, 36,* 1065–1079.

Johnston, C. (1996). Parent characteristics and parent–child interactions in families of nonproblem children and ADHD children with higher and lower levels of oppositional-defiant behavior. *Journal of Abnormal Child Psychology, 24,* 85–104.

Kendall, P. C. (Ed.). (2000). *Child and adolescent therapy: Cognitive-behavioral procedures* (2nd ed.). New York: Guilford Press.

Kendall, P. C., & Braswell, L. (1985). *Cognitive-behavioral therapy for impulsive children.* New York: Guilford Press.

Klein, R. G., & Mannuzza, S. (1991). Long-term outcome of hyperactive children: A review. *Journal of American Academy of Child and Adolescent Psychiatry, 30,* 383–387.

Lahey, B. B., Carlson, C. L., & Frick, P. J. (1997). Attention deficit disorder without hyperactivity: A review of research relevant to DSM-IV. In T. A. Wideger, A. J. Frances, H. A. Pincus, et al. (Eds.), *DSM-IV Sourcebook* (Vol. 3, pp. 189–209). Washington, DC: American Psychiatric Association.

Levy, F., Hay, D. A., McStephen, M., Wood, C., & Waldman, I. (1997). Attention-deficit hyperactivity disorder: A category or a continuum? Genetic analysis of a large-scale twin study. *Journal of the American Academy of Child and Adolescent Psychiatry, 36,* 737–744.

Luk, S. (1985). Direct observation studies of hyperactive studies of hyperactive behaviors. *Journal of the American Academy of Child Psychiatry, 24,* 338–344.

Mannuzza, S., Klein, R. G., Bessler, A., Malloy, P., & LaPadula, M. (1993). Adult outcome of hyperactive boys: Educational achievement, occupational rank, and psychiatric status. *Archives of General Psychiatry, 45,* 13–18.

Meichenbaum, D., & Goodman, J. (1971). Training impulsive children to talk to themselves: A means of developing self-control. *Journal of Abnormal Psychology, 77,* 115–126.

Miranda, A., & Presentacion, M. J. (2000). Efficacy of cognitive-behavioral therapy in the treatment of children with ADHD, with and without aggressiveness. *Psychology in the Schools, 37,* 169–182.

Murphy, K., & Barkley, R. A. (1996a). Attention deficit hyperactivity disorder in adults. *Comprehensive Psychiatry, 37,* 393–401.

Murphy, K., & Barkley, R. A. (1996b). Prevalence of DSM-IV symptoms of ADHD in adult licensed drivers: Implication for clinical diagnosis. *Journal of Attention Disorders, 1,* 147–161.

Pelham, W., Wheeler, T., & Chronis, A. (1998). Empirically supported psychosocial treatments for attention deficit hyperactivity disorder. *Journal of Clinical Child Psychology, 27,* 190–205.

Quay, H. C. (1997). Inhibition and attention deficit hyperactivity disorder. *Journal of Abnormal Child Psychology, 25,* 7–13.

Shapiro, E. S., & Cole, C. L. (1994). *Behavior change in the classroom: Self-management interventions.* New York: Guilford Press.

Shelton, T., Barkley, R., Crosswait, C., Moorehouse, M., Fletcher, K., Barrett, S., Jenkins, L., & Metevia, L. (1998). Psychiatric and psychological morbidity as a function of adaptive disability in preschool children with aggressive and hyperactive–impulsive–inattentive behavior. *Journal of Abnormal Child Psychology, 26,* 475–494.

Solomon, A., & Haaga, D. (in press). Cognitive theory and therapy of depression. In M. Reinecke & D. Clark (Eds.), *Cognitive therapy across the lifespan: Prospects and challenges.* Cambridge, UK: Cambridge University Press.

Streissguth, A. P., Bookstein, F. L., Sampson, P. D., & Barr, H. M. (1995). Attention: Prenatal alcohol and continuities of vigilance and attentional problems from 4 through 14 years. *Development and Psychopathology, 7,* 419–446.

Weiss, G., & Hechtman, L. (1993). *Hyperactive children grown up* (2nd ed.). New York: Guilford Press.

Zametkin, A. J., Norcross, T. E., Gross, M., King, A. C., Semple, W. E., Rumsey, J., Hamburger, S., & Cohen, R. M. (1990). Cerebral glucose metabolism in adults with hyperactivity of childhood onset. *New England Journal of Medicine, 323,* 1361–1366.

Zentall, S. (1985). A context for hyperactivity. In K. D. Gadow & I. Bialer (Eds.), *Advances in learning and behavioral disabilities* (Vol. 4, pp. 273–343). Greenwich, CT: JAI Press.

SUGGESTED READINGS

Anastopoulos, A. D., & Shelton, T. L. (2001). *Assessing attention-deficit/hyperactivity disorder.* New York: Kluwer Academic/Plenum.

Barkley, R. A. (1997). *Defiant children: A clinician's manual for assessment and parent training* (2nd ed.). New York: Guilford Press.

Barkley, R. A. (1998). *Attention-deficit hyperactivity disorder: A handbook for diagnosis and treatment* (2nd ed.). New York: Guilford Press.

DuPaul, G. J., & Stoner, G. (1994). *ADHD in the schools: Assessment and intervention strategies.* New York: Guilford Press.

Hinshaw, S. P. (2000). Attention-deficit/hyperactivity disorder: The search for viable treatments. In P. C. Kendall (Ed.), *Child and adolescent therapy: Cognitive-behavioral procedures* (2nd ed., pp. 88–128). New York: Guilford Press.

Pelham, W., Wheeler, T., & Chronis, A. (1998). Empirically supported psychosocial treatments for attention deficit hyperactivity disorder. *Journal of Clinical Child Psychology, 27,* 190–205.

Quay, H. C. (1997). Inhibition and attention deficit hyperactivity disorder. *Journal of Abnormal Child Psychology, 25,* 7–13.

3

Treatments for Oppositional Defiant Disorder

DUSTIN A. PARDINI
JOHN LOCHMAN

Although oppositional defiant disorder (ODD) was initially recognized as a diagnosable condition in third edition of the *Diagnostic and Statistical Manual of Mental Disorders* (DSM-III; American Psychiatric Association, 1980), there still is much debate about the nature and treatment of the disorder. Some of the more recent controversies have concerned issues like differentiating ODD from conduct disorder (CD) and attention-deficit/hyperactivity disorder (AD/HD), clarifying the key characteristics of the disorder, and differentiating ODD from normal rebelliousness in childhood. As conceptualizations of ODD and its etiology have become more refined in recent years, there has been a burgeoning research literature documenting successful family- and child-based treatments for the disorder. Some of the most successful treatments have coupled behavior management training for parents with child-based interventions aimed at correcting the maladaptive social-cognitive processes and problem-solving abilities found in children with ODD. The purpose of the current chapter is to describe recent research pertaining to the identification and etiology of oppositional defiant disorder, introduce some empirically validated techniques used to treat the disorder, and provide a case example of how these techniques can be used in clinical practice.

DEFINITIONAL ISSUES

In its initial conceptualization as part of DSM-III, the diagnosis of oppositional defiant disorder required that children have two of five symptoms, including violations of minor rules, temper tantrums, argumentativeness, defiance, provocativeness, and stubborness (American Psychiatric Association, 1980). Changes to the definition in the revised third edition, DSM-III-R, included expanding the symptom list to nine and adding the word "often" to each symptom in an attempt to differentiate them from normal childhood behaviors (American Psychiatric Association, 1987). Moreover, there was a passage added to DSM-III-R indicating that while many preschool-age children exhibit oppositional and defiant behaviors, these symptoms must be abnormal in either frequency or intensity, or persist into the school-age years where they normally begin to decline, in order to be considered indicative of ODD (Loeber, Lahey, & Thomas, 1991). The diagnostic symptom threshold was also increased so that three of the nine symptoms were required throughout a 6-month period.

During the DSM-IV (American Psychiatric Association, 1994) field trials, the diagnostic criterion of swearing or using obscene language was eliminated from the definition of ODD due to minimal support for its clinical utility in differentiating between ODD and conduct disorder and its poor association with other oppositional defiant disorder symptoms (Burns et al., 1997). In addition, a more conservative diagnostic threshold of four symptoms for ODD, rather than three symptoms as outlined in the DSM-III-R, was adopted. This more restricted diagnostic threshold was meant to identify a smaller, more severely impaired set of youth and to help reduce the number of false positives (Lahey et al., 1994). This decision was supported by recent research indicating that, in comparison to the DSM-III-R definition of ODD, the DSM-IV criteria seem to identify a more impaired group of children, while excluding only a few children with minimal impairments (Angold & Costello, 1996). As a result, the current definition of ODD requires that four of eight symptoms, including frequent loss of temper, argumentative and defiant behavior with adults, deliberate annoyance of others, irritability, anger, and vindictiveness, be present over a 6-month period at a level that is abnormal for the child's age or developmental level.

Although there has been significant progress in refining the definition of ODD in recent years, there are several issues that remain unresolved. For example, while the current definition stresses that the symptoms of ODD must occur "more frequently than is typically observed in individuals of comparable age and developmental level," the interpretation of what constitutes "typical" is under the discretion of the therapist (American Psychiatric Association, 1994). Since this ambiguity could lead to increased variability in the diagnosis of ODD, some investigators have begun collecting data on the frequency of ODD symptoms among children in the general population and recommend that this data be used to come up with guidelines for identifying clinically significant levels of ODD symptoms (Angold & Costello, 1996). In addition, findings from this study indicate that requiring only two or three symptoms of ODD, while maintaining the requirement for psychosocial impairment, might optimally identify a group of children in need of treatment. In fact, evidence suggests that these children, in comparison to those who met DSM-IV criteria for ODD, are just as likely to experience impairment at 1-year follow-up and go on to meet criteria for CD.

OPPOSITIONAL DEFIANT DISORDER VERSUS OTHER DISRUPTIVE BEHAVIOR DISORDERS

There has been substantial debate about the distinction between ODD and CD as two separate diagnostic entities (Lahey, Loeber, Quay, Frick, & Grimm, 1992; Loeber et al., 1991). A recent review of the literature from the DSM-IV field trials revealed that a vast majority of children who met criteria for CD before puberty also met criteria for ODD, and the two disorders share several correlates such as low socioeconomic status, parental antisocial behavior, and poor parenting (Lahey et al., 1994). Despite these common correlates, there are several other reasons why CD and ODD remain distinct disorders. Specifically, the former seems to be more strongly related to adverse environmental factors than the latter (Lahey et al., 1992), and there is a distinct group of children who meet criteria for ODD that do not go on to exhibit symptoms of CD. Moreover, the symptoms of ODD are more prevalent in preadolescent children than CD symptoms, even for children on the developmental trajectory leading toward CD. Along similar lines, there are youth who develop CD in adolescence that have not met criteria for ODD in childhood. Several factor-analytic studies also have indicated that symptoms of CD and ODD reliably separate into two clusters of intercorrelated behaviors (Frick et al., 1991, 1994). Finally, while most symptoms of ODD poorly predict a diagnosis of CD, symptoms of CD show high diagnostic utility in predicting an ODD diagnosis, with the symptoms of anger and spite showing the highest loading on the ODD factor regardless of gender and age (Frick et al., 1994).

There has also been some interest in looking at the overlap between ODD and AD/HD in an attempt to distinguish the unique and overlapping features of these disorders. Some investigations have shown that impulsive symptoms associated with AD/HD (e.g., interrupting others, blurting out) tend to overlap with several ODD symptoms (Burns et al., 1997), and may serve as risk factors for the disorder (Pillow, Pelham, Hoza, Molina, & Stultz, 1998). Despite this fact, there is some reason to believe that these symptoms may be fundamentally different in their etiology. For example, Pillow et al. (1998) noted that children with ODD tend to purposefully interrupt and intrude on others, while children with AD/HD engage in these behaviors out of restlessness and violate social norms unintentionally. The same investigators found evidence suggesting that CD and ODD are both forms of aggressive disorders that are related to, yet distinct from, symptoms associated with AD/HD. Moreover, there are some who believe that there are two types of ODD associated with AD/HD, one that precedes the development of CD by several years and another that is a subsyndromal form of CD that is not likely to develop into CD (Biederman et al., 1996).

ETIOLOGY OF OPPOSITIONAL DEFIANT DISORDER

Although there are several developmental theories that attempt to explain the development of childhood antisocial behavior in general, few investigators have attempted to document a developmental trajectory associated with the manifestation of ODD in particular (Rey, 1993). Given the previously mentioned controversies regarding the core behavior symptoms of ODD, as well as difficulties differentiating ODD from other disruptive behavior disorders, this gap in the literature is understandable. As the definition of ODD has become more refined, investigators have begun examining the role that etiological factors such as parenting and familial characteristics and social information-processing variables play in the development of the disorder. In addition, attempts have been made to differentiate risk factors for general psychopathology from those that are unique to the development of oppositional and defiant behaviors. Despite this progress, many studies still cluster children with ODD or CD into one group, making it difficult to discern the relative importance of various etiological factors in the development of these two disorders. Since several successful treatments for ODD are based upon research documenting factors placing children at risk for antisocial behavior, a brief overview of research documenting the etiology of oppositional and defiant symptoms will be reviewed here.

Parenting and Familial Factors

There is substantial evidence linking various parenting and familial characteristics to the development of ODD in children. For example, Boyle and Pickles (1998) found that oppositional and defiant symptoms are related to increased levels of familial dysfunction and lower levels of family income, while Rey and Plapp (1990) found that adolescents diagnosed with ODD or CD reported higher levels of authoritarian parenting and lower levels of parental warmth than normal control children, with no differences between the ODD and CD groups. Frick et al. (1992) found that the families of children with ODD reported levels of parental supervision and consistent discipline between those of families of children with CD and clinic control families. There is also evidence suggesting that preschool children with ODD are more likely to exhibit insecure attachment to their maternal caregiver (Speltz, DeKlyen, Greenberg, & Dryden, 1995), which may arise as the result of maternal depression or stress.

    Several other investigations have found that various characteristics of parents and other adult caregivers are associated with ratings of aggressive behavior in children. Since aggressiveness is often associated with ODD, some of the pertinent findings of this research will be reviewed here. For example, Lochman and Dodge (1990) found that parents of aggressive boys tended to use physical and verbal aggression to discipline their children and reported higher levels of marital hostility than parents of nonaggressive children. Evidence suggests that this heightened level of emotional conflict in the home leads children to become hypervigilant to hostile cues (O'Brien & Chin, 1998), thereby increasing the likelihood that children will react aggressively in ambiguous peer-conflict situations (Lochman & Craven, 1993). Moreover, parents of aggressive children tend to use unclear commands, rigid and controlling parenting strategies, ineffective monitoring, and exhibit low levels of parental warmth and support (for review see Lochman and Lenhart, 1993). Given the variable definitions of "aggressiveness" in these studies, it remains unclear what parenting factors are related to both ODD and aggressive behavior in children and what factors may be uniquely related to these two constructs.

Further complicating the link between parent characteristics and ODD are studies providing evidence for a genetic inheritance of deviant behavior. Specifically, data from a twin study suggests that there may be a general genetic liability for conduct problems like property violations, oppositional behavior, and aggression (Simonoff, Pickles, Meyer, Silber, & Maes, 1998). Results from a similar study indicate that ODD symptoms during adolescence seem to represent an early expression of genetic liability for adult antisocial personality in males, even more so than the behavioral criteria associated with CD (Langbehn, Cadoret, William, Troughton, & Stewart, 1998). While there is some evidence that the relation between childhood conduct problems and parental criminality can be accounted for by ineffective and/or harsh parenting (Laub & Sampson, 1988), other investigations have found that having a biological parent with antisocial personality disorder (APD) may be a more important risk factor than specific parenting behaviors (Frick et al., 1992). Despite this fact, the authors of the latter study concede that the link between parental APD and childhood conduct problems could be the result of modeling or reinforcement of antisocial behavior, rather than genetic factors. In addition, parental antisocial behavior may need to be addressed as part of an intervention because it tends to interfere with attempts to change dysfunctional behavior management strategies (Hanish, Tolan, & Guerra, 1996).

Social-Cognitive Processes

There has been a recent accumulation of research suggesting that children who exhibit deviant behaviors have problems with social information-processing and interpersonal problem solving. Crick and Dodge (1994) proposed that deviant children have difficulties at six different stages of social information-processing, including (1) encoding social cues, (2) making interpretations and attributions about social information, (3) identifying goals to be addressed in the social situation, (4) generating possible solutions to interpersonal problems, (5) deciding which plan to enact based on the perceived consequences, and (6) enacting the chosen plan. In support of this theory, a substantial amount of evidence indicates that children with conduct problems exhibit maladaptive social-cognitive processes at each of these stages. Unfortunately, many of these investigations have combined children with ODD and CD into a single group or looked at the difference between aggressive and nonaggressive children in term of their social-cognitive processing. Since most of these studies used definitions of aggression or conduct problems that included oppositional and defiant behaviors, and various forms of aggressive behavior have been associated with both ODD and CD (Frick et al., 1993, 1994), the major findings in this literature will be reviewed here.

There are a number of different social information-processing and problem-solving deficits that have been associated with antisocial behavior in children. Specifically, studies have found that children exhibiting antisocial behavior are more likely than normal children to attend to hostile cues (Gouze, 1987) and attribute hostile intentions to others (Lochman & Dodge, 1994) when involved in ambiguous conflict situations with peers. There is also evidence indicating that children who exhibit antisocial behavior are more likely to expect and value the positive consequences associated with aggression and less likely to expect and value the negative consequences associated with violent behavior (Pardini & Lochman, 2000; Perry, Williard, & Perry, 1990). Children exhibiting antisocial behavior are also more likely to endorse social goals that are damaging to interpersonal relationships when compared to normal peers (Lochman, Wayland, & White, 1993) and lack perspective-taking skills and emotional empathy during social interactions (Cohen & Strayer, 1996). In addition, youth with conduct problems have greater difficulty generating alternative solutions for resolving social conflicts (Lochman, Meyer, Rabiner, & White, 1991) and are less adept at enacting positive interpersonal behaviors than children without conduct problems (Dodge, Pettit, McClaskey, & Brown, 1986).

There are a few recent studies indicating that children with a diagnosis of either ODD or CD have significant problems with social problem-solving skills. One investigation found that children with ODD/CD tend to encode fewer social cues and generate fewer solutions to problems, and are more confident in their ability to enact aggressive responses across a variety of different problematic social situations in comparison to normal controls (Matthys, Cuperus, & Van Engeland, 1999). Moreover, when given the opportunity to choose from various responses in problem situations, they are also more likely to select an aggressive response, and less likely select a prosocial response, in comparison to normal controls. A similar study by Webster-Stratton and Lindsay (1999) examined a wide variety of social information-processing deficits in clinic-referred children (ages 4–7) who met criteria for ODD or CD using DSM-IV criteria. In comparison to normal controls, children with ODD/CD were more likely to attribute hostile intentions to others in hypothetical social situations, and they generated a smaller number of positive problem-solving strategies to resolve imaginary conflicts. During their play interactions with peers, children with ODD/CD tended to engage in parallel play, and they displayed fewer positive social skills and exhibited aggressive problem-solving skills more often than normal control children. Despite these obvious deficits across a wide variety of social information-processing variables, children with ODD/CD did not differ from controls in terms of their perceived social acceptance and feelings of loneliness. To explain this finding, the authors suggested that young children with conduct problems might overestimate their social competence and acceptance as a way to defend against feelings of loneliness. Consequently, clinical professionals may need to help children with ODD objectively evaluate how their behaviors impact interpersonal relations with others before attempting to teach them appropriate social skills.

Since many previously mentioned studies combined children with ODD and CD when examining their social-cognitive deficits, it is difficult to discern what areas of social competence are most relevant to children with ODD. To help answer this question, Dunn, Lochman, and Colder (1997) examined the differences between children with CD and those with ODD in terms of their social problem-solving skills when involved in conflicts with peers, parents, and teachers. Findings revealed that children with ODD and CD do not differ in the total number of solutions generated or the number of aggressive solutions generated when presented with a peer-conflict situation. Conversely, boys with CD proposed more aggressive solutions to teacher and parent conflicts, and generated fewer nonaggressive verbal solutions to peer conflicts, in comparison to boys with ODD. Taken together, these results suggest that children with ODD tend to generate and choose aggressive solutions as a means to resolve peer conflicts, but are less likely than children with CD to use aggression during conflicts with teachers and parents. Although this seems to support the previously mentioned notion that ODD is a subsyndromal form of CD, future studies should attempt to identify the social information-processing deficits associated with ODD by comparing them to normal controls.

COGNITIVE-BEHAVIORAL INTERVENTIONS FOR OPPOSITIONAL DEFIANT DISORDER

Recent efforts have been made to identify empirically supported treatments for a variety of developmental psychopathologies, including externalizing and conduct problems in children. While Kazdin and Weisz (1998) have identified three groups of promising treatments for children with externalizing behavior problems, there have not been any treatments validated for ODD per se. Many of the treatments found to produce significant reductions in aggressive and antisocial behaviors include parent training (Patterson, Reid, & Dishion, 1992) and cognitive problem-solving skills training (Kazdin, Esveldt-Dawson, French, & Unis, 1987). As part of a task force on effective psychosocial interventions, Brestan and Eyberg (1998) reviewed the intervention research on children with conduct problems and concluded that 2 parent training interventions had well-established empirical support, and 10 other programs were probably efficacious based on their outcome research reports. The "probably efficacious" treatments reviewed in the next sections represent interventions that have been designed to address antisocial behavior in youth at several different developmental levels, from preschool to early adolescence. For continuity purposes they are presented in order of the age group served and include Parent–Child Interaction Therapy, Dinosaur School with Parent Training, the Montreal Delinquency Prevention Program, Anger Coping and Coping Power programs, and Problem-Solving Skills Training.

Parent–Child Interaction Therapy

The most recent revision of Parent–Child Interaction Therapy (PCIT) was specifically tailored for preschool-age children meeting diagnostic criteria for ODD (Schuhmann, Foote, Eyberg, Boggs, & Algina, 1998). Treatment sessions occur 1 hour per week and continue until parents are able to master the skills taught and their child no longer meets criteria for ODD. All treatment sessions are implemented in the context of naturalistic play settings. Initially, parents are taught how to engage in child-directed interaction when having free play with their child. This includes using skills like reflecting the child's statements, describing and praising the child's behavior, ignoring undesirable behaviors, and answering his or her question, while avoiding the tendency to direct the play, question the child, or criticize the child. The purpose of this component is to strengthen the parent–child relationship and extinguish maladaptive behaviors that are reinforced by parental attention. Parents are asked to practice these skills in session with their child as the therapist provides feedback and suggestions for improvement. Once parents demonstrate mastery of child-directed play, they are instructed in parent-directed interaction, which is designed to increase low-rate positive behaviors and decrease maladaptive behaviors that are unresponsive to extinction procedures or are too harmful to be ignored. During this phase of treatment parents are taught to use clear and direct commands with their child, provide consistent reinforcement (i.e., praise) when their child is compliant, and use time-out as a way to deal with noncompliance. Similar to the child-directed interaction training, parents are asked to demonstrate these skills in session with their child while the therapist offers suggestions and feedback.

Families that have participated in Parent–Child Interaction Therapy have shown significant improvement in comparison to wait-list controls across a number of different studies (Eyberg, Boggs, & Algina, 1995; McNeil, Eyberg, Eisenstadt, Newcomb, & Funderburk, 1991; Schuhmann et al., 1998). One investigation looking at the relative effectiveness of the two components of PCIT found that families who received the parent-directed interaction therapy first showed faster behavioral improvements and lower levels of parent-reported conduct problems at posttreatment than families who received the child-directed interaction training first (Eisenstadt, Eyberg, McNeil, Newcomb, & Funderburk, 1993). Although both groups improved irrespective of treatment sequence, these results suggest that implementing the parent-directed interaction training first may serve to maximize treatment effects and increase parental satisfaction with treatment. A more recent study found that clinic-referred families who received PCIT showed lower levels of clinically significant child conduct problems and increased levels of child compliance following treatment in comparison to wait-list controls (Schuhmann et al., 1998). In addition, parents receiving treatment reported lower levels of personal distress, and child behavior gains were maintained at a 4-month follow-up.

Dinosaur School with Parent Training

This program consists of a parent and a child component and is designed for children ages 4–7 who have conduct problems significant enough to warrant a diagnosis of either ODD or CD. The child component, which is referred to as "Dinosaur School," consists of groups of five or six children who attend 22 sessions, each lasting approximately 2 hours, designed to address issues that young children with conduct problems frequently face. Since children in the program are so young, the intervention uses a performance-based treatment in which videotapes and life-size puppets are used to model ways of successfully dealing with interpersonal problems that are typically experienced by preschool and young school-age children. The topics addressed include making friends, emotionally empathizing with others, using perspective-taking skills, resolving conflicts successfully, cooperating with others, coping with teasing, and controlling feelings of anger. During the group sessions, children discuss and practice the social skills that are modeled in the videotaped vignettes and collaborate with one another on acceptable solutions to hypothetical problems. In addition, children are rewarded for using positive social skills while interacting with other members of the group. To help promote generalization of these skills, weekly letters are sent to parents and teachers explaining the issues being discussed for the week and encouraging them to reward the child for using positive social skills at home or school.

The Parent Training condition consists of groups of 10-12 parents who meet with a therapist on a weekly basis for approximately 22 sessions, each lasting 2 hours. Similar to the child component, parents watch approximately 17 different videotapes containing vignettes modeling appropriate ways for dealing with problematic parent–child interactions. The therapist leads group discussions pertaining to the topics depicted in the videos, and parents are encouraged to ask questions about the techniques being presented. The major topics presented during the parent training sessions include effective play techniques, limit setting, ways to handle misbehavior, and communication of emotions (Webster-Stratton, 1981). In order to lay a foundation for positive parent–child interactions, parents are initially encouraged to initiate non-threatening play sessions with their child in a manner that shows a genuine interest and appreciation for their ideas. Next, parents are taught to use consistent limit setting in various situations without being too permissive or inflexible. Another set of videotaped vignettes is designed to teach parents how to use positive attention and praise to reward compliant behaviors, while simultaneously employing strategies like ignoring and time-out to extinguish misbehavior. Finally, parents are shown ways in which they can verbally and nonverbally express acceptance, warmth, and caring toward their child. Examples show how critical and demanding parents may elicit rebelliousness in children, while parents who are accepting and enthusiastic produce children who are confident and creative.

Research findings regarding the effectiveness of the Dinosaur School and Parent Training interventions alone and in combination are promising. The Parent Training component has produced significant behavioral gains in comparison to wait-list controls across a number of different studies, even when the parenting videotapes were self-administered without the aid of a therapist (Webster-Stratton, 1984; Webster-Stratton & Hammond, 1997; Webster-Stratton, Kolpacoff, & Hollinsworth, 1988). In addition, overall improvements in parent reports of their children's behavior were still present at 3-year follow-up, with the intervention combining videotaped modeling with therapist-led discussion showing stable improvements (Webster-Stratton, 1990). A more recent investigation revealed that children who attended the Dinosaur School without Parent Training experienced a significant reduction in the amount of conduct problems reported in the home and increases in social problem-solving skills in comparison to wait-list controls (Webster-Stratton & Hammond, 1997). Moreover, at 1-year follow-up nearly two-thirds of children attending this group had parent ratings of behavioral problems in the normal rather than clinically significant range. Although the combination of child and parent training proved superior to each of the component pieces, this finding indicates that cognitive-behavioral treatments directed at young children can be effective in reducing disruptive behavior problems and could potentially be used when parents are unwilling or unable to participate in treatment.

The Montreal Delinquency Prevention Program

The Montreal Delinquency Prevention Program was designed as a preventive intervention for children in the early elementary school years exhibiting significant aggressive and oppositional behaviors. The intervention took place over the course of 2 years (second and third grades) and consisted of a parent-training component based on the strategy developed by the Oregon Social Learning Center (Patterson, 1982) and a child component consisting of social skills and self-control training groups (Tremblay, Masse, Pagani, & Vitaro, 1996). In order to reinforce the use of appropriate social skills and avoid stigmatization, the child groups consisted of an equal number of target children and teacher-nominated prosocial peers. Child groups met once a week for approximately 45 minutes with four to six children in each group. The first year of the child component consisted of nine sessions designed to teach participants a number of different social skills such as how to compliment and help others, appropriate ways to question authority figures, how to invite peers into a group, and ways to meet other children. During the second year of the child intervention, 10 additional sessions were conducted to teach participants how to use appropriate problem-solving strategies and self-control skills. Children were presented with several age-appropriate problem situations, such as being teased or rejected by another child, and then asked to analyze and solve the conflict. In particular, the children were asked to identify the problem, identify their feelings in the situation, analyze the intentions of the provocative peer, come up with potential solutions to the conflict, analyze the consequences of each solution, and choose a final plan. While these skills were initially taught through the use of verbal instructions, modeling, and role plays in-session, each week children were encouraged to use these skills at both home and school. Moreover, both teachers and parents were sent home letters describing the new skills learned each week, and they were encouraged to praise the child for using these new skills whenever possible.

The family intervention consists of a parent-training component based on a strategy developed by the Oregon Social Learning Center (Patterson, 1982). The topics addressed were similar to many of the successful interventions for disruptive behavior disorders. Initially, parents were taught how to effectively monitor and record problematic behaviors in their child and use positive reinforcement to increase the frequency of their child's prosocial behaviors. Sessions also focused on using nonabusive yet consistent methods of discipline to deal with disruptive behaviors. For example, parents were taught to use time-out or naturally occurring consequences for inappropriate behavior, such as making a child's bedtime earlier if her or she refuses to get up on time for school in the morning. Sessions also focused on teaching parents to use problem-solving strategies and negotiation techniques to manage crises within the family system. Finally, the treatment team worked with parents to help them generalize the skills they had learned to specific familial problems they were experiencing, and efforts were made to increase the level of collaboration between parents and their child's teacher. These parenting skills were taught using modeling, coaching, and handouts, while in-session role plays were used to practice and reinforce newly learned skills.

Several longitudinal studies have found that the Montreal Delinquency Prevention Program can successfully reduce antisocial behaviors during childhood and adolescence. Interestingly, evidence supporting the effectiveness of treatment for reducing antisocial behavior in children was not found until the 2-year follow-up, indicating that the benefits of the program maybe long-term rather than acute (Tremblay et al., 1991). Specifically, investigations indicated that by age 12, boys who received the intervention were less likely to have serious adjustment problems in school (Tremblay et al., 1992) and antisocial friends (Vitaro & Tremblay, 1994), and they reported fewer instances of trespassing and stealing (McCord, Tremblay, Vitaro, & Desmarais-Gervais, 1994) than untreated boys. During adolescence, individuals who received the treatment were less likely to be involved in gangs (Tremblay, Masse, Pagani, & Vitaro, 1996) and reported lower levels of delinquency and substance use (Tremblay, Kurtz, Masse, Vitaro, & Pihl, 1995) than the untreated controls. Since many of these treatment effects emerged at age 12 and remained stable up until age 15, the results of this preventive intervention provide substantial evidence that early cognitive-behavioral interventions in the elementary school years can produce effects that last throughout adolescence.

Anger Coping and Coping Power Programs

Although the Anger Coping Program was initially designed as a structured 18-session school-based intervention for fourth- through sixth-grade children exhibiting aggressive behaviors, it has been implemented in outpatient mental health clinics as a treatment for children with ODD and CD. Sessions typically last 45–60 minutes in school-based groups, and 60–90 minutes in outpatient groups. In the initial group session, the rules for conduct are discussed and a point system rewarding children for compliant behavior during sessions is introduced. Another facet of the treatment that is introduced early on and is continued throughout the program involves having each child identify and work on goals designed to improve his or her behavior. In order to help facilitate this process, group counselors typically meet with teachers or parents early on in treatment to identify four or five behavioral goals designed to reduce problematic behaviors. Since initial successes are important in motivating children to work on challenging issues, leaders help the children to initially select goals that are of low to moderate difficulty. Progress in meeting these goals is monitored through the use of weekly goal sheets, and children receive points for agreed-upon levels of goal completion, which are then used to earn certain privileges.

The remainder of the Anger Coping Program is designed to promote positive coping skills for dealing with anger and facilitate appropriate problem-solving abilities in social situations. The anger management portion consists of teaching children how to use calming self-thoughts and distraction techniques to deal with feelings of anger. In order to promote generalization, children then practice these skills as other group members are teasing them, first using puppets, and then directly role playing the responses to teasing. In addition, perspective-taking sessions are used to help participants understand how others can have a range of intentions in a given situation that are often unclear. This is done in an attempt to prevent children from assuming that other people are always trying to be cruel or mean in conflict situations. The longest section of the Anger Coping Program focuses on social problem solving, which involves integrating skills from the anger management and perspective-taking sessions. Specifically, children practice brainstorming multiple possible solutions to social problems and evaluating the long-term and short-term consequences of each solution. The last six sessions of the program are less structured and provide the opportunity to rehearse previously introduced skills (e.g., anger management) and role play and problem solve real life social difficulties that the children experience.

The Coping Power Program (Lochman, 2003; Lochman & Wells, 1996) is a lengthier, multicomponent version of the Anger Coping Program designed to enhance outcome effects and to provide for better maintenance of gains over time. The Coping Power Program (CPP) has added sessions to the Anger Coping framework to create a total of 33 group sessions addressing additional topics such as emotional awareness, relaxation training, social skills enhancement, positive social and personal goals, and dealing with peer pressure. Other elements of the CPP child component include regular individual sessions that take place every 4–6 weeks and are designed to increase generalization of the program to the children's actual social situations. In addition, periodic consultation is provided to the teachers of children who are making some progress in treatment sessions but who are still having recurrent behavior problems at school.

The Coping Power Program also has a parent component that consists of 16 parent group sessions that last approximately 2 hours each and are designed to cover the same 15- to 18-month period of time as the CPP child component. The 16 sessions are designed to address issues such as social reinforcement and positive attention, the importance of clear house rules, behavioral expectations and monitoring procedures, the use of appropriate and effective discipline strategies, family communication, positive connection to school, and stress management. Parents are also informed of the skills their children are working on during their sessions, and parents are encouraged to facilitate and reinforce children for using these new skills. The parent component also includes periodic individual contacts with parents through home visits and telephone contacts to promote generalization of skills.

Research on the effectiveness of the Anger Coping Program has produced some optimistic results in terms of short- and long-term behavior. One of the seminal studies found that aggressive boys randomly assigned to the treatment condition displayed less parent-reported aggressive behavior, fewer problems associated with disruptive and aggressive behavior in the classroom, and higher levels of self-esteem at posttreatment in comparison to minimal treatment and no-treatment conditions (Lochman, Burch, Curry, & Lampron, 1984). In addition, Lochman and Lampron (1988) found that children in the Anger Coping Program showed improved levels of on-task behavior at school at a 7-month follow-up. At a 3-year follow-up, boys who received the Anger Coping Program exhibited lower levels of substance use and maintained increases in self-esteem and problem-solving skills (Lochman, 1992), indicating the presence of long-term maintenance of social-cognitive gains and prevention effects in the area of onset of substance use. However, the boys in the Anger Coping Program did not have significant reductions in delinquent behavior at follow-up.

Two grant-funded studies are currently in process to examine the efficacy of the Coping Power Program. In the first of these studies (Lochman, 2003; Lochman & Wells, 1996; Lochman & Wells, 1999a), 183 boys who had high rates of teacher-rated aggression in fourth or fifth grade were randomly assigned to either a school-based CPP child component, a combination CPP including both child and parent components, or an untreated control condition. Initial outcome analyses indicate that the CPP intervention has had broad effects at postintervention on boys' social competence, social-information processing, locus of control, temperament, and aggressive behavior, and on parents' parenting practices, anger, and marital relationships. In analyses of the 1-year follow-up assessment for the first of the two cohorts, most of these effects were maintained. Most intervention effects, especially in the arena of children's social competence, social information-processing, and school behavior were apparent in both intervention cells, indicating the influence of the child intervention. Despite this fact, certain effects—such as parents' sense of efficacy and satisfaction with their parenting, aspects of their marital relationship, and reductions in children's aggressive behavior in the home at follow-up—were evident only in the combined intervention cell, indicating the importance of multicomponent interventions impacting both children's social-cognitive processes and parents' parenting practices. In the second ongoing study, we are examining whether the effects of the CPP can be enhanced by combining the indicated intervention with a universal prevention intervention randomly offered to half of the fifth-grade teachers and the parents of the students in these classrooms. Initial midintervention analyses with 245 aggressive children indicate that both the universal and indicated interventions produce significant effects on children's social competence and behavior and on parents' positive involvement with their children (Lochman & Wells, 1999b). Early findings from these two studies indicate the effects of this form of cognitive-behavioral intervention can be enhanced by including both child and parent intervention components, and that the intervention effects are evident as early as midintervention and maintained at 1-year follow-up.

Problem-Solving Skills Training and Parent Management Training

Kazdin's problem-solving skills training (PSST) and parent management training (PMT) are two of the most extensively researched cognitive-behavioral treatments for conduct problems in childhood. Although the program is designed for children from 7 to 13 years of age with a wide variety of antisocial behaviors, much of the research on its effectiveness has included a nearly equal number of children with either ODD or CD. The primary focus of the child component is teaching and reinforcing prosocial problem-solving skills in order to promote a child's ability to effectively manage potentially volatile interpersonal situations. The children attend 25 individually administered sessions once per week, with each session lasting approximately 50 minutes. During treatment, children are presented with potentially volatile interpersonal situations that are congruent with the environment in which they are having problems (e.g., home, school, peers, siblings). The therapist then assists the child in objectively evaluating the situation, developing prosocial goals, and generating alternative solutions to meet these goals. These problem-solving skills are practiced and refined in session through the use of modeling, role plays, corrective feedback, and reinforcement. In order to promote the generalization of these skills to settings outside of therapy, children are assigned "super-solver" tasks in which they apply newly learned skills to real-life interpersonal situations of increasing complexity. Moreover, parents are taught to cue and assist the child in the use of these problem-solving strategies at home and in the community.

The parent management component of this program consists of 16 individual treatment sessions that occur over the course of 6–8 months, with each session lasting approximately 2 hours. In general, the program is designed to instruct parents how to apply various behavioral principles like reinforcement and shaping when identifying and modifying problematic behavior in their children. During the sessions, the therapist uses a combination of didactic instruction, modeling, and role plays to teach parenting skills like the appropriate use of time-out, verbal reprimands, negotiation, and behavioral contracting. After a home behavioral program is started, the therapist works with the parents to begin a school-based reinforcement program to help improve the child's academic and behavioral compliance. The school program consists of negotiating certain school goals and monitoring the child's progress in meeting these goals through the use of a home–school behavioral report card. At both home and school, the child is given reinforcement (e.g., special activities, privileges) for achieving specific goals and the child is frequently given feedback regarding his or her behavioral progress.

Several research studies have provided support for the effectiveness of the problem-solving training and parent management training independently, as well as a combination of the two treatments for oppositional and defiant behaviors. Specifically, the child component was shown to be superior to nondirective relationship therapy and control conditions in reducing global externalizing and internalizing problems, increasing social activities, and improving overall school adjustment (Kazdin et al., 1987). In addition, problem-solving skills training was effective in reducing disruptive behaviors and increasing prosocial activities at both home and school in comparison to nondirective behavior therapy, and these effects remained at 1-year follow-up (Kazdin, Bass, Siegel, & Thomas, 1989). Although another study indicated that both problem-solving skills training and parent management training in isolation produce significant improvements in global dysfunction, social competence, and deviant behavior at 1-year follow-up, PSST was superior to PMT in terms of improving children's social competence at school and reducing self-reports of aggression and delinquency (Kazdin, Seigel, & Bass, 1992). Since long-term outcomes for treatment of childhood conduct problems have been poor, it seems that a combination of PSST and PMT may be optimal for children with ODD.

Summary of Treatments for Oppositional Defiant Disorder

Although each of the empirically supported treatments previously discussed differed in terms of age group targeted, length of treatment, and method of instruction, there are substantial common factors across the programs discussed. For example, the parent training component of each intervention focused on teaching parents how to use the behavioral principles of positive reinforcement and shaping to increase the frequency of prosocial behaviors in their children, while using various extinction procedures like time-out and selective ignoring to reduce the occurrence of oppositional and defiant behaviors. In addition, parents are instructed in how to be firm yet flexible with their children, and they are encouraged to engage their children in warm and supportive interactions on a regular basis. Many of the programs also utilized a behavioral program at home and school in which the child earns points for achieving various behavioral goals of increasing difficultly. For those programs with a child component, there is a focus on teaching children systematic ways to solve interpersonal problems by helping them identify the intentions of others, generate prosocial solutions, evaluate the consequences of their behavior, and practice implementing prosocial solutions through the use of role plays in session. Moreover, many of the child programs seek to generalize the skills learned by having teachers and parents reinforce their use and assigning behavioral homework for the child. Another common factor across many treatment studies is that parent training alone seems to produce more beneficial effects than child training alone, while a combination of the two seems optimal.

Identifying the common factors across successful interventions for oppositional and defiant children is important for several reasons. First, it gives practicing clinicians a firm theoretical and empirical base from which to build when treating children with ODD in the community. In fact, some prominent professionals have gone so far as to argue that if an empirically supported treatment for a certain disorder exists, it is unethical to initially offer treatments that do not have empirical support (Chambless, 1996; Meehl, 1997). This assertion is validated by studies indicating that newly developed or untested treatments for children with behavioral problems can produce negative, rather than positive, outcomes (Dishion & Andrews, 1995). Unfortunately, many practicing clinicians seem to support the use of empirically supported treatments, but they do not routinely use them in their practice (Plante, Andersen, & Boccaccini, 1999). It seems that clinical practitioners may view manualized treatments as too rigid to be implemented in the "real-world" setting, but it is important to recognize that many of the techniques used in these treatments can be used in clinical practice with minimal modification. While some have stressed that you "get what your pay for" (Durlak, 1999, p. 6) when you begin implementing portions of programs, the use of consistently validated empirical techniques in a systematic fashion can produce positive results. The remainder of this paper presents a case in which many common factors of the previously mentioned treatments, as well as techniques unique to some programs, were used to treat a child with ODD in an outpatient psychology clinic.

CASE EXAMPLE

Presenting Problem

Zaine S., a 10-year-old male, was brought to the psychology clinic by his mother, Ms. Hill, at the suggestion of the principal at his elementary school. Ms. Hill noted that Zaine had been sent to principal's office several times during the school year for fighting with other students and being disrespectful of and defiant toward his teacher, Ms. Rudd. During a telephone interview, Ms. Rudd noted that Zaine frequently refused to do his work in class, and he was constantly irritating other students. She mentioned that few children in the classroom liked Zaine, and that his only friend was another boy with similar behavioral problems. Despite these problems, Ms. Rudd noted that Zaine usually was able to calm down after his tantrum and would sometimes apologize for his behavior. Although Ms. Rudd noted that Zaine was a bright and capable student, she mentioned that his "bad attitude" and "short temper" kept him from achieving academically.

At home, Ms. Hill noted that Zaine threw temper tantrums and was argumentative on a regular basis. She also noted that Zaine frequently lied to get out of doing his chores and was always fighting with his younger brother, Anthony. According to Ms. Hill, Zaine was jealous of the attention that his younger brother received, and he would start "pitching a fit" if she focused her attention on Anthony for an extended period of time. When asked what Zaine did well, Ms. Hill answered "he hasn't been doing anything good for a while." Although Ms. Hill described Zaine as a "hateful child," she acknowledged that he would occasionally apologize for his aggressive behavior. In general, Ms. Hill seemed overwhelmed by Zaine's current problems at home and school, and she partially blamed herself for his defiance. She explained that she had let Zaine "get away with murder" for a long time, and now she had to "teach him to respect authority." Despite this fact, Ms. Hill mentioned that it was difficult to consistently discipline Zaine because she was a single working mother who was often too tired to deal with his behavior problems when she got home. Although Ms. Hill occasionally disciplined Zaine by sending him to his room, she admittedly resorted to spanking and yelling on a regular basis, especially when tired or frustrated. She explained that spanking Zaine typically improved his behavior for a couple of days, but then he was "back to his old self." In general, Ms. Hill seemed motivated to learn how to effectively deal with Zaine's behaviors and understood that in order to produce long-lasting change she needed to be more consistent.

Zaine, a child of below average height for his age, was neatly dressed during our initial therapy sessions. When asked about his current problems at school, Zaine stated, "My teacher hates me. She blames me for things that other kids do." In addition, Zaine mentioned that it seemed like his mom was "always yelling" at him, and he was "always in trouble." Upon further questioning, Zaine acknowledged that he sometimes had a "bad attitude" with others and tended to "get mad easily." Moreover, Zaine explained that he typically fought with other students at school when they called him names like "elf" or "shorty." In general, Zaine seemed very eager to make a good impression and expressed a desire for special attention. He frequently asked what his mom had said about him, and several times he inquired if we would get to meet together on a regular basis.

As the result of the initial clinical interviews, Zaine met criteria for oppositional defiant disorder. His current behavioral problems were not severe enough to warrant a diagnosis of conduct disorder, and he did not seem to have significant symptoms associated with attention-deficit/hyperactivity disorder. It was clear that adult attention was important to Zaine. He seemed to use defiant behaviors to elicit attention from his mother, especially when she spent time with his younger brother. In addition, Zaine and his mother had become involved in a predominately negative interaction pattern, with little parental warmth and support. Finally, Zaine was having difficulty controlling his anger when teased at school. He used aggression as the primary means for resolving conflicts, indicating deficits in his basic problem-solving abilities. He also lacked some basic communication skills, which prevented him from interacting with peers in an appropriate manner and limiting his ability to resolve conflicts verbally.

Course of Treatment

Therapy sessions were divided between individual sessions with Zaine and parent training sessions with his mom. Skills taught during the parenting sessions were identical to those used in several empirically validated parent-training programs for children exhibiting aggressive and oppositional behavior (Eisenstadt et al., 1993; Kazdin et al., 1992; Lochman & Wells, 1996; Tremblay et al., 1996; Webster-Stratton & Hammond, 1997). The initial parenting sessions focused on teaching Ms. Hill some basic behavioral principals associated with learned behavior in children, especially positive reinforcement and extinction. Since Zaine seemed to place high value on adult attention, we discussed how giving him negative attention for oppositional and defiant behavior may inadvertently reinforce these actions. Ms. Hill acknowledged that Zaine often seemed "starved for attention" and that many of their interactions had been of a punitive nature. At this point, we discussed the importance of designating at least 15 minutes each day as Zaine's special playtime. I explained that these sessions were an opportunity for her to build a more positive relationship with Zaine by attending to him in a supportive, but nondirective, manner. We also talked about other ways positive attention could be used to shape Zaine's behavior on a regular basis. For example, Ms. Hill was instructed to praise Zaine verbally whenever he was compliant or well behaved and ignore his behavior, as much as possible, when he became defiant or oppositional. We agreed that a good rule of thumb was to give Zaine more attention for his positive behaviors than for negative behaviors. Consistency in implementing these strategies was stressed as the key to making them work. Ms. Hill was amenable to trying these new parenting techniques, and she was hopeful that they would help improve Zaine's behavior.

During the course of treatment, several problems arose as Ms. Hill attempted to implement the previously mentioned parenting skills. Specifically, she had a hard time consistently spending time with Zaine. She mentioned that she was extremely tired after work and was often too over-whelmed with both children to set aside time for Zaine. After brainstorm-ing some solutions to this problem, Ms. Hill agreed that she could engage in special time with Zaine after Anthony had gone to bed. In addition, there were several sessions wherein Ms. Hill became frustrated with the Zaine's slow behavioral progress. Specifically, Ms. Hill would say things like "therapy is not working" or "spanking is the only thing that works." During these episodes, we would review the gains that Zaine had made since the beginning of therapy or discuss the potential negative conse-quences associated with the use corporal punishment, such as modeling aggressive behavior and damaging Zaine's self-esteem. Most importantly, Ms. Hill was continually praised for her hard work and persistence in deal-ing with a very difficult home situation. After these discussions, Ms. Hill typically had renewed faith in the positive parenting practices learned dur-ing therapy sessions, and she would admit being negativistic due to elevated stress levels.

As the result of verbally reinforcing Zaine's compliant behaviors, ignoring his maladaptive behaviors, and spending time engaging him in a supportive manner, many of Zaine's disruptive behaviors dissipated. Ms. Hill reported that he was more likely to respond to requests at home and he had fewer emotional outbursts when she was interacting with his younger brother. In addition, she reported feeling more competent as a parent and less overwhelmed about caring for her children. Because Zaine was still having some problems following rules at school and performing his duties around the house, we devised a behavioral schedule that targeted two prob-lem areas at both home and school. Zaine earned points for achieving behavioral goals on a daily basis, which he could use at the end of the week to earn privileges like going out to dinner with his mother or buying a small toy. We started with behavioral goals that would be fairly easy for Zaine to achieve during the first couple of weeks to help build his sense of compe-tence and self-efficacy. For example, one of his initial goals at home was to refrain from calling his little brother names and one of his first goals at school was to stay out of the principal's office. We also formed a list of be-haviors that were severe enough to warrant immediate consequences, such as hitting his younger brother. Ms. Hill set up a time-out chair in her home, which was away from any potentially rewarding stimuli, and she began us-ing it as a consequence for more serious behaviors.

Individual sessions with Zaine initially focused on teaching him effec-tive problem-solving strategies and social skills to help him deal with inter-personal conflicts. Many of the techniques used during these sessions came from several empirically validated child-based treatments for children exhibiting aggressive and oppositional behaviors (Kazdin et al., 1992; Lochman & Wells, 1996; Tremblay et al., 1996; Webster-Stratton & Hammond, 1997). Specifically, Zaine was presented with simple yet realistic vignettes about interpersonal conflicts between children and then asked to analyze the situation and come up with potential solutions. Early on, Zaine had particular difficulty coming up with prosocial verbal solutions to problems. For example, one vignette asked Zaine what a boy named Jeff should do if he allowed some children to borrow his soccer ball during lunchtime at school, but they failed to return it by the end of the day. Zaine's initial responses were all direct action solutions:

> "He could have just took the soccer ball without playing with them. He could have went home and next morning seen them playing with it and gone up to them and taken it without asking. Next morning if it's in the locker room he could have went in the locker room and took it out."

Further questioning revealed that Zaine had a tendency to attribute negative intentions to others, making him focus on retaliation rather than communication when brainstorming solutions to peer problems. As a result, sessions focused on generating alternative intentions besides malice that peers may have during conflicts. In addition, Zaine learned ways to address problems with peers using assertive verbal communication rather than nonverbal direct actions that frequently provoked conflict. As Zaine progressed in therapy, we began talking about problems he was having with other peers at school, and we would role play ways to handle the situation. On a few occasions during treatment, Zaine was involved in physical fights with other children at school. These episodes were treated as learning experiences rather than failures, and we would discuss what Zaine could do next time to avoid physical confrontation.

Skills included as part of the Anger Coping Program were used to teach Zaine how to deal with feelings of anger in a prosocial manner (Lochman & Lenhart, 1993). Zaine acknowledged that in order to effectively solve many of his social problems, he needed to prevent his anger from escalating to the point where he felt out of control. During our initial session on anger management, Zaine was asked to list how his body sensations changed as his anger progresses, starting with signs of low-level frustration and ending with signs of extreme anger. Zaine's anger hierarchy was as follows: (1) My face feels hot; (2) I clench my fist; (3) I make a mad face; (4) I think about doing something bad (e.g., hitting or yelling); (5) I yell and call others names; and (6) I hit someone. We talked about the importance of doing something to reduce his anger before it got out of control and resulted in punishment. Zaine agreed that when he found himself making mean faces or thinking about doing something bad, it would be a good time to try and calm down. We then began talking about specific techniques that could be used to reduce his anger levels. Initially, Zaine learned how to use slow, deep breaths to reduce his physiological arousal. After trying this skill in session Zaine stated, "That was cool. It made me real tired." In addition, Zaine brainstormed his own self-coping statements that could help reduce his anger when ridiculed by his peers. Zaine's favorite self-soothing statement was "I am not your puppet. You're just trying to get me into trouble. I am the puppet master. " He also found that imagining he was inside a "cement cellar" that protected him from taunting prevented his anger from escalating.

As Zaine mastered various problem-solving skills and anger management techniques in session, he was encouraged to begin using them at home and school. Ms. Hill and Ms. Rudd were updated about the new skills Zaine had learned, and they were encouraged to reinforce him for using these techniques at home and school. In fact, Ms. Hill began practicing the deep breathing techniques with Zaine at home and often prompted him to use his anger coping skills when he became upset. She also began giving Zaine extra points on his behavioral sheets for resolving conflicts at home and school by using effective verbal communication rather than physically provocative behaviors. In general, Zaine's behavior at home and school improved substantially. He still had occasional outbursts of anger, but these were typically short-lived. His got along better with his peers at school, and Ms. Rudd noted that it was easier to focus Zaine on his work. Since Ms. Hill was satisfied with Zaine's behavioral progress, and summer was approaching, we agreed to terminate our therapy sessions. We discussed the importance of consistently using the parenting practices learned over the past few months and maintaining close contact with Zaine's teacher during the following school year. Ms. Hill agreed to call to schedule additional therapy sessions at the psychology clinic if future assistance was needed.

REFERENCES

American Psychiatric Association. (1980). *Diagnostic and statistical manual of mental disorders* (3rd ed.). Washington, DC: Author.

American Psychiatric Association. (1987). *Diagnostic and statistical manual of mental disorders* (3rd ed., rev.). Washington, DC: Author.

American Psychiatric Association. (1994). *Diagnostic and statistical manual of mental disorders* (4th ed.). Washington, DC: Author.

Angold, A., & Costello, J. (1996). Toward establishing an empirical basis for the diagnosis of oppositional defiant disorder. *Journal of the American Academy of Child and Adolescent Psychiatry, 35,* 1205–1212.

Biederman, J., Faraone, S. V., Milberg, S., Jetton, J. G., Chen, L., Mick, E., Greene, R. W., & Russell, R. L. (1996). Childhood oppositional defiant disorder a precursor to adolescent conduct disorder? Findings from a four-year follow-up study of children with ADHD. *Journal of the American Academy of Child and Adolescent Psychiatry, 35,* 1193–1204.

Boyle, M. H., & Pickles, A. R. (1998). Strategies to manipulate reliability: Impact on statistical associations. *Journal of the American Academy of Child and Adolescent Psychiatry, 37,* 1077–1084.

Brestan, E. V., & Eyberg, S. M. (1998). Effective psychosocial treatments of conduct-disordered children and adolescents: 29 years, 82 studies, and 5,272 kids. *Journal of Clinical Child Psychology, 27,* 180–189.

Burns, G. L., Walsh, J. A., Patterson, D. R., Holte, C. S., Sommers-Flanagan, R., & Parker, C. M. (1997). Internal validity of the disruptive behavior disorder symptoms: Implications from parent ratings for a dimensional approach to symptom validity. *Journal of Abnormal Child Psychology, 25,* 307–319.

Chambless, D. L. (1996). In defense of dissemination of empirically supported psychological interventions. *Clinical Psychology: Science and Practice, 3,* 230–235.

Cohen, D., & Strayer, J. (1996). Empathy in conduct-disordered and comparison youth. *Developmental Psychology, 62,* 366–374.

Crick, N. R., & Dodge, K. A. (1994). A review and reformulation of social information-processing mechanisms in children's social adjustment. *Psychological Bulletin, 115,* 74–101.

Dishion, T. J., & Andrews, D. W. (1995). Preventing escalation in problem behaviors with high-risk young adolescents: Immediate and 1-year outcomes. *Journal of Consulting and Clinical Psychology, 63,* 538–548.

Dodge, K. A., Pettit, G. S., McClaskey, C. L., & Brown, M. M. (1986). Social competence in children. *Monographs of the Society for Research in Child Development, 51*(2, Serial No. 213).

Dunn, S. E., Lochman, J. E., & Colder, C. R. (1997). Social problem-solving skills in boys with conduct and oppositional defiant disorder. *Aggressive Behavior, 23,* 457–469.

Durlak, J. A. (1999). Principles related to successful school-based prevention programs. *Clinical Child Psychology Newsletter, 14,* 4–6.

Eisenstadt, T. H., Eyberg, S., Mc Neil, C. B., Newcomb, K., & Funderburk, B. (1993). Parent–child interaction therapy with behavior problem children: Relative effectiveness of two stages and overall treatment outcome. *Journal of Child Clinical Psychology, 22,* 42–51.

Eyberg, S. M., Boggs, S., & Algina, J. (1995). Parent–child interaction therapy: A psychosocial model for the treatment of young children with conduct problem behavior and their families. *Psychopharmacology Bulletin, 31,* 83–91.

Frick, P. J., Lahey, B. B., Loeber, R., Stouthamer-Loeber, M., Christ, M. A. G., & Hanson, K. (1992). Familial risk factors to oppositional defiant disorder and conduct disorder: Parental psychopathology and maternal parenting. *Journal of Consulting and Clinical Psychology, 60,* 49–53.

Frick, P. J., Lahey, B. B., Loeber, R., Stouthamer-Loeber, M., Green, S., Hart, E. L., & Christ, M. A. G. (1991). Oppositional defiant disorder and conduct disorder in boys: Patterns of behavioral covariation. *Journal of Clinical Child Psychology, 20,* 202–208.

Frick, P. C., Van Horn, Y., Lahey, B. A., Christ, M. A. G., Loeber, R., Hart, E. A., Tannenbaum, L., & Hanson, K. (1993). Oppositional defiant disorder and conduct disorder: A meta-analytic review of factor analyses and cross-validation in clinic sample. *Clinical Psychology Review, 13,* 319–340.

Frick, P. J., Lahey, B. B., Applegate, B., Kerdyk, L., Ollendick, T., Hynd, G. W., Garfinkel, B., Greenhill, L., Biederman, J., Barkley, R. A., McBurnett, K.,

Newcorn, J., & Waldman, I. (1994). DSM-IV field trials for the disruptive and attention deficit disorders: Diagnostic utility of symptoms. *Journal of the American Academy of Child and Adolescent Psychiatry, 33,* 529–539.

Gouze, K. R. (1987). Attention and social problem solving as correlates of aggression in preschool males. *Journal of Abnormal Child Psychology, 15,* 181–197.

Hanish, L. D., Tolan, P. H., & Guerra, N. G. (1996). Treatment of oppositional defiant disorder. In M. A. Reinecke, F. M. Dattilio, & A. Freeman (Eds.), *Cognitive therapy with children and adolescents: A casebook for clinical practice* (pp. 62–78). New York: Guilford Press.

Kazdin, A. E., Bass, D., Siegel, T., & Thomas, C. (1989). Cognitive-behavioral therapy and relationship therapy in the treatment of children referred for antisocial behavior. *Journal of Consulting and Clinical Psychology, 57,* 522–535.

Kazdin, A. E., Esveldt-Dawson, K., French, N. H., & Unis, A. S. (1987). Problem-solving skills training and relationship therapy in the treatment of antisocial child behavior. *Journal of Consulting and Clinical Psychology, 55,* 76–85.

Kazdin, A. E., Siegel, T. C., & Bass, D. (1992). Cognitive problem-solving skills training and parent management training in the treatment of antisocial behavior in children. *Journal of Consulting and Clinical Psychology, 60,* 733–747.

Kazdin, A. E., & Weisz, J. R. (1998). Identifying and developing empirically supported child and adolescent treatments. *Journal of Consulting and Clinical Psychology, 66,* 19–36.

Lahey, B. B., Applegate, B., Barkley, R. A., Garfinkel, B., McBurnett, K., Kerdyk, L., Greenhill, L., Hynd, G. W., Frick, P. J., Newcorn, J., Biederman, J., Ollendick, T., Hart, E. L., Perez, D., Waldman, I., & Shaffer, D. (1994). DSM-IV field trials for oppositional defiant disorder and conduct disorder in children and adolescents. *American Journal of Psychiatry, 151,* 1163–1171.

Lahey, B. B., Loeber, R., Quay, H. C., Frick, P. J., & Grimm, J. (1992). Oppositional defiant disorder and conduct disorder: Issues to be resolved for DSM-IV. *Journal of the American Academy of Child and Adolescent Psychiatry, 31,* 539–546.

Langbehn, D. R., Cadoret, R. J., William, Y. R., Troughton, E. P., & Stewart, M. A. (1998). Distinct contributions of conduct and oppositional defiant symptoms of adult antisocial behavior: Evidence from an adoption study. *Archives of General Psychiatry, 55,* 821–829.

Laub, J. H., & Sampson, R. J. (1988). Unraveling families and delinquency: A reanalysis of the Gluecks' data. *Criminology, 26,* 355–380.

Lochman, J. E. (1992). Cognitive-behavioral interventions with aggressive boys: Three-year follow-up and preventive effects. *Journal of Consulting and Clinical Psychology, 60,* 426–432.

Lochman, J. E. (2003). Preventive intervention with precursors to substance abuse. In W. J. Bukoski & Z. Sloboda (Eds.), *Handbook of drug abuse theory, science, and practice* (pp. 307–326). New York: Plenum Press.

Lochman, J. E., Burch, P. P., Curry, J. F., & Lampron, L. B. (1984). Treatment and generalization effects of cognitive-behavioral and goal setting interventions with aggressive boys. *Journal of Consulting and Clinical Psychology, 52,* 915–916.

Lochman, J. E., & Craven, S. V. (1993). *Family conflict associated with reactive and proactive aggression at two age levels.* Paper presented at the Biennial meeting of the Society for Research in Child Development, New Orleans, LA.

Lochman, J. E., & Dodge, K. A. (1990). *Dysfunctional family and social-cognitive process with aggressive boys.* Paper presented at the annual meeting of the Society for Research in Child and Adolescent Psychopathology, Costa Mesa, GA.

Lochman, J. E., & Dodge, K. A. (1994). Social-cognitive processes of severely violent, moderately aggressive, and nonaggressive boys. *Journal of Consulting and Clinical Psychology, 62,* 366–374.

Lochman, J. E., & Lampron, L. B. (1988). Cognitive behavioral intervention for aggressive boys: Seven month follow-up effects. *Journal of Child and Adolescent Psychotherapy, 5,* 15–23.

Lochman, J. E., & Lenhart, L. A. (1993). Anger coping intervention for aggressive children: Conceptual models and outcome effects. *Clinical Psychology Review, 13,* 785–805.

Lochman, J. E., Meyer, B. L., Rabiner, D. L., & White, K. J. (1991). Parameters influencing social problem solving of aggressive children. In R. Prinz (Ed.), *Advances in behavioral assessment of children and families* (Vol. 5, pp. 31–63). Greenwich, CT: JAI Press.

Lochman, J. E., Wayland, K. K., & White, K. K. (1993). Social goals: Relationship to adolescent adjustment and to social problem solving. *Journal of Abnormal Child Psychology, 21,* 135–151.

Lochman, J. E., & Wells, K. C. (1996). A social-cognitive intervention with aggressive children: Prevention effects and contextual implementation issues. In R. D. Peters & R. J. McMahon (Eds.), *Prevention and early intervention: Childhood disorders, substance use and delinquency* (pp 111–143). Thousand Oaks, CA: Sage.

Lochman, J. E., & Wells, K. C. (1999a, June). *Effects of an indicated intervention with aggressive boys.* Paper presented at the International Society for Research in Child and Adolescent Psychopathology Ninth Scientific Meeting, Barcelona, Spain.

Lochman, J. E., & Wells, K. C. (1999b, October). *Preventive intervention with preadolescent aggressive children and their parents: The Coping Power Program.* Paper presented at the American Academy of Child and Adolescent Psychiatry annual meeting, Chicago, Illinois.

Loeber, R., Lahey B. B., & Thomas, C. (1991). Diagnostic conundrum of oppositional defiant disorder and conduct disorder. *Journal of Abnormal Psychology, 100,* 379–390.

Matthys, W., Cuperus, J. M., & Van Engeland, H. (1999). Deficient social problem-solving with ODD/CD, with ADHD, and with both disorders. *Journal of the American Academy of Child and Adolescent Psychiatry, 38,* 311–321.

McCord, J., Tremblay, R. E., Vitaro, F., & Desmarais-Gervais, L. (1994). Boys' disruptive behavior, school adjustment, and delinquency: The Montreal prevention experiment. *International Journal of Behavioral Development, 17,* 739–752.

McNeil, C. B., Eyberg, S., Eisenstadt, T. H., Newcomb, K., & Funderburk, B. W. (1991). Parent–child interaction therapy with behavior problem children: Generalization of treatment effects to the school setting. *Journal of Child Clinical Psychology, 20,* 140–151.

Meehl, P. (1997). Credentialed persons, credentialed knowledge. *Clinical Psychology: Research and Practice, 4,* 91–98.

O'Brien, M., & Chin, C. (1998). The relationship between children's reported exposure to interparental conflict and memory biases in the recognition of aggressive and constructive conflict words. *Personality and Social Psychology Bulletin, 24,* 647–656.

Pardini, D. A., & Lochman, J. E. (2000, March). *Social-cognitive processes of serious and non-serious juvenile offenders.* Poster presented at the 46th annual meeting of the Southeastern Psychological Association, New Orleans, LA.

Patterson, G. R. (1982). *Coercive family process.* Eugene, OR: Castalia.

Patterson, G. R., Reid, J. B., & Dishion, T. J. (1992). *Antisocial boys.* Eugene, OR: Castalia.

Perry, D. G., Williard, J. C., & Perry, L. C. (1990). Peers' perceptions of the consequences that victimized children provide aggressors. *Child Development, 61,* 1310–1325.

Pillow, D. R., Pelham, W. E., Hoza, B., Molina, B. S. G., & Stultz, C. H. (1998). Confirmatory factor analyses examining attention deficit hyperactivity disorder symptoms and other childhood disruptive behaviors. *Journal of Abnormal Child Psychology, 26,* 293–309.

Plante, T. G., Andersen, E. N., & Boccaccini, M. T. (1999). Empirically supported treatments and related contemporary changes in psychotherapy practice: What do clinical ABPPs think? *Clinical Psychologist, 52,* 23–31.

Rey, J. M. (1993). Oppositional defiant disorder. *American Journal of Psychiatry, 150,* 1769–1778.

Rey, J. M, & Plapp, J. M. (1990). Quality of perceived parenting in oppositional and conduct disordered adolescents. *Journal of the American Academy of Child and Adolescent Psychiatry, 29,* 157–162.

Schuhmann, E. M., Foote, R., Eyberg, S. M., Boggs, S. R., & Algina, J. (1998). Efficacy of parent–child interaction therapy: Interim report of a randomized trial with short-term maintenance. *Journal of Child Clinical Psychology, 27,* 34–45.

Simonoff, E., Pickles, A., Meyer, J., Silber, J., & Maes, H. (1998). Genetic and environmental influences on subtypes of conduct disorder behavior in boys. *Journal of Abnormal Child Psychology, 26,* 495–509.

Speltz, M. L., DeKlyen, M., Greenberg, M. T., & Dryden, M. (1995). Clinic referral for oppositional defiant disorder: Relative significance of attachment and behavioral variables. *Journal of Abnormal Child Psychology, 23,* 487–507.

Tremblay, R. E., Kurtz, L., Masse, L. C., Vitaro, F., & Pihl, R. O. (1995). A bimodal preventive intervention for disruptive kindergarten boys: Its impact through mid-adolescence. *Journal of Consulting and Clinical Psychology, 63,* 560–568.

Tremblay, R. E., Masse, L. C., Pagani, L., & Vitaro, F. (1996). From childhood physical aggression to adolescent maladjustment. In R. D. Peters & R. J. McMahon (Eds.), *Preventing childhood disorders, substance abuse and delinquency* (pp. 268–289). Thousand Oaks, CA: Sage.

Tremblay, R. E., McCord, J., Boileau, H., Charlebois, P., Gagnon, C., LeBlanc, M., & Larivee, S. (1991). Can disruptive boys be helped to become competent? *Psychiatry, 54,* 148–161.

Tremblay, R. E., Vitaro, F., Bertrand, L., LeBlanc, M., Beauchesne, H., Boileau, H., & David, H. (1992). Parent and child training to prevent early onset of delinquency: The Montreal longitudinal–experimental study. In J. McCord & R. E. Tremblay (Eds.), *Preventing antisocial behavior: Interventions from birth through adolescence* (pp. 117–138). New York: Guilford Press.

Vitaro, F., & Tremblay, R. E. (1994). Impact of a prevention program on aggressive-disruptive children's friendships and social adjustment. *Journal of Abnormal Child Psychology, 22,* 457–475.

Webster-Stratton, C. (1981). Videotape modeling: A method of parent education. *Journal of Clinical Child Psychology, 10,* 93–97.

Webster-Stratton, C. (1984). Randomized trial of two parent-training programs for families with conduct-disordered children. *Journal of Consulting and Clinical Psychology, 52,* 666–678.

Webster-Stratton, C. (1990). Long-term follow-up of families with young conduct-problems children: From preschool to grade school. *Journal of Consulting and Clinical Psychology, 19,* 1344–1349.

Webster-Stratton, C., & Hammond, M. (1997). Treating children with early-onset conduct problems: A comparison of child and parent training interventions. *Journal of Consulting and Clinical Psychology, 65,* 93–109.

Webster-Stratton, C., Kolpacoff, M., & Hollinsworth, T. (1988). Self-administered videotape therapy for families with conduct problem children: Comparison with two cost effective treatments and a control group. *Journal of Consulting and Clinical Psychology, 56,* 558–566.

Webster-Stratton, C., & Lindsay, D. W. (1999). Social competence and conduct problems in young children: Issues and assessment. *Journal of Clinical Child Psychology, 28,* 25–43.

SUGGESTED READINGS

Brestan, E. V., & Eyberg, S. M. (1998). Effective psychosocial treatments of conduct-disordered children and adolescents: 29 years, 82 studies, and 5,272 kids. *Journal of Clinical Child Psychology, 27,* 180–189.

Crick, N. R., & Dodge, K. A. (1994). A review and reformulation of social information-processing mechanisms in children's social adjustment. *Psychological Bulletin, 115,* 74–101.

Frick, P. J., Lahey, B. B., Loeber, R., Stouthamer-Loeber, M., Christ, M. A. G., & Hanson, K. (1992). Familial risk factors to oppositional defiant disorder and conduct disorder: Parental psychopathology and maternal parenting. *Journal of Consulting and Clinical Psychology, 60,* 49–53.

Lochman, J. E., & Lenhart, L. A. (1993). Anger coping intervention for aggressive children: Conceptual models and outcome effects. *Clinical Psychology Review, 13,* 785–805.

Peters, R. D., & McMahon, R. J. (1996). *Preventing childhood disorders, substance abuse and delinquency.* Thousand Oaks, CA: Sage.

Rey, J. M. (1993). Oppositional defiant disorder. *American Journal of Psychiatry, 150,* 1769–1778.

Webster-Stratton, C., & Lindsay, D. W. (1999). Social competence and conduct problems in young children: Issues and assessment. *Journal of Clinical Child Psychology, 28,* 25–43.

4

Recovery Maintenance and Relapse Prevention with Chemically Dependent Adolescents

HENRY O. PATTERSON
DAVID F. O'CONNELL

Cognitive-behavioral therapy has attracted a considerable following in the helping professions. The proliferation of research and clinical evidence supporting cognitive-behavioral therapy increasingly supports its effectiveness in a wide range of clinical settings and with a broad spectrum of disorders and dysfunctions.

However, as we reported in the first edition of this book (O'Connell & Patterson, 1996), the literature on cognitive-behavioral therapy has gaps, notably in the area of recovery maintenance and relapse prevention with chemically dependent adolescents. Because cognitive-behavioral techniques were developed with adults, most of the early literature deals with the treatment of various adult disorders and dysfunctions, including some attention to adult substance abuse (e.g., Beck, Wright, & Newman, 1992; Beck, Wright, Newman, & Liese, 1993). With growing evidence of effectiveness, therapists began adapting methods for use with adolescents and children, especially targeting depression and anxiety. Still, cognitive-behavioral therapists have given little attention to one of the most common problems of childhood and adolescence—substance abuse.

The purpose of this chapter is to focus attention of the use of cognitive-behavioral techniques with adolescents in the treatment of substance abuse, with an emphasis on relapse prevention—a central concern in treatment programs. After a brief review of the literature on the use of cognitive-behavioral therapy with substance-abusing adolescents, we compare cognitive-behavioral therapy with traditional addiction treatment programs, offer some practical suggestions on using cognitive-behavioral therapy with this population, and conclude with a case study (expanded from the first edition) from outpatient therapy sessions with a recovering 16-year-old male.

REVIEW OF THE LITERATURE

Compared with the fairly extensive clinical and empirical literature on the techniques and outcomes of cognitive-behavioral therapy with adults, relatively little literature exists for adolescents. A search in PsycINFO revealed more than 7,400 publications since 1983 dealing with cognitive-behavioral therapy and related cognitive techniques. Only about 790 of these publications focus on adolescents and, among these, only 44 publications focus specifically on cognitive-behavioral therapy and substance abuse. Narrowing the focus to issues of relapse and relapse prevention involving drug or alcohol abuse treatment, only two articles are cited: the first edition of this chapter (O'Connell & Patterson, 1996) and a recent article by Crome (1999). Given the high rates of relapse in adolescent substance abuse treatment programs, it is surprising that cognitive-behavior therapy has not been more widely discussed or recommended in the literature. The conclusion we drew in 1996 still appears to be valid: Cognitive-behavioral therapy has been ignored as a strategy for maintaining recovery and preventing relapse with substance-abusing adolescents.

Because we could not locate any clinical or empirical research publications on cognitive-behavioral therapy and recovery and relapse prevention in adolescents for the previous edition of this chapter, we undertook a review of the literature in several related areas: rational-emotive therapy (RET), delinquency, child and adolescent therapy, depression, anxiety, obsessive–compulsive disorder, attention-deficit/hyperactivity disorder (AD/HD), anger and aggression, sexual offenders, and acting-out. We will not revisit that literature review here, but the general conclusion we drew from those somewhat disparate publications also appears to be valid today: Because research, albeit limited, has generally supported positive outcomes from the use of cognitive-behavioral therapy with a wide range of adolescent disorders and problems, it is reasonable to assume that this approach would also be effective in treating adolescent substance abusers and in helping to maintain their recovery.

Although not specifically addressing the issue of relapse, there is a small but growing literature on the use of cognitive-behavioral treatment for substance-abusing adolescents that has appeared since our literature search for the first edition and that supports the preceding conclusion. We briefly review that literature here.

Three empirical studies related to cognitive-behavioral treatment of adolescent substance abuse appear in the literature. A series of reports by Kaminer et al. (Kaminer, Blitz, Burleson, Kadden, & Rounsaville, 1998; Kaminer & Burleson, 1999; Kaminer, Burleson, Blitz, Sussman, & Rounsaville, 1998) summarizes an outcome study of 32 dually diagnosed adolescent substance abusers given either cognitive-behavioral therapy or interactional treatment. After 3 months, the cognitive-behavioral group showed a significant reduction in substance abuse severity, although at 15 months gains did not appear to be related to therapy type. Both groups, however, did maintain gains. A more recent outcome study of 114 substance-abusing adolescents conducted by Waldron, Slesnick, Brody, Charles, and Thomas (2001) reports that cognitive-behavioral therapy, family therapy, and combined family and individual therapy all reduced use levels from pretreatment to 4 months. Although not outcome research, a third study by Hogue et al. (1998) investigates treatment adherence and differentiation in cognitive-behavioral and family therapy with adolescent substance abusers and finds that therapists used techniques unique to each model. The implications for advancing the treatment of adolescent drug users is discussed.

Although not empirical studies, several publications discuss cognitive-behavioral techniques with adolescent substance abusers. Kaminer and Bukstein (1992) discuss cognitive-behavioral therapy with adolescent substance abusers in an inpatient facility. Nay and Ross (1993) advocate using cognitive-behavioral strategies to change adolescents' beliefs and attributions about themselves and drugs. Wagner, Myers, and Brown (1994) discuss cognitive-behavioral interventions with adolescents and provide some approaches to design and implementation. Hollon and Beck (1994) discuss underlying processes in both cognitive therapy and cognitive-behavioral therapy, and relate both to adolescent disorders and substance abuse. Many of the practical aspects of using cognitive-behavioral intervention strategies with adolescents with drug problems—including the importance of assessment—are discussed by Myers, Wagner, and Brown (1998). In their discussion of cognitive-behavioral therapy with adolescents, van Bilsen and Wilke (1998) argue that the techniques are no different from other client groups; they also describe motivational interviewing techniques. Winters, Latimer, and Stinchfield (1999) describe four theoretical approaches used in the United States for treating adolescent substance abusers: cognitive-behavioral therapy, family-based approaches, therapeutic communities, and the Minnesota model. Crome (1999) reviews treatment interventions used with adult substance abusers and makes suggestions for a comprehensive treatment of adolescents—including recovery maintenance. Curry, Wells, Lochman, Craighead, and Nagy (2001) report the successful treatment of an adolescent case of comorbid depression and substance abuse using cognitive behavior therapy. Finally, Barrett-Waldron, Brody, and Slesnick (2001) discuss a model integrating family systems therapy and cognitive-behavioral therapy in the treatment of adolescent substance abuse.

Notwithstanding this relatively small literature on cognitive-behavioral therapy with substance-abusing adolescents and the paucity of empirical outcome studies, we concur with two recent literature reviews that this approach has shown effectiveness in reducing drug use and improving interpersonal functioning (Sudderth, 2000) and that it has great promise as a treatment modality (Deas & Thomas, 2001). Given the high relapse rates observed in adolescent treatment programs (35–85%), and the resurgence in drug use (Weinberg, Rahdert, Colliver, & Glantz, 1998), clearly the need for more effective treatment techniques is great. Today a growing number of therapists are promoting cognitive-behavioral therapy as a supplement to more traditional approaches with adolescents; however, in the absence of extensively tested clinical directives for applying cognitive-behavioral therapy to the problem of adolescent chemical dependency—especially recovery maintenance and relapse prevention—we must continue to rely on clinical judgment in selecting and utilizing cognitive-behavioral therapy techniques that have been found useful and effective with adult addicts. A growing number of therapists have found, as we have, that cognitive-behavioral therapy approaches can be easily adapted to the adolescent population, and we believe this a testament to the flexibility and universality of cognitive-behavioral therapy.

In the remainder of this chapter, we describe our experience and give an example of how we have used cognitive-behavioral therapy to prevent relapse and to maintain recovery in adolescent substance abusers.

APPLYING COGNITIVE-BEHAVIORAL THERAPY TO RECOVERY MAINTENANCE AND RELAPSE PREVENTION

Based on our review of the treatment literature, it appears that cognitive therapeutic approaches to addiction treatments are underutilized in the substance dependence field (see also Weinberg et al., 1998). Typically, traditional treatment for chemical dependency occurs first on an inpatient basis. This type of treatment focuses on the identification and expression of feelings that are held to be repressed, suppressed, or anesthetized by the use of psychoactive substances. Along with this focus, which usually occurs in a group context, is an emphasis on the identification and lowering of defenses that block the patient's capacity to deal with troubling feelings and to develop a more intimate relationship with self and others. Traditional chemical dependency treatment for adolescents also relies heavily on psychoeducational interventions and programs. Most programs have a strong didactic component to teach patients about the process of addiction. Many of these psychoeducational approaches are consonant with the cognitive model of treatment. Educational interventions are designed to modify the perceptions, attitudes, and beliefs of chemically dependent patients. Typically, patients are exposed to information on the psychological, physiological, and spiritual effects of addictive use of psychoactive substances. From a physiological perspective, they learn how the various psychoactive agents produce neurophysiological and neuropsychological impairment and lead to decreased adaptive functioning. From the psychological perspective, patients learn how drugs of abuse affect the thinking and perceiving processes, distort values, and modify painful feeling states. From the spiritual perspective, which is generally based on the Alcoholics Anonymous (AA), Narcotics Anonymous (NA), and other 12-step philosophies, patients see how the process of addiction alienates a person from him- or herself, others, and his or her higher power or sense of transcendence.

Although not typically acknowledged, 12-step programs appear to rely on approaches designed to modify the cognitions and perceptions of patients. Common aphorisms such as "There's nothing so bad that a drink won't make it worse," "Bring your body (to the meeting) and your mind will come," "First things first," "One day at a time," "Poor me, poor me, pour me a drink," all have obvious cognitive components to them. Twelve-step approaches to addictions treatment also emphasize a daily program of recovery and encourage adherents to read awareness-expanding, attitude-modifying, and meditative and contemplative literature on a regular basis. Implicit in the 12-step approaches to treatment are cognitive-behavioral therapy techniques such as rational restructuring, reframing, countering, perceptual shifting, shame attacking, turning adversity to advantage, and exaggeration.

This rather extensive, although often implicit, cognitive focus in traditional chemical dependency treatment makes formal cognitive-behavioral therapy, in our opinion, a natural treatment of choice for recovery maintenance and relapse prevention. Patients are drawn to this type of therapy and it often potentiates the existing recovery mechanisms. A psychologist or other cognitive psychotherapist typically comes in contact with an adolescent patient after he or she has already completed a 28-day inpatient program. The patient also probably has been exposed to AA and NA and may be participating in a daily program, although he or she may vary in level of commitment to 12-step activities. The cognitive therapist is unlikely to see an adolescent patient for the primary treatment of chemical dependency on a strictly outpatient basis, so cognitive-behavioral therapy will likely be used in concert with other approaches to addiction treatment. Cognitive-behavioral therapy is recommended, however, as the primary approach to relapse prevention.

Practical Suggestions for Clinical Management of Patients

Based on our experience treating adolescents with cognitive-behavioral therapy, we offer the following advice and suggestions:

1. Don't dispute the disease model of addictions. Most adolescent patients coming to treatment with a cognitive therapist have been taught that addiction is a genetically transmitted, physical disease with psychological, social, and spiritual manifestations. Patients exposed to the "medical model" of addiction will have an even more rigidly restricted view of addictive disorders and may view them as entirely physical in their origin and manifestation. The cognitive model can be used effectively with the disease model, although there are alternative views (Lawson & Lawson, 1992). It is usually nonproductive to attempt to change the patient's model of addiction or to dispute the utility of the medical or disease model; such discussions can confuse the patient and alienate the addictions treatment community within which the therapist operates. Rather, we suggest the concept of utilization; that is, we suggest the therapist become thoroughly familiar with the disease/medical model of addiction and build on existing cognitive techniques and ideas present in these approaches.

2. Don't avoid or downplay spirituality. Many therapists are uncomfortable with or unaccustomed to dealing directly with spiritual issues with patients. However, chemically dependent patients, especially 12-step participants, view spirituality as an important area for focus in therapeutic sessions. For example, many patients use the therapeutic alliance for fourth- and fifth-step work. According to the 12-step philosophy, a "spiritual awakening" is the basis for recovery from addictive diseases. The components of a spiritual experience can be operationalized, however, into cognitive-behavioral terms. Whatever the exact nature of a spiritual awakening, it has direct effects on the perceptions, attitudes, beliefs, and behaviors of patients who undergo it, and in many ways it can be viewed as a cognitive and perceptual shift in a person's relationship with self and the environment. For example, one 19-year-old patient was able to reframe the pain and struggle of her addiction as a rite of passage to spiritual maturity and as an opportunity for growth and development. In general, cognitive-behavioral therapy can assist the patient in achieving a sense of freedom and love that is at the very heart of the spiritual experience. The spiritual awakening rarely occurs suddenly or abruptly; it is rather a gradual, cumulative process that unfolds as the patient matures in recovery. Once the spiritual experience is operationalized within a cognitive framework, the therapist can proceed with this aspect of the patient's treatment as with any other issue brought up in therapy.

3. Be aware of the phase of recovery and the stage of change. The developmental model of recovery (Brown, 1985) depicts the recovery process

as a developmental phenomenon. As in other areas of human development, over time the patient gradually acquires abilities and capacities and therapeutic work is accomplished. In practical terms, patients in initial stages of recovery look and act very different from patients who are drug-free for a significant period of time (6 months or more), and cognitive interventions should be geared toward the style of functioning of the patient in his or her stage of recovery process. For example, patients in early phases of recovery typically are plagued by cravings and urges to use psychoactive chemicals, and the therapist may need to provide the patient with cognitive and behavioral approaches to cope with these impulses. Patients in the middle phase of recovery generally do not suffer from conscious urges to use drugs, but have difficulty dealing with the management of emotions—particularly hostility and anger—and need assistance dealing with life in a drug-free fashion. (See Miller, 1995, for suggestions on strategies for anger management.) Patients in this phase also may begin questioning whether they are chemically dependent and whether they can use substances in a controlled fashion. In the later phase of recovery, patients appear to the therapist more and more like their non–substance-dependent clientele. Neurotic conflicts, personality problems, adjustment issues, and interpersonal difficulties all come to the foreground after the patient has gained a significant amount of time in abstinence from psychoactive drug use. Here the therapist can shift the focus of therapy to psychological issues that predate the addiction and may be blocking the patient's personal development.

Related to the developmental concept of recovery is the transtheoretical stage theory of change proposed by Prochaska, DiClemente, and Norcross (1992; see also Freeman & Dolan, 2001). Because patients in recovery typically relapse and recycle through the five stages of Precontemplation, Contemplation, Preparation, Action, and Maintenance, the approach and focus of treatment should take into consideration the patient's stage.

4. Avoid extensive "homework." In our experience, adolescent patients equate therapeutic homework with schoolwork, show an aversion to it, and often do not complete it. We have found that focusing on the patient's lack of completion of homework assignments as resistance in the therapeutic process is not productive. Typically, the adolescent patient may be involved in daily NA or AA meetings and also concurrent traditional outpatient addictions therapy. This leaves little time for homework assignments. As an alternative, we suggest expanding the therapeutic hour to 1½ hours and allowing the patient to read brief, summarized literature on cognitive-behavioral therapy, and if written techniques are to be utilized (e.g., the triple-column technique, see Burns, 1989, and Beck, 1995) that they be performed with the therapist's assistance within the therapeutic session. Work on specific social skills, adaptive coping, and affect regulation

as proposed by Monti and his colleagues might also be considered (Monti, Abrams, Binkoff, & Zwick, 1990; Monti, Gulliver, & Meyers, 1994; Monti, Rohsenow, Colby, & Abrams 1995).

5. Be active and challenging. Perhaps because of the cognitive development of the adolescent patient, specifically the development of "metacognition," we have found that adolescent patients enjoy the polemics and debate that can be involved in cognitive-behavioral therapy. We suggest a very active, challenging, and, when appropriate, confrontational style for the therapist, so as to engage the often passive and at times taciturn adolescent in the treatment process. At the same time, it is important to be mindful of the cognitive limitations of some adolescents. Many have not fully developed Jean Piaget's stage of formal operational thought, and are not capable of highly abstract thinking about their own mental processes or the external world. Adolescent egocentrism is often a hindrance to objective self-reflection. The therapist should keep sessions as structured and concrete as possible, frequently checking to see if the patient fully grasps the concepts being discussed.

6. Anticipate several relapses. Relapse rates for adolescent chemically dependent patients remain very high (Catalano, Hawkins, Wells, Miller, & Brewer, 1990; Henry, 1989), often over 90% following discharge from a 28-day inpatient program. Therapists should expect that their adolescent patients will relapse one or several times in the course of therapy, and will recycle through stages of change (Prochaska et al., 1992). Therapists should also expect that they will be manipulated and lied to. Often the patient will seem to be doing very well in therapy and "look good," all the while abusing substances outside of the therapeutic environment. Random urinalysis is often helpful in dealing with the issue of relapse, and we suggest it be utilized along with the cognitive approach.

7. Dual diagnosis. Previous research (Bukstein, Brent, & Kaminer, 1989; Curry et al., 2001; O'Connell, 1989, 1990; Pierce, 1991) has shown that chemically dependent patients are a heterogenous population, with a large proportion of patients showing a concurrent Axis I or Axis II diagnosis. Often the therapist has at least two diagnoses with which to contend, significantly complicating treatment. Again, we feel that the cognitive approach emerges as the treatment of choice for this population because cognitive-behavioral therapy has been found to be effective for a wide spectrum of emotional and behavioral disorders with adolescents.

8. Address issues of social culture. Because social influence is a significant factor in the initiation of substance use for adolescents, some attention should be given to social networks and the power of peer pressure. Adolescents need to understand the importance of choosing friends and associates who value and support adaptive behaviors over those who do not.

OVERVIEW OF TREATMENT

Initial work with chemically dependent adolescents involves educating patients about the cognitive model of treatment and operationalizing their problems in cognitive terms (Beck et al., 1992). The standard approach to conceptualizing problems in cognitive terms has been portrayed in many excellent books (e.g., Burns, 1989; Beck, 1995) and will not be repeated here. In general, clients are taught that their thoughts, beliefs, or schemas are responsible for negative emotions and behaviors. The therapist tells the patient that the bulk of therapy will be focusing on those thoughts and beliefs that are causing problems for the patient and may result in a relapse to active addiction or other emotional difficulties in the recovery process.

In addition to this general discussion of the cognitive model, several important points developed by Marlatt and Gordon (1985) should be included. First of all, the adolescent patient is told that recovery can be understood as a journey and that, like any journey, it involves continual discovery, dealing with novel situations, improvising when things do not go well, and learning new and useful ways to cope with problems along the way. Cognitive-behavioral therapy provides a map for the journey and also the skills necessary to negotiate the journey in the most effective way. It is useful to tell young patients that recovery from substance dependence usually proceeds along unremarkably until the adolescent encounters what is termed a *high-risk* situation. This could be anything that threatens the adolescent, such as an awkward, stressful social situation or an internal affective state, such as extreme anger, anxiety, or depression. When an adolescent encounters a high-risk situation, the chances for picking up a drink or a drug increase significantly. The patient is then told that handling high-risk situations in an adaptive way is the key to ongoing recovery and relapse prevention, and that how he or she perceives, interprets, and understands a high-risk situation can directly affect the outcome.

Here, the idea of automatic thoughts and cognitive distortions can be introduced. We have found that an explanation of common cognitive distortions in addictions is useful in conceptualizing the patient's problems. For each of the following distortions identified by Marlatt and Gordon (1985), we offer patients common examples associated with the relapse process.

- *Overgeneralization.* With this cognitive error the patient seems to be saying "If it happened in this situation, it's going to happen in any situation that is even remotely like it." For example, the patient has one slip by taking a drag on a marijuana cigarette and uses this as evidence that he or she is not "working a recovery program" and will not be able to avoid slips again.
- *Selective abstraction.* Similar to overgeneralization, with this error

the patient measures him- or herself in terms of failure or mistakes. When committing this distortion, the patient focuses excessively on a negative situation to the exclusion of all previous positive experiences. For example, a patient with 6 months of continuous sobriety became obsessed with the idea that he had inhaled some nitrous oxide with a friend at a party. He was seized with the idea that all of his treatment and efforts at recovery were in vain.

• *Excessive responsibility.* With this error, the patient assumes more responsibility than he or she actually has for a relapse or other problem in his or her life. In the case of a relapse, patients may feel that they lack willpower, are constitutionally defective, or just do not have what it takes to remain abstinent. Patients making this error see themselves as the sole cause of their problems without giving consideration to the many other causes or variables that affect any given behavior or situation.

• *Assumption of temporal causality.* This cognitive error is the temporal equivalent to overgeneralization. The patient seems to be saying, "It was true in the past and its always going to be true." With this error a slip is viewed as "the beginning of the end," and all future attempts at coping and staying sober are seen as abortive.

• *Self-reference.* Here, patients show adolescent egocentric thinking and the imaginary audience, common cognitive traits associated with adolescence (Elkind, 1967), and feel that the world is watching them and is overly concerned with their problems. As in excessive responsibility, patients see themselves as the cause of their problems and anticipate that others are blaming them and looking down on them. Patients who are unable to stay sober often suffer extreme guilt and shame due to this distortion.

• *Catastrophizing.* With this error, patients anticipate the worst happening. In our experience, it is probably the most common cognitive error. One patient was convinced that after he had one beer or snort he would turn into a homeless drug addict, roaming from crackhouse to crackhouse, finally ending up on the streets dying from exposure to the elements.

• *Dichotomous thinking.* This is black-and-white thinking. For example, patients committing this error may see themselves either actively pursuing recovery and doing everything they can to stay sober or being irresponsible and "not working a program." They approach their sobriety with an either/or mentality.

Describing common cognitive distortions in addictive thinking, along with concrete examples from the patients' lives, is highly effective in helping adolescents to understand the cognitive model and apply appropriate cognitive interventions.

In initial therapeutic sessions, patients should be apprised of the "abstinence violation effect" (AVE). This effect, described by Marlatt and Gordon (1985), can occur when the adolescent patient picks up a drink or a drug, and has two components: (1) a cognitive attribution as to the per- ceived cause of the relapse and (2) an affective reaction to this attribution. Typically, patients experience this response when they see themselves as the cause of a lapse and feel an overwhelming sense of guilt, shame, or other negative affect. Patients experience the AVE when they attribute a lapse to internal, stable, and global factors that are viewed as uncontrollable (e.g., having the gene for alcoholism, lacking willpower, being mentally defi- cient). The AVE can be decreased in intensity by assisting the patient to see that a lapse can be caused by external, unstable, changeable factors such as acquired coping skills level. The patient is then told that learning cognitive coping skills can decrease the probability of a full-blown relapse when a slip occurs.

Another useful concept to consider is the "biphasic response." Typi- cally, the adolescent does not consider both the long- and short-term effects of a drug when deciding whether to again use substances. Most patients show what is termed "positive outcome expectancies" when they pick up a drink or a drug. What they forget is that only the short-term or initial phase of the drug effect is positive. This is followed by a negative phase when the drug begins to wear off and the patient experiences physical discomfort, followed by emotional discomfort from feelings such as guilt and anxiety. In the cognitive approach to treatment, patients are encouraged to antici- pate the biphasic response and to consider both the positive and negative immediate consequences of picking up a drink or a drug and also the delayed consequences, positive or negative, that can come from drug or alcohol use.

Emery (1988) has developed a structured program, Dependency Free, that can also be quite useful in the initial stages of treatment with chemi- cally dependent adolescents. One of the useful components of Dependency Free includes the concept of "psychological reversal," a psychological state that renders the patient highly vulnerable to relapse. At such a time, patients become more concerned with seeking *pleasure* than gaining long- term results and focusing on *happiness*. Pleasure provides an immediate escape, and the person does not have to work for it; pleasure experiences are acquired. Happiness, on the other hand, involves letting go. It is a deeper, more subtle, more powerful experience and is the hallmark of psy- chological maturity. Happiness comes spontaneously and automatically when one stops fighting life and moves toward accepting everything life has to offer. Dropping one's need to be important is integral to creating happi- ness. It is achieved when one becomes involved in life in the *here and now*. Pleasure can come from the use of drugs or alcohol, but happiness can never be derived from substances.

Several dysfunctional beliefs are identified for the patient in Depend- ency Free. We typically offer these to patients to help them dissolve the fol- lowing beliefs and substitute more rational ones: "I need others' approval to prove I am worthy"; "I need to achieve to prove that I am good enough"; "I need to be in control to avoid feeling helpless"; "I am powerless to get what I want."

Substance-abusing adolescent patients typically harbor one or more of these beliefs. A good deal of exploration and active direction by the therapist may be necessary to draw out these beliefs. Once they are brought to the surface, the therapist can employ the full spectrum of cognitive interventions to challenge them and supplant them with more rational assumptions.

Using a similar approach in his book *Healing the Addictive Mind*, Jampolsky (1991) lists 13 core beliefs of the addictive thought system, followed by 13 beliefs that serve as the rational counterpart. He sees chemically dependent patients as developing a thought system based on fear and a past or future orientation that robs them of love and serenity. In Jampolsky's approach to therapy, the addictive core beliefs are to be supplanted by a rational, love-based thought system. For example, the irrational belief that "the past and the future are real and need to be constantly evaluated and worried about" is countered with the belief that "only the present is real, the past is over, and the future is not yet here." The belief that "other people are responsible for how I feel; the situation is the determiner of my experience," is replaced with "I am responsible for the world I see, and I choose the feelings that I experience; I decide upon the goal I will achieve." The view that "I need something or someone outside of myself to make me complete and happy" is countered with "I am complete right now."

Finally, it is important for cognitive therapists to keep in mind that patients typically view the recovery process as a spiritual as well as psychological growth process. But the emphasis on rationality of beliefs provides an interesting and useful mix with the more traditional intuitive focus on love and spirituality. In practice, we have found these techniques to be more useful with older adolescents who have typically developed higher levels of abstraction and self-insight, and a more articulated sense of self.

CASE EXAMPLE

The following case is typical of the clinical scenario a cognitive therapist might encounter. Justin is a 16-year-old male who presents with a concurrent Axis I diagnosis, and comes from a family in which the father is an active alcoholic. Since age 12, he has had a history of alcohol, cannabis, and inhalant dependence, and has been through two previous inpatient stays at a midsized, free-standing, specialized inpatient treatment center for chemically dependent adolescents. Previously he was diagnosed with conduct disorder, undifferentiated type. Justin is repeating the 10th grade in high school and was active in athletics, but he discontinued his involvement as his addiction progressed. The patient was evaluated previously as part of a routine evaluation when he was admitted to treatment.

Clinically, Justin presents as a somewhat anxious but open and affable young man. Around adults he is polite and endearing. He is rather talkative and likes to discuss topics such as politics and religion, but around his age-mates it is a different story. He becomes more defiant and critical and enjoys being the focus of attention. Justin was referred for cognitive-behavioral therapy because of his inability to stay sober for more than a few months. He enjoyed his previous inpatient stays and NA/AA meetings, but he had difficulty with outpatient therapy. He could not stay out of trouble and became bored with standard outpatient addictions therapy because he had "heard it all before."

The case portrays a rather tight focus on specific problems generated by the patient and those cognitive interventions drawn from the larger pool of cognitive techniques that we have found particularly useful in dealing with recovery and relapse in chemically dependent teenagers. Several cognitive techniques are illustrated, along with some sample therapeutic dialogue. However, as indicated earlier, all of the cognitive approaches and techniques developed over the past two decades can be applied to chemical dependency treatment (Freeman, Simon, Beutler, & Arkowitz, 1989).

Initial Assessment

Justin was administered the Drug Taking Confidence Questionnaire (DTCQ), developed by Annis and Martin (1985; see also Annis & Davis, 1988). This is a 50-item self-report questionnaire designed to assess Bandura's concept of self-efficacy in relation to the patient's perceived ability to cope effectively with drugs/alcohol. Eight subscores are obtained, five for personal states (unpleasant emotions, physical discomfort, pleasant emotions, testing personal control, urges and temptations to use), and three for situations involving other people (conflict with others, social pressure to use, and pleasant times with others). The subscores are obtained by the patient's response to 50 statements in which the patient rates him- or herself as zero ("Not at All Confident") to 100 ("Very Confident") in the ability to resist the urge to use alcohol or drugs. There are two versions of the DTCQ: one for alcohol only, and another for all other drugs. The eight subscales generate eight separate confidence levels that can then be graphed on a confidence profile. Figure 4.1 shows Justin's DTCQ confidence profile. The results reveal his lowest confidence scores to be in two areas: social pressure and unpleasant emotions. On the social pressure subscore, Justin rated himself as low in confidence in his ability to refuse drugs when they were offered to him if he were socializing with friends and they suggested that the group use drugs, or if he were with a group of friends who were using

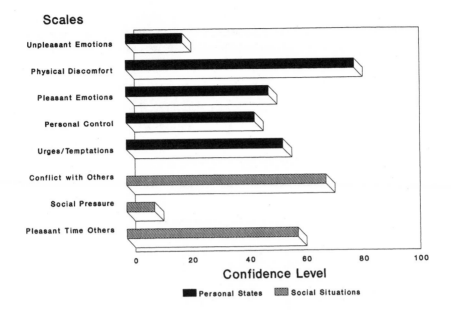

FIGURE 4.1. DTCQ profile for Justin.

drugs. With regard to unpleasant emotions, Justin rated himself as low in confidence in his capacity to resist drug use if he was depressed, bored, lonely, anxious, angry, or confused.

We have organized this case report around these two problem areas. Each section includes clinical comments and transcripts of therapeutic sessions that illustrate the various cognitive interventions we have found useful with adolescent addicts. Many presentations on cognitive therapeutic techniques use a one-technique-at-a-time case excerpt method to illustrate the technique. This approach can be quite artificial. Therapy rarely proceeds in a compartmentalized, structured, point-by-point fashion—one technique after the next. Many cognitive techniques are similar and can be used at any given choice point in the therapeutic process; thus, the case excerpts illustrate our style of cognitive-behavioral therapy and each session transcript illustrates a number of cognitive interventions.

Social Pressure: Fourth Session

THERAPIST: Looking at your relapse profile and based on your discussions thus far, you seem to have lots of concerns about social pressures to use drugs and alcohol again.

JUSTIN: Yeah, I'm really OK at meetings and in school for the most part, or hanging out with recovering friends. It's when I go to parties, especially if some of the cooler people at school are there and especially if they're smoking pot or drinking.

THERAPIST: So what happens when you go to one of these parties?

JUSTIN: Well, it actually starts before I get there. I start thinking about who's going to be there and how they're going to treat me.

THERAPIST: So you've gotten pretty good at this. You start upsetting yourself even before you get there.

JUSTIN: Well, yeah. But I don't do this on purpose.

THERAPIST: You mean you don't do it consciously with a goal in mind of making yourself nervous, but you've gotten quite good at it.

JUSTIN: OK, yeah, it's automatic.

THERAPIST: All right, so you're tense and now you've walked into the party. Now what happens?

JUSTIN: Well, I see several of the cooler dudes and I start thinking, well, you know, they know I've been through a rehab and here comes "reformed Jus." Here's "Mr. Recovery" or something. I feel I start making them nervous.

THERAPIST: And how do you know all this?

JUSTIN: I don't know, I can just tell.

THERAPIST: You can read their minds?

JUSTIN: Well, of course not. They just act differently toward me.

THERAPIST: So there's an appropriate, specific way to act toward you.

JUSTIN: I don't know, they just seem different when I'm there.

THERAPIST: So you're causing them to act different.

JUSTIN: Maybe.

THERAPIST: Wow, you must have a lot of power over these fellows! How cool can they be?! Sounds to me like you don't have a heck of a lot of information in this situation so your mind begins making stuff up and you project it on to these people. Some of this is psychological, you know. Our brains don't like incomplete or vague information that is not readily understandable, and our minds go about the process of making sense out of situations. This is all right, but we all have distorted thinking and this can take a neutral or positive situation and make it negative. You're just beginning to become aware of the ways you do this. So far I see you *mind reading* and *personalizing*. (*Proceeds to discuss these distortions and to help the patient identify examples in other situations.*) Remember we talked before about rational counters. You've got a lot of distorted thinking in these social pressure situations. Part of an effective way of dealing with it is to identify your thinking errors. The other part is to develop a rational counter to your automatic negative thought. Now remember the principle here is that when you argue against an irrational thought repeatedly, that thought becomes progressively weaker over time. These thoughts have a grip on you now, but they won't always. (*Therapist and Justin work together to come up with a list of counters to offset irrational automatic thinking Justin experiences in high-pressure social situations.*) So let's write some of these down.

1. These people are more concerned with getting high than with my social status.
2. They don't know what they are doing, but *I do.*
3. There's no evidence that they think I'm a wimp. Maybe they're just curious.
4. Just because I feel nervous and I have thought of using doesn't mean I *have to.*
5. Well, let's say I take a toke and blow my sobriety. Will these people be there for me to help me?

JUSTIN: (*Practices the counters subvocally.*)

In this therapeutic exchange a number of cognitive techniques were utilized: reframing, examining the evidence, listing cognitive distortions, challenging labels, and rational countering. The therapist also took the opportunity to provide information to the patient to raise his level of self-awareness and to help him understand his thought process.

Because social pressure situations figured so prominently in Justin's history of relapse, considerable time in therapy was spent in addressing it. This focus on social pressure continues in the next excerpt.

Social Pressure: Sixth Session

THERAPIST: One of the things that I've noticed about you, Justin, is that you've gotten *so good* at putting others' opinions of you before your own and worrying about how they think! I want you to teach me how to do that.

JUSTIN: What?!

THERAPIST: No, really, I really want you to teach me how to do that. I think I have the opposite problem. I'm not concerned enough with how people view me or think of me. I want you to be my teacher. I want you to teach me how to become preoccupied with how other people view me.

JUSTIN: But I don't do this on purpose, I—

THERAPIST: I didn't say you did it on purpose, I'm just saying you're good at it, and I want you to teach me. OK, you be my trainer, you be my coach. What's Step number 1? When I walk into a party and I see drug abusing, "cool" people there, what's the first thing I should do to get myself worked up?

JUSTIN: (*Laughs.*) Well I don't know. I feel a little silly. Well, let me see, first you look around the room and see who's there.

THERAPIST: To find the coolest people?

JUSTIN: Yeah, you know, to sort of find your place.

THERAPIST: OK, and then what?

JUSTIN: Well, then I guess you start talking to yourself and say things like, "Oh God, there's Steve, I know he's going to ask me about the rehab."

THERAPIST: Good, great. So I start to monologue with myself. Telling myself exactly what's going to happen before it starts.

JUSTIN: Yeah, that's right.

THERAPIST: So what do I do when I actually go up and start talking with these people?

JUSTIN: Uh, pretend you're not nervous.

THERAPIST: Okay, so now I introduce tension by pretending I don't feel a certain way.

JUSTIN: Yeah, I guess that's what I do.

THERAPIST: And then what? (*Continues eliciting a step-by-step process of how Justin creates the problem of social pressure to use drugs.*) Well, I'm really starting to get the knack of this, but I just realized you have to teach me your underlying beliefs and assumptions. I've got some ideas on them. How about "One should be more concerned with others' opinions than one's own," and "It's terrible not to be in complete emotional control in social situations"? How about "Being a recovering person is an insurmountable, everlasting, social handicap"? You see, you have to teach me these beliefs that are behind your problem here.

JUSTIN: You know, I never really thought of this like that. There is so much involved.

In this exchange the therapist relies on a cognitive intervention developed by McMullin (1986), a variation of a paradoxical technique titled

Teach Thyself. This technique allows the therapist to dramatically illustrate the components of the patient's problem in social situations, including assumptions, behavioral sequence, and distorted thinking. In addition to being a powerful cognitive intervention, it can be a lot of fun for both the therapist and patient.

Unpleasant Emotions: Eleventh Session

THERAPIST: You have a really low level of confidence dealing with unpleasant emotions based on your test [DTCQ].

JUSTIN: Yeah, I know. That is really tough for me. Like when I get depressed or when I get really angry, especially, I just say, "Screw it." I guess I'm pretty moody. And then if I do pick up a drug or drink, it makes it even worse, because then I figure, what the hell, I may as well keep going.

THERAPIST: Yeah, I've heard recovering patients say that one of the worst things is to have a head full of AA and a belly full of booze.

JUSTIN: Yeah, I know what they mean. And once that happens, I'm gone and things get worse.

THERAPIST: The weird thing about relapsing is that at the time you make the decision to use, you act as if there's not going to be any negative consequences. You forget about the biphasic drug response and stay focused exclusively on a positive outcome.

JUSTIN: Yeah, you know it happens so quickly.

THERAPIST: Yes, drugs are very predictable and very reliable, both in the positive and negative effects.

JUSTIN: But at the time it just seems to come over so quickly. It's like I don't even think, it's just automatic.

THERAPIST: Yes, well, that's where the therapy comes in—to help you keep your thinking, your perceptions, and your behavior from being so automatic. Now, when you get into these negative moods, I want you to focus on what you're telling yourself, what self-talk you're engaging in. Remember you can't have an emotion without also having a thought and perception of the feeling and the situation you are involved in. Since you go through so many moods, this is going to be important. So when you realize what you're telling yourself, I want you to pick out the negative thoughts and then the distortions, and I want you to ask what evidence you have for the particular thought. Then I want you to do your countering. Above all, I want you to *do* something in these situations. Remember to be action-oriented. We talked about psychological reversal. You've got to keep moving in these situations. I've found that getting out of a situation by leaving it or doing something physical, like taking a brisk walk, is really helpful in dealing with moods. I get a lot of them myself. (*Discusses how the physiology affects moods and how to use meditation to normalize mood and reduce anxiety and depression.*) Remember, moods come and go, so detach from them. Thousands of thoughts go through your mind everyday, and you might go through a dozen or more moods. So what? Why should you be concerned? Your job is to keep moving, to keep growing, and enjoy yourself.

Later in the same session:

JUSTIN: What's really hard for me is dealing with my dad, you know, his drinking. Seeing him come home drunk really pisses me off. He's just a mess. He just ruins everything at home. I can't talk to him, he's so moody. At times he jumps on me and screams at me for no reason. It's like everything at home revolves around how drunk he is.

THERAPIST: Yeah, this could be a difficult situation, and along with your anger, I also sense a lot of hurt, seeing your father so dysfunctional.

JUSTIN: (*Tears well up in his eyes.*) I never thought of it as hurt, but it really does hurt and there's nothing I can do for him.

THERAPIST: Well, I imagine you're feeling all sorts of feelings, perhaps shame, anger, hurt, sadness, frustration. Maybe the anger is the easiest one for you to deal with. This can be a tough situation, having all of these feelings at one time. It's obviously overwhelming for you. Now let's look at what you tell yourself during these situations. When your father comes home drunk, what kind of self-talk do you have?

JUSTIN: Well, let me see. I say to myself, "What the hell is wrong with him, can't he see what he is doing, and what it's doing to us? Why can't he get his act together? He acts like he knows everything and doesn't have a problem."

THERAPIST: I hear a lot of shoulds here. That he should be aware of his problems, that he should be able to stop drinking, that he should be in control of himself. It's very understandable how you would think this. But let's look at addiction. Consider your own experiences getting sober. You've had to go through a lot of hard knocks until you really got any significant clean time. Your dad's in the same boat. But it may not always be this way. *You've* changed and you have all sorts of beliefs about your dad that may not be realistic, and we'll deal with these, but what about you? What do you say to yourself in these situations?

JUSTIN: Well, I guess I just feel like "I can't handle this." I can't stand it, and then I leave, and then I pick up.

THERAPIST: Well, getting out of there may be good sometimes, but it seems to me you rush right to chemicals. There seems to be a belief here that you can't experience a feeling and let it run its course. This is a time when you are reversed. You need to accept the situation and that you can't do anything right away to change your father, and then you need to let the feelings take their course, and then you need to do what we're doing here: Slow down, look at your thinking errors, stand back from the situation. You feel compelled to pick up a drug because you feel you don't have any options, but, as you're learning, that is clearly not the case.

In this session, the therapist took the opportunity to teach the patient about needs and feelings and how to deal with them. Helping an adolescent patient deal with an actively alcoholic parent is always difficult. There has been a considerable focus on the children of alcoholics syndrome over the past decade, and we feel it can be effectively addressed through cognitive interventions.

SUMMARY AND CONCLUSIONS

We have found cognitive-behavioral therapy to be an important and effective primary component of recovery maintenance and relapse prevention with chemically dependent adolescents, a finding consistent with the extant literature on effectiveness of cognitive-behavioral therapy with adults and adolescents suffering from a variety of disorders. Moreover, we believe that it can be used in a complementary fashion with other educational, medical, social, and psychological approaches to addictions treatment, as opposed to a sole approach.

Cognitive therapists who treat adolescent chemically dependent patients should possess a knowledge of the process of relapse and, in particular, cognitive relapse determinants. A knowledge of both the disease model and the developmental model of addiction is also strongly recommended.

In considering future research and directions for treatment, it is clear that empirical outcome research must be done on the effectiveness of cognitive-behavioral strategies to maintain recovery with substance-abusing adolescents. We also believe that research needs to be done on the issue of how to most effectively fuse these strategies not only with traditional approaches such as the 12-step programs, but also with newer, nontraditional approaches such as meditation. Cognitive-behavioral therapists have long recognized the utility of meditation and relaxation exercises as an adjunct to cognitive-behavioral therapy (e.g., Freeman & Dattilio, 1992; Kendall, 1991; Meichenbaum, 1977). Of all the methods of meditation available, transcendental meditation (TM) appears to have the most potential (see Chalmers, Clements, Schenklun, & Weinless, 1987, 1989, 1990; Eppley, Abrams, & Shear, 1989; O'Connell, 1989, 1991; O'Connell & Alexander, 1994; Orme-Johnson & Farrow, 1976). To our knowledge, no comprehensive outcome study has combined TM with cognitive-behavioral strategies; we believe such a combination would be well worth studying.

In summary, in this chapter we have reviewed the literature on cognitive approaches to the treatment of adolescent substance abuse, compared cognitive-behavioral therapy with traditional treatment programs for addicted adolescents, provided some practical suggestions on using cognitive-behavioral therapy with adolescents, and illustrated their use in relapse prevention with a typical case. We agree with a growing number of practitioners that cognitive therapeutic approaches should be standard components in both inpatient and outpatient treatment for chemical dependency with both adolescents and adults. Armed with the knowledge and skills of cognitive-behavioral therapy, addiction treatment professionals can become much more vital, potent agents of change and change maintenance in the lives of chemically dependent patients.

REFERENCES

Annis, H., & Davis, C. (1988). Self efficacy and the prevention of alcoholic relapse: Initial findings from a treatment trial. In T. Baker & D. Cannon (Eds.), *Addictive disorders: Psychological research on assessment and treatment* (pp. 88–112). New York: Praeger.

Annis, H., & Martin, G. (1985). *Inventory of drug taking situations.* Toronto: Addiction Research Foundation of Ontario.

Barrett-Waldron, H., Brody, J. L., & Slesnick, N. (2001). Integrative behavioral and family therapy for adolescent substance abuse. In P. M. Monti, S. M. Colby, & T. A. O'Leary (Eds.), *Adolescents, alcohol, and substance abuse: Reaching teens through brief interventions* (pp. 216–243). New York: Guilford Press.

Beck, A. T., Wright, F. D., & Newman, C. F. (1992). Cocaine abuse. In A. Freeman & F. M. Dattilio (Eds.), *Comprehensive casebook of cognitive therapy* (pp. 185–192). New York: Plenum Press.

Beck, A. T., Wright, F. D., Newman, C. F., & Liese, B. S. (1993). *Cognitive therapy of substance abuse.* New York: Guilford Press.

Beck, J. (1995). *Cognitive therapy: Basics and beyond.* New York: Guilford Press.

Brown, S. (1985). *Treating the alcoholic: A developmental perspective.* New York: Wiley.

Bukstein, O. G., Brent, D. A., & Kaminer, Y. (1989). Comorbidity of substance abuse and other psychiatric disorders in adolescents. *American Journal of Psychiatry, 146*(9), 1131–1141.

Burns, D. D. (1989). *The feeling good handbook: Using the new mood therapy in everyday life.* New York: Morrow.

Catalano, R. F., Hawkins, J. D., Wells, E. A., Miller, J., & Brewer, D. (1990). Evaluation of the effectiveness of adolescent drug abuse treatment, assessment of risks for relapse, and promising approaches for relapse prevention. *International Journal of the Addictions, 25*(9A & 10A), 1085–1140.

Chalmers, R., Clements, G., Schenklun, H., & Weinless, M. (Eds.). (1987). *Scientific research on Maharishi's transcendental mediation and TM-Sidhi programme* (Vol. 2). Vlodrop, The Netherlands: MIU Press.

Chalmers, R., Clements, G., Schenklun, H., & Weinless, M. (Eds.). (1989). *Scientific research on Maharishi's transcendental mediation and TM-Sidhi programme* (Vols. 3–4). Vlodrop, The Netherlands: MIU Press.

Chalmers, R., Clements, G., Schenklun, H., & Weinless, M. (Eds.). (1990). *Scientific research on Maharishi's transcendental mediation and TM-Sidhi programme* (Vol. 5). Vlodrop, The Netherlands: MIU Press.

Crome, I. B. (1999). Treatment interventions: Looking towards the millennium. *Drug and Alcohol Dependence, 55*(3), 247–263.

Curry, J. F., Wells, K. C., Lochman, J. E., Craighead, W. E., & Nagy, P. D. (2001). Group and family cognitive behavior therapy for adolescent depression and substance abuse: A case study. *Cognitive and Behavioral Practice, 8*(4), 367–376.

Deas, D., & Thomas, S. E. (2001). An overview of controlled studies of adolescent substance abuse treatment. *American Journal on Addictions, 10*(2), 178–189.

Elkind, D. (1967). Egocentrism during adolescence. *Child Development, 38*, 1025–1034.

Emery, G. (1988). *Dependency free: Rapid cognitive therapy of substance abuse.* Santa Monica, CA: Association for Advanced Training in the Behavioral Sciences.

Eppley, K., Abrams, A., & Shear, J. (1989). Differential effects of relaxation techniques on trait anxiety: A meta-analysis. *Journal of Clinical Psychology, 45*, 957–974.

Freeman, A., & Dattilio, F. M. (Eds.). (1992). *Comprehensive casebook of cognitive therapy.* New York: Plenum Press.

Freeman, A., & Dolan, M. (2001). Revisiting Prochaska and DiClemente's stages of change theory: An expansion and specification to aid in treatment planning and outcome evaluation. *Cognitive and Behavioral Practice, 8*(3), 224–234.

Freeman, A., Simon, K. M., Beutler, L. E., & Arkowitz, H. (1989). *The comprehensive handbook of cognitive therapy.* New York: Plenum Press.

Henry, P. B. (1989). *Practical approaches in treating adolescent chemical dependency: A guide to clinical assessment and intervention.* New York: Haworth Press.

Hogue, A., Liddle, H. A., Rowe, C., Turner, R. M., Dakof, G. A., & LaPann, K. (1998). Treatment adherence and differentiation in individual versus family therapy for adolescent substance abuse. *Journal of Counseling Psychology, 45*(1), 104–114.

Hollon, S. D, & Beck, A. T. (1994). Cognitive and cognitive-behavioral therapies. In A. E. Bergin & S. L. Garfield (Eds.), *Handbook of psychotherapy and behavior change* (4th ed., pp. 428–466). New York: Wiley.

Jampolsky, L. (1991). *Healing the addictive mind.* Berkeley, CA: Celestial Arts.

Kaminer, Y., Blitz, C., Burleson, J. A., Kadden, R. M., & Rounsaville, B. J. (1998).

Measuring treatment process in cognitive-behavioral and interactional group therapies for adolescent substance abusers. *Journal of Nervous and Mental Disease, 186*(7), 407–413.

Kaminer, Y., & Bukstein, O. G. (1992). Inpatient behavioral and cognitive therapy for substance abuse in adolescents. In V. B. Van Hasselt & D. J. Kolko (Eds.), *Inpatient behavior therapy for children and adolescents* (pp. 313–339). Boston: Allyn & Bacon.

Kaminer, Y., & Burleson, J. A. (1999). Psychotherapies for adolescent substance abusers: 15-month follow-up of a pilot study. *American Journal on Addictions, 8*(2), 114–119.

Kaminer, Y., Burleson, J. A., Blitz, C., Sussman, J., & Rounsaville, B. J. (1998) Psychotherapies for adolescent substance abusers: A pilot study. *Journal of Nervous and Mental Disease, 186*(11), 684–690.

Kendall, P. C. (Ed.). (1991). *Child and adolescent therapy: Cognitive-behavioral procedures.* New York: Guilford Press.

Lawson, G., & Lawson, A. (1992). *Adolescent substance abuse: Etiology, treatment and prevention.* Gathersberg, MD: Aspen.

Marlatt, G. A., & Gordon, J. R. (Eds.). (1985). *Relapse prevention: Maintenance strategies in the treatment of addictive behaviors.* New York: Guilford Press.

McMullin, R. (1986). *Handbook of cognitive therapy techniques.* New York: Norton.

Meichenbaum, D. (1977). *Cognitive-behavior modification: An integrative approach.* New York: Plenum Press.

Miller, D. B. (1995). Treatment of adolescent interpersonal violence: A cognitive-behavioral approach. *Journal of Child and Adolescent Group Therapy, 5*(4), 191–200.

Monti, P., Abrams, D., Binkoff, J., & Zwick, W. (1990). Communication skills training, communication skills training with family, and cognitive behavioral mood management training for alcoholics. *Journal of Studies on Alcohol, 51,* 263–270.

Monti, P., Gulliver, S., & Meyers, M. (1994). Social skills training for alcoholics: Assessment and treatment. *Alcohol and Alcoholism, 29,* 627–637.

Monti, P., Rohsenow, D., Colby, S., & Abrams, D. (1995). Coping and social skills training. In R. Hester & W. Miller (Eds.), *Handbook of alcoholism treatment approaches: Effective alternatives* (2nd ed., pp. 221–241). Boston: Allyn & Bacon.

Myers, M. G., Wagner, E. F., & Brown, S. A. (1998). Substance abuse. In V. B. Van Hasselt & M. Hersen (Eds.), *Handbook of psychological treatment protocols for children and adolescents: The LEA series in personality and clinical psychology* (pp. 381–411). Mahwah, NJ: Erlbaum.

Nay, W. R., & Ross, G. R. (1993). Cognitive-behavioral intervention for adolescent drug abuse. In A. J. Finch & W. M. Nelson (Eds.), *Cognitive-behavioral procedures with children and adolescents: A practical guide.* Boston: Allyn & Bacon.

O'Connell, D. F. (1989). Treating the high risk adolescent: A survey of effective programs and interventions. In P. B. Henry (Ed.), *Practical approaches in treating adolescent chemical dependency: A guide to clinical assessment and intervention* (pp. 49–69). New York: Haworth Press.

O'Connell, D. F. (Ed.). (1990). *Managing the dually diagnosed patient: Current issues and clinical approaches.* New York: Haworth Press.

O'Connell, D. F. (1991). The use of Transcendental Meditation in relapse prevention counseling. *Alcoholism Treatment Quarterly, 8*(1), 53–68.

O'Connell, D. F., & Alexander, C. (Eds.). (1994). *Self-recovery: Treating addictions using Transcendental Meditation and Maharishi Ayur-ved.* New York: Haworth Press.

O'Connell, D. F., & Patterson, H. O. (1996). Recovery maintenance and relapse prevention with chemically dependent adolescents. In M. A. Reinecke, F. M. Dattilio, & A. Freeman (Eds.), *Cognitive therapy with children and adolescents: A casebook for clinical practice* (pp. 79–102). New York: Guilford Press.

Orme-Johnson, D. W., & Farrow, J. T. (Eds). (1976). *Scientific research on the Transcendental Meditation: Collected papers* (Vol. 1). Vlodrop, The Netherlands: MIU Press.

Pierce, T. (1991). Dual disordered adolescents: A special population. *Journal of Adolescent Chemical Dependency, 1*(3), 11–28.

Prochaska, J. O., DiClemente, C. C., & Norcross, J. C. (1992). In search of how people change: Applications to addictive behaviors. *American Psychologist, 47*(9), 1102–1114.

Sudderth, L. K. (2000). What works in treatment programs for substance-abusing youth. In M. P. Kluger, G. Alexander, & P. A. Curtis (Eds.), *What works in child welfare* (pp. 337–344). Washington, DC: CWLA Press.

van Bilsen, H., & Wilke, M. (1998). Drug and alcohol abuse in young people. In P. J. Graham (Ed.), *Cognitive-behaviour therapy for children and families* (pp. 246–261). New York: Cambridge University Press.

Wagner, E. F., Myers, M. G., & Brown, S. A. (1994). Adolescent substance abuse treatment. In L. VandeCreek & S. Knapp (Eds.), *Innovations in clinical practice: A source book* (Vol. 13, pp. 97–121). Sarasota, FL: Professional Resource Press/ Professional Resource Exchange.

Waldron, H. B., Slesnick, N., Brody, J. L., Charles, W. T., & Thomas, R. P. (2001). Treatment outcomes for adolescent substance abuse at 4- and 7-month assessments. *Journal of Consulting and Clinical Psychology, 69*(5), 802–813.

Weinberg, N. Z., Rahdert, E., Colliver, J. D., & Glantz, M. D. (1998). Adolescent substance abuse: A review of the past 10 years. *Journal of the American Academy of Child and Adolescent Psychiatry, 37*(3), 252–261.

Winters, K. C., Latimer, W. L., & Stinchfield, R. D. (1999). Adolescent treatment. In P. J. Ott & R. E. Tarter (Eds.), *Sourcebook on substance abuse: Etiology, epidemiology, assessment, and treatment* (pp. 350–361). Boston: Allyn & Bacon.

SUGGESTED READINGS

Beck, A. T., Wright, F. D., Newman, C. F., & Liese, B. S. (1993). *Cognitive therapy of substance abuse.* New York: Guilford Press.

Beck, J. (1995). *Cognitive therapy: Basics and beyond.* New York: Guilford Press.

Emery, G. (1988). *Dependency free: Rapid cognitive therapy of substance abuse.* Santa Monica, CA: Association for Advanced Training in the Behavioral Sciences.

Marlatt, G. A., & Gordon, J. R. (Eds.). (1985). *Relapse prevention: Maintenance strategies in the treatment of addictive behaviors.* New York: Guilford Press.

Nay, W. R., & Ross, G. R. (1993). Cognitive-behavioral intervention for adolescent drug abuse. In A. J. Finch & W. M. Nelson (Eds.), *Cognitive-behavioral procedures with children and adolescents: A practical guide* (pp. 315–343). Boston: Allyn & Bacon.

Sudderth, L. K. (2000). What works in treatment programs for substance-abusing youth. In M. P. Kluger, G. Alexander, & P. A. Curtis (Eds.), *What works in child welfare* (pp. 337-344). Washington, DC: CWLA Press.

van Bilsen, H., & Wilke, M. (1998). Drug and alcohol abuse in young people. In P. J. Graham (Ed.), *Cognitive-behaviour therapy for children and families* (pp. 246–261). New York: Cambridge University Press.

Wagner, E. F., Myers, M. G., & Brown, S. A. (1994). Adolescent substance abuse treatment. In L. VandeCreek & S. Knapp (Eds.), *Innovations in clinical practice: A source book* (Vol. 13, pp. 97–121). Sarasota, FL: Professional Resource Press/ Professional Resource Exchange.

Winters, K. C., Latimer, W. L., & Stinchfield, R. D. (1999). Adolescent treatment. In P. J. Ott & R. E. Tarter (Eds.), *Sourcebook on substance abuse: Etiology, epidemiology, assessment, and treatment* (pp. 350–361). Boston: Allyn & Bacon.

5

Modular Therapy for Adolescents with Major Depression

JOHN F. CURRY
MARK A. REINECKE

Depression is a term that can refer to a single negative emotion, a cluster of symptoms that accompanies such an emotion, or a psychiatric disorder. In this chapter we discuss the treatment of depressive symptoms and depressive disorders among adolescents. Depressive disorders are defined by the presence of a set of symptoms lasting for a certain period of time, and representing a negative change from the adolescent's usual level of functioning. The depressive disorders include major depression (MDD) and dysthymia (DD) (American Psychiatric Association, 1994). The diagnosis of MDD in adolescents requires at least one episode lasting 2 weeks or longer in which the teen has had five or more of the following symptoms, including one of the first two: (1) depressed or irritable mood, (2) loss of interest or pleasure in activities, (3) appetite or weight loss or gain, (4) difficulty sleeping or excessive sleep, (5) psychomotor agitation or retardation, (6) fatigue or energy loss, (7) feelings of worthlessness or excessive guilt, (8) decreased ability to think, concentrate, or decide, (9) repetitive thoughts of death or suicide or a suicide plan or actual attempt. The diagnosis of DD is given if depressed or irritable mood is present most days for a year or more, accompanied by two or more of these six symptoms: poor appetite or excessive eating, insomnia or hypersomnia, low energy or fatigue, low self-esteem, poor concentration or difficulty making decisions, or feelings of hopelessness. MDD and DD are not mutually exclusive. Some adolescents experience a long-standing DD, upon which an episode of MDD has been super-imposed ("double depression").

Depression is one of the most common forms of psychopathology among adolescents. Lewinsohn and his colleagues found that depressive disorders, anxiety disorders, and substance use disorders were the three most frequent diagnoses in a community sample of American teenagers (Lewinsohn, Hops, Roberts, Seeley, & Andrews, 1993). Based on diagnostic interviews with over 1,500 U.S. high school students, anxiety disorders had higher point prevalence than depression, substance use, or disruptive behavior disorders, but depression had higher lifetime prevalence. The point prevalence for MDD was 2.57% and the lifetime prevalence rate was 18.48% in this study. The point prevalence rate for DD was 0.53% and the lifetime prevalence rate was 3.22%.

Depression during adolescence tends to recur. It is often a chronic disorder and is associated with an increased risk of depression and psychosocial impairment in adulthood (Essau, Conradt, & Petermann, 1999). Depression is associated with age and with gender (Birmaher et al., 1996). Rates of MDD are higher in adolescents than in children. A number of symptoms, including anhedonia, hypersomnia, weight change, and lethal suicide attempts are more common among adolescents than children. Among depressed children there is equal gender representation, but in adolescents the ratio is about two females to one male, similar to the pattern among adults (Essau & Dobson, 1999).

There is wide variability in the duration of depressive episodes during adolescence. Lewinsohn and colleagues (1993) reported a range from 2 weeks to 10 years. About one-third of adolescents who recovered from MDD had a second episode within 4 years, indicating that the disorder is often recurrent. The widespread experience of depression among teenagers and the chronic course of the disorder suggest that it may be important to develop interventions to relieve the suffering and functional impairment associated with this condition.

PSYCHOTHERAPEUTIC TREATMENT
FOR ADOLESCENT MAJOR DEPRESSION

To date, both psychotherapeutic and pharmacological interventions have proven to be efficacious for acute treatment of adolescent depression (Brent et al., 1997; Emslie et al., 1997; Harrington, Whittaker, Shoebridge, & Campbell, 1998; Lewinsohn & Clarke, 1999; Stark, Swearer, Kurowski, Sommer, & Bowen, 1996). Among psychotherapeutic interventions, there is accumulating evidence that cognitive-behavioral therapy (CBT) helps to reduce depressive symptoms and to reduce the risk of relapse or recurrence. Reinecke, Ryan, and DuBois (1998) reviewed six CBT studies, finding that

CBT significantly reduced depressive symptoms and that the intervention had a moderate to large effect size when compared to control conditions. At follow-up, which in most of the studies was 3 months or less, a moderate effect size of treatment was maintained.

VARIETIES OF COGNITIVE-BEHAVIORAL THERAPY

Although all cognitive behavior therapies share an underlying assumption that therapeutic change can be effected by assisting patients to modify their thoughts and behaviors, different forms of CBT emphasize varying techniques to bring about therapeutic gains (Lewinsohn & Clarke, 1999). For example, primarily behavioral techniques include training in social skills, participation in pleasant activities, or social problem solving. Primarily cognitive techniques include setting and monitoring progress toward goals, identifying cognitive distortions, and formulating realistic thoughts to counter depressive cognitions. Two recent reviews of empirically supported treatments for childhood or adolescent disorders examined the common techniques that appeared to characterize successful CBT interventions (Kaslow & Thompson, 1998; Kazdin & Weisz, 1998). These reviews indicated that efficacious forms of psychotherapy included therapeutic methods designed to increase participation in pleasant, mood-enhancing activities; increase and improve social interactions; improve conflict resolution and social problem-solving skills; reduce physiological tension; and modify depressive thoughts.

Two cognitive-behavioral traditions for treating MDD have been successfully applied with adolescents and warrant further discussion: the cognitive therapy tradition identified with Aaron Beck and his colleagues and the more behavioral tradition identified with Peter Lewinsohn and his colleagues. We will briefly summarize the applications of these CBT traditions to adolescents with MDD, and attempt to identify both common and unique elements of each approach.

Cognitive Therapy

Cognitive therapy is based on Beck's cognitive model of depression and its treatment. In this model depression is viewed as a function of maladaptive thoughts, including rapid automatic thoughts that occur so quickly as to elude notice. These thoughts are supported by systematic cognitive or perceptual biases that distort information, and by underlying, tacit negative beliefs. The cognitive therapist forms a collaborative alliance with the patient and focuses on identifying and modifying these negative thoughts, distortions, and beliefs (Beck, Rush, Shaw, & Emery, 1979). Behavioral techniques form a part of cognitive therapy, particularly at the beginning of the treatment, but they play a secondary role, since they are viewed primarily as experiments for the patient to perform in order to bring forth and identify associated maladaptive thoughts.

Brent and his colleagues adapted cognitive therapy for use with adolescents. Their adaptation placed relatively more emphasis than the original model on family and adolescent psychoeducation, on exploring issues of adolescent autonomy, and on the acquisition of skills in problem solving, social interactions, and affect regulation skills. In their clinical trial, 107 adolescents with major depression were randomly assigned to one of three psychosocial treatments of 12–16 weeks' duration: CBT, systemic behavioral family therapy (SBFT), or nondirective supportive therapy (NST) (Brent et al., 1997). SBFT emphasized identification of dysfunctional family behavior patterns, family communication, and problem-solving skills. NST did not include skills training, but emphasized an empathic relationship, emotion expression, and problem discussion. Remission from the episode of MDD was greatest with CBT, with 60% of CBT adolescents, versus 38% of SBFT and 39% of NST adolescents, in remission by the end of acute treatment. Adolescents who had received CBT showed more rapid reductions in symptoms than the other two groups. Parents also found CBT a more credible treatment for depression than the other interventions.

Cognitive therapy can be highly individualized. As a routine part of each session, the patient's current mood is monitored; the patient is expected to generate an agenda of items to be worked on in the session with the assistance of the therapist; and efforts are made by the therapist to check with the patient to assure that key points are understood and can be summarized by the patient.

Behavioral Therapy

What we are describing as more behavioral studies with adolescents have been based on Lewinsohn's model of depression and on the Coping with Depression Course (Lewinsohn, Antonuccio, Steinmetz-Breckenridge, & Teri, 1984), a psychoeducational group intervention. Lewinsohn's model emphasizes the role of low rates of positive reinforcement, especially of social reinforcement, as a causal or maintaining variable in depression. However, attention is also directed toward negative, depressive thinking. In the Adolescent Coping with Depression Course (Clarke, Lewinsohn, & Hops, 1990), the reciprocally influential role of behaviors, thoughts, and emotions is a core concept taught to teenagers. Positive thoughts may lead to positive behavior and positive affect in an "upward spiral" with euthymic mood, while negative thoughts may lead to negative behavior and negative affect in a "downward spiral" with depressed mood. Treatment is conceptualized as skills training, with behavioral and cognitive skills included in the overall treatment program, along with the affect regulation skill of relaxation.

Lewinsohn and colleagues (1990) initially randomly assigned 59 depressed adolescents to the Adolescent Coping with Depression Course (CWD-A; Clarke et al., 1990), CWD-A with concurrent parent group (CWD-A+P), or a wait-list condition. Treatment consisted of 14 2-hour group sessions over 7 weeks, augmented by seven 2-hour parent groups in the CWD-A+P condition. Skills that were covered in CWD-A included mood monitoring, learning the association between activities and mood, increasing pleasant activities, relaxation, identifying and modifying depressive thoughts, problem solving, communication, and social interaction. Parent groups were psychoeducational, focusing on the skills that the teenagers were learning in their groups. At the end of treatment, remission from the depressive episode had occurred for 43% of CWD-A and 48% of CWD-A+P adolescents, but for only 5% of wait-list teens. More recently, with treatment extended to 8 weeks, rates of improvement paralleled these initial findings but with higher rates of recovery. By the end of treatment, 65% of CWD-A and 69% of CWD-A+P adolescents no longer met criteria for a diagnosis of depression, versus 48% of wait-list adolescents.

The more behavioral treatment for adolescent depression emphasizes skills training as an end in itself, and not primarily as a means to elicit negative cognitions. In keeping with the emphasis on learning new skills, however, the structure of the more behavioral intervention is less flexible and less individualized than that of cognitive therapy. Each session is devoted a priori to the learning of one or more skills. Although there is no reason such treatment could not be conducted individually, it has been conducted in a group modality and appears well suited to such a modality: The presence of multiple group members can enhance opportunities for direct and vicarious practice, for learning from mistakes, and for role playing. However, there is more limited time for the expression of individual concerns, and there is not provision for setting individualized agendas.

Common Components of Efficacious Treatments

Even restricting our comparison to these two streams of CBT, it is evident that they have many features in common. For example, both emphasize the adolescent's need to monitor mood, both focus on identifying and modifying maladaptive cognitions, both teach problem solving, social skills, and affect regulation skills. Finally, both emphasize the importance of psychoeducation about depression and its treatment. It seems evident that CBT for adolescents with MDD, if it is to be evidence-based, should include these common components of successful interventions.

MODULAR COGNITIVE-BEHAVIORAL THERAPY

Many forms of CBT include skills-based interventions that are presented in a set sequence. Each session is constructed so as to include training in one or more specific skills. This is true, for example, of the Adolescent Coping with Depression Course (Clarke et al., 1990). In this psychoeducational group approach to treatment, each session has sections of time devoted to training in specific skills, and sequential sessions are interlaced. For example, one approach to relaxation is covered in a given session, followed in a subsequent session by a second approach to relaxation. Consistent with a psychoeducational approach, the sequence of sessions is set and ordered in such as way that a given session builds upon material learned in earlier sessions. For this reason it would be inconsistent with the psychoeducational treatment approach to deviate from the order of sessions or to attempt to teach one particular session in isolation from the others.

However, it is not necessary for modules to be organized in a set sequence, nor is it necessary for modular forms of CBT to be group-oriented or highly structured. Next, we will describe seven advantages of a modular approach to CBT that is tailored for individual therapy.

Within-Session Flexibility

A criticism of "manualized" treatments is that they lack flexibility. How can the therapist respond to the immediate needs of the patient if the therapist is required to "cover" certain material that may or may not be related to those needs? However, modules can be organized in such a way as to promote flexibility within a session. Required skills training can be embedded within a context that promotes the active involvement of the individual patient in the treatment process. It is possible to develop treatment protocols that are modular but moderately structured. Each session focuses on learning a specific skill, but each session is also divided into distinct parts, only one of which is the skills training component. Parts of the session may be used to elicit the patient's particular concerns and to review homework, whereas the final third of the session may involve working on the patient's specific concerns and formulating a new, individualized homework assignment. Embedded in the middle of the session is training in a specific skill. This session structure enables the therapist to elicit the patient's agenda and to work on that agenda, but also assures that skills training takes place. In perhaps an ideally integrated session of this type, the newly learned skill can be applied immediately to concerns or issues that the patient brings to the session. However, even if this proves not to be feasible, previously learned skills can be applied during that third of the session in which the patient's immediate concerns are the focus of attention.

A session structure that combines agenda setting and skills training in this way appears to build upon strengths of both of the CBT traditions reviewed earlier, which have been applied successfully to treating adolescent MDD. Required skills training in each session is a characteristic of the Lewinsohn tradition, and agenda setting is a characteristic of the Beck tradition.

Flexibility between Sessions

If each treatment module in a CBT manual is written such that it can function as a "stand-alone" session, maximum flexibility between sessions can be attained. In order to serve as a "stand-alone" session, a module should contain one skill to be taught within that session, in such a way that no previous training in other skills is required. There is an associated loss with this approach, namely, the loss of a linear sequence of interlaced sessions in which some sessions build upon previously covered material. However, the corresponding advantage lies in the therapist's ability to choose a module for a given treatment session that appears directly relevant to the needs of the patient and to omit modules that appear unnecessary for this particular patient. This type of flexibility between sessions leads to the remaining advantages of a modular approach.

Designation of Core versus Non-Core Modules

CBT interventions for various disorders share many common components. For example, training in interpersonal problem solving is a component of the Adolescent Coping with Depression Course (Clarke et al., 1990) and of Lochman's Anger Coping Program for childhood aggression (Pardini & Lochman, Chapter 3, this volume). On the other hand, some CBT skills are particularly relevant to specific disorders. For example, parents of substance-abusing adolescents may be given training in the skill of monitoring their adolescent's leisuretime activities, but this would not typically be part of the treatment for adolescent depression.

What CBT skills are essential components of a treatment package for depression is an empirical question that has no definitive answer at this time. However, as noted earlier, Kazdin and Weisz (1998) and Kaslow and Thompson (1998), on the basis of reviews of empirically supported treatments, identified common key components of protocols that have been found effective to date. Likewise, we have identified components that are common to cognitive therapy and to the more behavioral therapy for adolescent MDD. Such components may be designated as core components of CBT for adolescent depression and as "required" elements of an adequate CBT intervention. In writing a treatment manual, then, these constitute the core modules that should be covered in the treatment of each patient. Other modules, however, may be viewed as "non-core" or "optional," and are used only when the therapist judges the skill to be relevant for the adolescent. An example would be the module on rekindling the affectionate attachment between the adolescent and parents. For many families this was unnecessary and was, therefore, omitted from the treatment plan. For others it was a critical component of treatment and a virtual prerequisite for any further progress.

Individualized Pace of Treatment

Adolescents arrive at treatment varying greatly along such dimensions as motivation, trust, and cooperativeness. Low levels of any of these characteristics can impede the speed and progress of treatment. Simply forging ahead with skills training without regard to issues of trust and therapeutic alliance is likely to doom treatment to failure. In a modular CBT, however, in which certain skills are designated as core and others as non-core or optional, the therapist has greater freedom to adjust the pace of skills training while establishing a trusting alliance. Only those modules designated as core to the treatment need to be covered in order for the intervention to be considered complete.

Similar considerations pertain to the variability among adolescents in their speed of learning. For reasons having to do with learning ability, processing speed, or general intellectual functioning, some adolescents proceed at a slow pace through skills training modules. For teenagers with this cognitive style, more than one session can be devoted to learning the material contained in a single module. The speed of progress through the skills training modules can be adjusted to meet the needs of the patient.

Individualized Sequence of Treatment

Kazdin and Weisz (1998) noted that many adolescents drop out of treatment before the full "package" of an empirically supported intervention can be completed. For example, if treatment is designed to take 12 weeks but the adolescent drops out after 6 weeks, as much as half of the proposed treatment has been missed. For this reason they proposed presenting the core or most important elements of the treatment early in the sequence of intervention. This can be accomplished in modular CBT by placing the core modules in the first part of the sequence of treatment.

However, there are circumstances in which a non-core module would need to be moved up to a point early in treatment. Consider, for example, the adolescent whose depression is accompanied by emotion dysregulation and self-cutting. This teenager would need the CBT treatment to include the skill of affect regulation: A module teaching one or more methods of self-regulation would be essential to his or her treatment, even though it might not be designated as a core module for all depressed adolescents. Because other core skills, such as problem solving or formulating realistic counterthoughts, are likely to be completely "forgotten" by this particular teenager under conditions of high affect arousal (Brent & Poling, 1997), it is essential to teach the module on affect regulation relatively early in treatment. In this way affective control can be maintained as other skills are learned and utilized in stressful circumstances.

Flexible Involvement of Parents and Family Members in Treatment

Data on the optimal role of parents or other family members in the treatment of adolescent depression are relatively lacking, and what findings exist suggest a complicated picture. In acute treatment, the involvement of parents in parallel psychoeducational groups has not been shown to convey an advantage over adolescent group CBT alone. Moreover, systemic behavioral family therapy (SBFT) appears to be less credible as a treatment for MDD among adolescents than individual cognitive therapy. On the other hand, a 2-year follow-up of the latter sample revealed no significant difference in remission rates between the SBFT and CBT groups (Birmaher et al., 2000). Over the 2-year course of the study, 84% of all adolescent participants experienced a remission from the presenting episode of MDD, suggesting that any of the three study treatments (nondirective supportive therapy was the third treatment) could be considered ultimately efficacious. However, recurrence of MDD during the 2-year follow-up period was associated with parent–child or family discord. This finding suggests the need for some type of family intervention during the course of treatment to prevent relapse.

Modular CBT permits at least two types of parent involvement in treatment: psychoeducational and interactive. Psychoeducational parent modules are designed to educate the parents about the nature of MDD, its symptoms, possible course, and efficacious treatments. Psychoeducation also describes for parents what CBT is like as well as their role and that of other family members in treatment sessions. Psychoeducation can have indirect therapeutic value by describing for parents some types of family interactions that are likely not to be helpful to a depressed teenager, such as elevated rates or intensity of criticism. Other parent or family modules are written for interactive family therapy sessions. For example, after the teenager learns a method for problem solving, the parents can learn the method and practice it along with the teenager in an interactive family problem-solving session.

Flexibility of treatment is maintained by minimizing the number of interactive family sessions that are required in the acute treatment package and by allowing the therapist or the therapist and family together to decide what skills are most pertinent for their particular family to learn.

Psychoeducational sessions, on the other hand, which characterized both the individual cognitive therapy intervention of Brent and Poling (1997) and the parent intervention of Clarke and Lewinsohn (1989), appear to be essential elements of efficacious treatment for individual adolescents and thus, core components of CBT. Psychoeducation explains the disorder and the treatment process to adolescents and their parents, thus demystifying the process and facilitating cooperation and active engagement.

Adaptations to Address Comorbidity

Comorbidity is the rule rather than the exception in adolescents with MDD. Angold and Costello (1993) reviewed studies that have shown that depression (either MDD or DD) in young people is very often accompanied by oppositional or conduct disorders (20–80% across samples) and the various anxiety disorders (30–70% across samples). Comorbidity of depression with other psychiatric disorders can present the clinician with a number of challenges insofar as depressed youth with a comorbid psychiatric disorder are at an increased risk for additional episodes of depression and manifest a wider range of psychosocial deficits than do depressed children without a coexisting disorders (Asarnow, 1988; Hughes et al., 1990; Keller et al., 1988; Reinecke, 1995). Lifetime substance use disorders occur in about 20% of adolescents with MDD or DD (Lewinsohn et al., 1993). One of the major challenges in transferring treatment efficacy research to broad-based community settings is the challenge of comorbidity. The adolescents with MDD who present to clinics or to private practitioners are frequently more complicated to treat than those who participate in university "laboratory" studies of treatment efficacy, because of their higher rates of comorbid disorders. Adolescents with comorbid disorders are frequently excluded from efficacy studies in order that the focus of the study can be maintained on the treatment of the target disorder. This in turn can lead practitioner therapists to the view that manualized efficacy treatments are irrelevant for the more complex sample of young people seen in actual practice.

Modular CBT can address comorbid disorders provided that the primary target disorder is indeed the adolescent's primary disorder. The core modules required to treat the MDD, generally presented first in sequence, can be supplemented later in treatment with other modules that address comorbidity. For example, adolescents with certain comorbid anxiety disorders may benefit by including a module on relaxation training in the treatment. Those with oppositional disorder may benefit by including a family module on contingency management or one on clear and effective family communication. In this way, comorbidity can be incorporated in treatment as one of the individualized concerns that drive selection of treatment modules.

CASE EXAMPLE

Theresa G., a 16-year-old Hispanic female, was referred for psychotherapy by her mother due to concerns about her mood, low self-esteem, and academic difficulties. Theresa is the eldest of five children and is in the 11th grade at a public high school. Although the results of standardized intelligence and academic achievement tests were within the normal range, she was earning Ds and Fs in all of her classes and had little motivation to attend school. Theresa's mother reported that she had "seemed sad" and had "shown little will to thrive" for several years. Theresa's home environment is quite chaotic. She lives in an impoverished, dangerous neighborhood, and has moved frequently during recent years due to financial problems. Her family lived in shelters on several occasions after her mother left her father due to physical abuse at home.

Presenting Problems

Theresa's mother reported that she has always "been a good child" but that she has not been happy for many years. Theresa has never met her father, and her relationship with her stepfather is strained. Her father abandoned her mother before she was born and moved to Central America. Her mother divorced Theresa's stepfather when she was 9 years old due to his volatile anger. He reportedly was physically and verbally abusive toward Mrs. G. and was verbally abusive toward Theresa. Theresa and her siblings changed schools frequently during her childhood, making it difficult for her to develop stable friendships.

Theresa meets DSM-IV criteria for major depression (MDD). Both she and her mother endorse the following criteria as being subjectively severe: depressed, irritable, anhedonic, lack of reactivity to positive stimuli, insomnia, hypersomnia, fatigue, low self-esteem, trouble concentrating, psychomotor retardation, and hopelessness. She experiences occasional suicidal ideations, but has not developed a plan. As Theresa stated, "I hate life, it sucks . . . why do I have to live?" There is no history, however, of suicidal gestures or attempts. Theresa's depressive symptoms first emerged at approximately 8 years of age, and worsen depending on the presence or absence of her stepfather.

Theresa enjoys few activities other than sitting in her room listening to alternative rock music. She typically declines invitations to go out with friends, and is not allowed out of the house alone due to gang activity on their street. She feels self-conscious around her peers, and is reluctant to speak in class. Theresa's mother is unemployed and suffers from a disabling medical condition. Theresa is fearful for her mother's health.

Theresa has struggled academically since elementary school. Although standardized achievement test scores reportedly have been within the normal range, her grades consistently are Ds and Fs. Theresa noted, nonetheless, that she loves to read. She attributes her poor performance to having changed schools on an almost annual basis. Theresa was retained in the sixth grade, but was promoted to the seventh when she transferred to a new school at midyear.

With the exception of allergies and mild asthma, Theresa's medical history is unremarkable. There is no history of serious illnesses, accidents, or injuries. She denied any history of alcohol or substance use, and reported that she "tried a cigarette once, but hated it." Theresa's father reportedly has a history of alcohol abuse and her mother has a history of depression. There is no other reported history of psychological difficulties among Theresa's immediate relatives. Theresa's specific symptoms include the following:

Affective: Dysphoria, sadness, embarrassment, anhedonia, anxiety, pessimism, frustration, anger (at herself), fear, discouragement, boredom, impatience, irritability.
Cognitive: Impaired concentration, indecisiveness, low self-esteem, fearful anticipation, self-critical, negligible sense of control over events.
Physiological: Insomnia, fatigue, psychomotor retardation.
Behavioral: Social withdrawal, avoids eye contact, speaks quietly, avoids challenging tasks, irritable toward siblings.

Initial Assessment

A review of Theresa's responses on a battery of self-report questionnaires, summarized in Table 5.1, indicates that she was experiencing moderately severe feelings of depression, anxiety, and pessimism at the time of her referral. Her responses on the Automatic Thoughts Questionnaire suggest that she experiences a large number of negative thoughts about herself, her world, her relationships with others, and her future. Mild elevations were apparent on the Social Undesirability and Fear of Abandonment subscales of the Young–Brown Schema Questionnaire. Theresa views herself as "dull and boring," "stupid," "very self-conscious," and "hypersensitive to criticism and rejection." She acknowledged that she often doubts that important relationships will last and that she expects that people she cares about will leave her. These beliefs are understandable given her father's having abandoned the family, her frequent moves, and her mother's history of depression and chronic illness.

Case Formulation

A number of cognitive, social, behavioral, and environmental factors appear to contribute to Theresa's current difficulties. She comes from a cha-

TABLE 5.1. Objective Rating Scales

Measure	Score	Severity
Beck Depression Inventory	21	Moderate
Reynolds Adolescent Depression Scale		Moderate
Beck Anxiety Inventory	18	Moderate
Hopelessness Scale	15	Significant
Automatic Thought Questionnaire		Moderate
Young–Brown Schema Questionnaire		Mild elevations on two subscales

otic home environment that is characterized by criticism, arguing, inconsistent and punitive discipline, and severe financial stress. Moreover, she lives in a dangerous, stressful neighborhood. She has few stable friendships or supports outside of the family due to their frequent moves, and is sensitive to criticism by her classmates due to her poor academic performance. She desires relationships with others, but is sensitive to rejection, criticism and abandonment. Her tendency to withdraw from others exacerbates her feelings of isolation and frustration. Her social supports, as such, are quite limited.

Theresa manifests negative views of herself, her world, and the future. She is quite self-critical and manifests a number of cognitive distortions (including overgeneralization, selective attention, and magnifying the severity of negative events). Theresa's perceptions of personal efficacy are limited. She is discouraged about her future and acknowledges feeling that she cannot influence important outcomes in her life. Theresa tends, as a result, to simply give up when challenged (either socially or academically). Although Theresa's rational problem-solving skills appear to be reasonably well developed, she maintains a negative, avoidant approach to solving problems. She tends to put off making decisions, and avoids addressing problems directly. In addition, Theresa manifests several maladaptive schemas. She believes, for example, that important relationships will end, and that people she cares about will die or leave her. Theresa tends, as well, to view herself as socially undesirable. Her self-concept is poor. She characterized herself as self-conscious, and noted that she is dull, cannot carry on a conversation, and never knows what to say in social situations. This observation is consistent with her mother's comment that Theresa was shy as a toddler. Although Theresa tends to dwell on her concerns when alone, she does not appear to demonstrate a globally negative attributional style. Her relationship with her mother is close, but conflicted. They argue frequently, typically about Theresa's choice of friends. Theresa's negotiation and conflict resolution skills, as such, may be weak. Moreover, her affect regulation skills appear to be developing slowly. This may be due, at least in part, to the lack of effective modeling and reinforcement of adaptive problem solving and mood regulation by her parents.

Theresa has a number of strengths. She is an attractive and kind teenager and has reasonably well-developed verbal skills. She is motivated to address her difficulties and to overcome her academic problems. Moreover, her social skills are good—she is a likable teen.

Course of Treatment

Developing Goals

Theresa was seen on 16 occasions over an 8-month period. As in cognitive therapy with depressed adults, modular CBT sessions follow a fairly standard format (J. Beck, 1995; Reinecke, 2002). Flexibly maintaining a strategic problem-focus can be reassuring to teenagers, and, equally important, can assist them in understanding and gaining a sense of control over emotional experiences that are, in some ways, inexplicable and overwhelming to them. An emphasis is placed not so much on expressing one's concerns and feelings during sessions as on gaining a sense of mastery over them. As Rehm, Kaslow, and Rabin (1987) note, effective forms of psychotherapy (1) provide patients with a clear and credible rationale for understanding their depression and the mechanisms of therapeutic change, (2) are highly structured and offer patients a viable course of action for addressing their concerns, (3) are active and problem-focused, and (4) encourage self-monitoring and the assessment of progress. Modular CBT meets each of these criteria. An overview of the structure of sessions is presented in Table 5.2.

During our first session we worked to clarify Theresa's primary concerns and to provide her and her mother with an overview of the cognitive therapy model. In addition to gathering a developmental history and completing a diagnostic interview, this session had a number of psychoeducational components. We worked, for example, to provide Theresa and her mother with information about (1) the nature of clinical depression, (2) factors that have been found to contribute to depression among youth, (3) skills that may be helpful in managing these feelings, and (4) a rationale for cognitive-behavioral psychotherapy. We noted that the dysphoria, irritability, and moodiness that characterize clinical depression represent a disease, and that they are not volitional. That is to say, they are not intentional and do not appear to be under Theresa's conscious control. This can be important insofar as parents often view their depressed teens as willful, petulant, and lazy. We attempted to demonstrate, using experiences and events described by Theresa, how her social withdrawal, reduced activity, tendency to ruminate unproductively about her concerns, and negativistic beliefs might exacerbate her feelings of depression and anxiety. We next described how cognitive and behavioral skills may be helpful in alleviating her dis-

TABLE 5.2. Structure of the Cognitive Therapy Session

1. Assess mood (using objective and subjective report) and review recent events.
2. Collaboratively set an agenda for the session.
3. Review homework from the previous session; reinforce progress.
4. Discuss "issues and incidents" on the agenda.
5. Introduce or review a specific skill or "module" to address these concerns.
6. Formulate a homework task, identify factors that may interfere with successful completion.
7. Help patient to summarize the main points and conclusions.
8. Discuss thoughts and feelings about the session.

tress. By having this discussion with her mother in the room, Theresa observed that her mother was interested in her well-being and was motivated to help her. We attempted, from the first session, to include Theresa's mother in the treatment process by encouraging her to support her daughter in practicing new skills, and by addressing parental beliefs that may interfere with treatment compliance.

During this session Theresa noted that she "is always tired and never has energy" and that she "feels sad and down. . . . I have a give-up attitude." When asked to elaborate, Theresa noted that she "always feels [she] just has to give up. . . . I don't try, and I don't know why . . . no matter what it is, I just feel I can't do it." Theresa was not able to identify how she had come to feel this way, but recalled that these feelings first became apparent when she was 12 years old. Theresa's father reportedly had been physically and verbally abusive toward her mother and a younger sister. Theresa recounted how she and her siblings had gone with her mother to a shelter to escape her father, and that they had lived on the streets for several weeks. Hearing this, Theresa's mother commented that she was "like that, too. . . . I sabotage myself and give up. . . . I don't have fun and I'm always really negative about life." Theresa's early home environment, as such, appears to have been chaotic and unpredictable. It was characterized by abuse, severe financial hardship, and episodic neglect. The possibility exists, as well, that Theresa's feelings of helplessness, negativity, and self-doubt have been inadvertently modeled and reinforced by her mother.

Theresa noted that her feelings of depression become more severe when she experiences academic and social disappointments. She reported, for example, that she becomes depressed when she falls behind in class, when she is unable to visit her boyfriend, and when a friend tells her she may not be able to participate in an enjoyable activity. Theresa noted, however, that her mood is responsive to environmental events. Her mood improves, for example, when she is able to visit with friends, while playing with her band, and while window shopping at a local mall.

Theresa's goals for treatment were to (1) not feel as depressed, (2) have more energy, (3) get a more positive attitude, and (4) work out problems with her mother. Interestingly, she did not identify improving her academic performance—a factor that had contributed to her depression—as a goal for treatment. Mrs. G.'s goals for Theresa included (1) developing a sense of self-confidence and "believing in herself," (2) being happy and having more energy, (3) developing plans for her future, and (4) making better life choices. Theresa and her mother agreed that their goals for treatment were complementary and sensible.

The importance of developing a warm and trusting rapport with both the teenager and his or her caregiver cannot be underestimated. Theresa initially was reluctant to attend therapy, and had told her mother that she "was gonna be mean" to her therapist. As she stated, "Who cares what he says? He can't do anything about my life." We were able, by carefully listening to the narrative of her experiences, by providing her with a sense that she was understood, and by developing a shared rationale for understanding her distress, to build a trusting foundation for our subsequent work.

Mood and Event Monitoring

As in cognitive therapy with adults, depressed adolescents are taught to monitor their moods, to identify situations that trigger negative affect, and to identify associated automatic thoughts. This skill or "module" can take the form of a diary or a formal Dyfunctional Thought Record (DTR; J. Beck, 1995). During our second session we discussed events during the past week that had been upsetting to Theresa, as well as thoughts that had gone through her mind at the time. She noted that she had been dropped from a band (for not playing well), and that this had made her "really depressed . . . because I'd wanted to do it for so long." When asked her thoughts at the time, she recalled thinking "I can't believe it. . . . I don't know what I'm gonna do. . . . There's nothing I can do . . . even my friends wanted to drop me." Upon inquiry it became apparent that Theresa was not upset so much by her poor playing or by the fact that her friends had wanted to drop her from the band. Rather, she was upset by the fact that this had been a long-term goal and that she saw no other enjoyable activities in her life. As she stated, "Now what? There's really *nothing* I can do." Theresa was able to see that this thought—"There's nothing I can do"—was followed almost immediately by an increase in her feelings of dysphoria and pessimism.

With this in mind, Theresa was asked to write down, prior to going to bed each night, the best and worst events of the day. She was then to briefly note what she had felt at these times, how strong these feelings had been (on a 0–100 scale), and what her thoughts were at the time. An example of one of her entries is presented in Figure 5.1.

Whereas standard approaches to cognitive therapy for depression focus upon monitoring negative events and automatic thoughts, we have elected to balance this by an attention to positive events, emotions, and cognitions. Rather than attending only to automatic thoughts (i.e., the spontaneous steam of negative self-referential thinking about the self, the world, and the future), we advocate monitoring the broader range of cognitive "contents" and "products" (Kendall, 2000; Kendall & MacDonald, 1993), including images, attributions, memories, goal and value statements, and perceptions which occur at these times. This serves to address depressed teenagers' tendency to selectively attend to and remember negative events in their lives, as well as their tendency to magnify the severity of stressful life events. It is important as well for adolescents to become adept at discriminating and labeling affective states, as emotions have been found to have broad effects on motivation, cognitive processes, and adaptive behavior. The usefulness of this exercise was noted by Theresa who, during the second week of treatment, recounted that she "had gone to a pizza parlor, which was fun, and . . . school was actually all right, and I got As on two exams." She spontaneously observed that "I didn't realize there were so many good things in my day!" and that she "feels worse when I think that things can't change . . . but that's not true." This skill—the ability to monitor events, cognitions, and moods—serves as a foundation for each of the performance-based techniques that will be introduced during subsequent weeks.

Pleasant Activities

Providing Theresa and her mother with a sense of support, developing a rationale for understanding her distress, and providing a treatment plan for

---

Wednesday

Negative Event:
    Situation: "I'm sitting in bed and I realize I didn't do any homework tonight."
    Feeling: Upset, disappointed, tired
    Amount: 45%
    Thoughts: "I never have energy. . . . I should just give it up."

Positive Event:
    Situation: "I got an 88% on a test."
    Feeling: Glad, really happy!
    Amount: 90%
    Thoughts: "I'm feeling smart. . . . I'm slowly accomplishing something. . . . I'd thought
                 I didn't have a chance but I pulled it off."

FIGURE 5.1. Mood and event monitoring.

addressing her depression were quickly effective in reducing her dysphoria. Theresa's Beck Depression Inventory (BDI) score dropped 11 points during the second week of treatment and by our third session she reported that she had "really improved" and that her energy level was "a lot better." Theresa's mother concurred, noting that she was "smiling and laughing more, and wasn't as irritable with the other kids." This observation—of rapid early gains in treatment—is consistent with research on the course of clinical improvement among depressed adults who benefit from cognitive therapy, and boded well for further progress (Tang & DeRubeis, 1999).

Participation in enjoyable, rewarding activities has been found in numerous studies to be associated with improvements in mood. With this in mind, we worked during our third session to develop a list of pleasant activities that Theresa could participate in that were active, inexpensive, available, and "not harmful." Theresa made a list of 17 potentially enjoyable activities. Among these were playing the guitar with her band, going to concerts, driving, going to the park, swimming, playing computer games, reading magazines, playing with pets, and trying "crazy" things (e.g., hang gliding, parachuting, scuba). As can be seen, several of these were solitary activities and a number were not readily available to teens in an urban environment. With this in mind, she selected five activities she would be able to do during the following week. We developed a baseline of how many of these activities she had engaged in during the past week, as well as ratings of her mood while she was doing them. We next developed a schedule of pleasurable activities she would like to pursue. These included (1) practicing her guitar with friends, (2) going shopping or to a movie with friends, (3) going to a concert, and (4) driving. Theresa felt that hang gliding would have a "high impact" on her mood, but that it was not a viable alternative for her to pursue.

This intervention also was quite effective. Theresa visited with friends on a daily basis, practiced her guitar, and drove with her mother several times. On each occasion she noted that her mood improved significantly.

Social Activities

Depression occurs in a social context (Coyne, 1976). Our moods influence our social behavior, and our social environment influences our mood. This is nowhere more important than among adolescents, for whom identification with the peer group and the maintenance of social relationships play a central role in normative development. Making and sustaining relationships with peers, while at the same time changing the rules, expectations, and values that define their relationships with parents, are a central task of adolescence. Rejection by family, friends, and peers can contribute to acute feelings of depression and hopelessness among youth (Kistner, Balthazor, Risi, & Burton, 1999; Panak & Garber, 1992; Vernberg, 1990). It is worth noting that relationships between rejection and mood appear to be transactional, and that it is the *perception* of rejection or abandonment that mediates the relationship between the quality of social relationships and mood.

During our third session we focused upon developing positive social relationships and on addressing Theresa's tendency to withdraw from others. In addition to encouraging social activity, we directly attempted to address her belief that her peers were rejecting, critical, and uncaring. She was encouraged, for example, to identify situations where friends had been supportive, and to note how her *perception* that they were uncaring might influence her reaction to them. During the following week she visited with friends after class, spent time with her cousins during the weekend, and invited her brother to play a board game with her. On each occasion she observed that her mood improved. Just as important, she accepted an invitation to go to a party with a classmate (something she would have rejected in the past) and to go to a movie at the mall with a friend. In sum, rejection by family and peers is a risk factor for depression among youth. Depressed mood, cognitions, and behavior contribute to a breakdown in social support. Modularized CBT addresses these factors directly by encouraging social activity, practicing social skills, and alleviating maladaptive beliefs that may interfere with teens' attempts to develop supportive relationships with peers and family members.

Parent Sessions

Parents play an important role in the development of social, cognitive, and behavioral skills during adolescence, and serve to maintain a positive, secure, and supportive home environment. Moreover, they are able to facilitate therapeutic progress by assisting their teenager in using cognitive therapy techniques between sessions. As such, parents can play an important role in the treatment process.

Our first goals when working with parents are to help them to feel understood; to address maladaptive beliefs, attributions, and expectations that might interfere with treatment process; and to provide them with a rationale for the treatment. A parent who does not feel understood and who does not accept the rationale and goals of psychotherapy may prematurely discontinue the treatment. A trusting and collaborative therapeutic rapport must be developed with the parent as well as with the teen. Parental beliefs and attributions that may interfere with treatment progress are presented in Table 5.3. During our initial therapy session, for example, Theresa's mother remarked that she felt her daughter was "just plain lazy" and that she "needed to get a better attitude." She felt that Theresa's depression was "due to her father" and that she "just wanted to make me mad" at home. On other occasions, Mrs. G. acknowledged that she felt frustrated and angry toward her daughter. When asked to elaborate, she remarked, "I'm sick of having to kick her a—. I'm sick of her. . . . She's a spoiled tyrant." These beliefs and attributions led Mrs. G. to resent her daughter and contributed to a conflicted, tense environment at home. Moreover, they reduced her motivation to assist Theresa with completing therapeutic tasks (such as participation in pleasant activities). As she stated, "Why should she be doing fun stuff with her friends when she's failing her classes and isn't cleaning her room?" Much as we would explore maladaptive beliefs held by a depressed teenager, we discussed these statements with her, how they led her to feel about her daughter and the treatment, whether they were necessarily true, and whether there was a more adaptive way of understanding her daughter's irritable, withdrawn behavior. Mrs. G. was able to see that Theresa's behavior was not malicious or intentional, and that her attempts to "force her to get going" had been ineffective. Adopting a Socratic stance, we asked whether there was any risk in approaching her daughter's depression differently. Mrs. G. acknowledged that assisting her daughter with therapeutic homework "was worth a try" and that addressing the depression might allow her to develop the motivation to confront her academic difficulties.

As during our sessions with Theresa, we asked Mrs. G. to summarize what she had learned from our meeting. She noted that she now felt "there's hope . . . and I can turn [to the therapist] for support," that it was "important not to blame and criticize Theresa," that she should "try to solve the problem when Theresa is struggling, and not just yell," and that "it's good for her to get out and do some pleasant things."

Parent and family sessions also focus on encouraging the use of positive behavior management techniques, reducing conflict at home, and developing feelings of competence, efficacy, and hope as a parent. Like her daughter, Mrs. G. was regularly given homework assignments—that is, tasks she could attempt during the week to assist Theresa to overcome her depression.

TABLE 5.3. Maladaptive Parental Beliefs

"It's really not a problem/my problem."
"She'll just outgrow it."
"It's her responsibility to change."
"Treatment shouldn't involve me."
"Depression is biological. . . . It can't be treated by talk."
"You're blaming me for my child's problems."
"She's doing it on purpose."
"She could change if she wanted to."
"I've tried everything . . . nothing can help."
"She can never change."

Rational Problem Solving

Evidence suggests that depression may stem, at least in part, from deficits in rational problem solving (Nezu, 1987; D'Zurilla & Nezu, 2001). Studies with children and adolescents indicate that deficits in social problem solving may be associated with an increased risk for both depression and suicide (Asarnow, Carlson, & Guthrie, 1987; Fremouw, Callahan, & Kashden, 1993; Rotheram-Borus, Trautman, Dopkins, & Shrout, 1990; Sadowski & Kelley, 1993; Spirito, Overholser & Stark, 1989). D'Zurilla and Nezu (2001) proposed that transactional relationships exist between the occurrence of stressful life events, the use of rational problem solving skills, and depressive symptoms. Following work by Nezu (1987), we view adaptive problem solving as including five components: (1) maintaining an adaptive problem-solving focus and motivation, (2) identifying and defining problems, (3) generating alternative solutions, (4) rational decision making, and (5) solution implementation and reinforcement.

Theresa approached problems in a passive, unfocused manner, and tended not to believe that her efforts would be successful. We attempted, with this in mind, to develop Theresa's rational problem-solving skills and endeavored to improve her problem-solving motivation. She was encouraged to approach problems optimistically, to think them through in a systematic, rational manner, to persist in the face of difficulties, and to inhibit impulsive attempts to avoid her problems. We presented this approach to Theresa in the form of an acronym—RIBEYE—and practiced it during sessions using both written vignettes of problems experienced by other teenagers and problems from her life. The steps in this approach are (R) Relax, (I) Identify the problem, (B) Brainstorm alternative solutions, (E) Evaluate each possible solution, (Y) Say "Yes" to one, and (E) Evaluate outcomes and reward success.

After successfully completing several vignettes, Theresa noted that she remained very concerned about her poor grades, particularly in math. She had failed math for several years and, although she was in high school, was completing arithmetic problems at a fifth-grade level. Her fear that she might fail once again was reasonable, and her tendency to avoid class only exacerbated the problem. In applying the RIBEYE model, Theresa was quickly able to identify the problem and recognized how her past attempts to cope with it had failed. When asked to "brainstorm" solutions, she was able (with assistance) to develop a range of alternatives. These included (1) get a tutor, (2) bribe the teacher, (3) get extra books and study, (4) ask another student for help, (5) sneak in and change the grade book, (6) take the class again in summer school, (7) sign up for an ACT study course, and 8) just give up and not graduate. She evaluated these possible courses of action, examining the short- and long-term benefits and consequences of each, and elected to get a tutor and to sign out extra books and study materials from the library.

It is worth noting that depressed teens may have reasonably strong rational problem-solving skills, yet fail in their attempts to resolve problems due to a negative problem orientation. They do not believe that their efforts will be successful, or tend to approach problems in an impulsive, haphazard, or avoidant manner (Reinecke, DuBois, & Schultz, 2001). This was of particular concern with Theresa given her rather pervasive sense that she "might as well give up" when she was disappointed or challenged. We were concerned then, that she might not follow through on her chosen course of action. This concern was well-founded. During the next week she did not initiate any of the solutions she had considered. When asked why, she noted that she would be embarrassed if other students found out she had seen a tutor. This expectation—that others will ostracize her for her efforts—was the basis of her negative problem orientation and undermined her attempts to pass her class. We examined this belief during our next meeting and developed a "rational plan" for determining whether it was true. We also agreed to a reward for her (she would get tickets for a concert with a friend) if she attended a tutoring session before our next meeting. Theresa began participating in tutoring that week and (contrary to her expectation) none of her peers commented on her receiving tutoring for math.

Identifying Maladaptive Thoughts

Identifying maladaptive thoughts plays a prominent role in cognitive therapy for depression among adults. So too in modular CBT with adolescents. As we have seen, Theresa was highly self-critical, was pessimistic about her future, maintained negative expectations about how others would act toward her, and was sensitive to possible rejection. Her thoughts, as such, were dominated by negative beliefs, attributions, and expectations. Before Theresa would be able to identify relationships between life events, thoughts, feelings, and behaviors, she would need to become more aware of her tendency to think negatively about herself and her life.

This is accomplished through psychoeducation, reviewing upsetting events that had occurred during the week and asking her to "step through" her thoughts and feelings on a moment-by-moment basis, and by noting shifts of affect during the therapy session. The latter approach is particularly powerful. By simply asking "What was going through your mind right then?" it is possible to identify thoughts associated with negative moods. During one session, for example, Theresa unexpectedly began crying while discussing her boyfriend, Sal. When asked her thoughts, she remarked, "I've hurt him and made him feel bad . . . like he's not good enough for me." She continued by noting that she was "100% sure she didn't want to date him anymore" and that she "always felt you shouldn't hurt someone."

It was not the breakup of their relationship that upset her so much as the thought that she was responsible for hurting him. These thoughts became the focus of our session. Once Theresa was able to identify automatic thoughts in session, we began monitoring them on a daily basis at home. A Dysfunctional Thought Record, or DTR, triple-column technique was used (J. Beck, 1995). A sample of a representative DTR completed by Theresa (after she had failed a math test) is presented in Figure 5.2.

Realistic Counterthoughts

The focus of this module is on assisting the teenager to become adept at developing adaptive ways of thinking about problematic situations. These are referred to as "realistic counterthoughts" and allow the teenager to respond to stressful events in a more adaptive manner. This approach is based upon cognitive restructuring or rational responding techniques used in cognitive therapy with depressed adults. Although automatic thoughts are, in many situations, based on legitimate concerns (Theresa had, in fact, failed an exam), the conclusions drawn from these experiences and the meanings attached to them may not be reasonable or adaptive. Put another way, some automatic thoughts, though valid, may not be "useful" (J. Beck, 1995).

Theresa was provided with five questions to ask when reflecting on events and thoughts that have been upsetting to her. These are (1) What is the *specific* thought that is upsetting me? (2) What is the evidence for and against this? (3) Is there another, more reasonable, way of looking at this? (4) So what? Is it really so big a deal? (decatastrophize), and (5) What can I do about it? What's the solution? After practicing this approach by applying these questions to vignettes of upsetting thoughts experienced by other teenagers we directed our attention to events in Theresa's life. In the preceding example, Theresa was quite concerned that her friends would know she had failed yet another exam and that they would think she was "stupid." Using the five questions, she was able to develop several realistic counterthoughts. These included (1) "I have nothing to be embarrassed about. The problem is that I have a hard time with math, but I haven't had the right teaching" and (2) "I *can* be persistent. It's like learning my guitar. . . . If I get a good teacher and practice, and start with basics, I can pick it up." Theresa noted that, when she thought of the event in these terms, her feelings of embarrassment and dread declined from 100% to 50%.

Using these techniques on a regular basis and maintaining an active solution-focus is particularly important in work with depressed teenagers. Nolen-Hoeksema (1987, 1990), in developing a model to account for the increased incidence of depression among adolescent females, proposed that individuals who ruminate unproductively on negative feelings and events are more likely to become clinically depressed than adolescents who do not.

Situation	Automatic thought	Emotion	Amount
Walking into school	"I've failed . . . they'll know it."	Embarrassed	100%
		Dread	95%
	"They'll make fun of me."	Embarrassed	90%
	"I'll have to take it again."	Sad, frustrated	60%
	"My life is unfair."	Frustrated	50%
	"Nobody can help me [with school]."	Hopeless	40%

FIGURE 5.2. Dysfunctional Thought Record.

A "ruminative" response set exacerbates feelings of depression by increasing access to negative memories, by interfering with adaptive behavior, and by increasing the likelihood that an individual will consider the depression a result of personal defects or flaws. Each of these considerations applied to Theresa. Theresa tended when depressed to withdraw from others and to ruminate unproductively on her predicament. Rather than seeking solutions for her difficulties, she tended to reflect on how unfair it was and on how she could not change the situation. With this in mind we practiced asking "What's the solution?" whenever she noticed her mood beginning to worsen. Rather than dwelling on problems, she was encouraged to "keep 'em in perspective" and to reflect on possible solutions. She was able to use this "radical solution focus" and found it both novel (as she quipped, "It's not the way I do things") and helpful.

Attachment

A growing body of evidence suggests that relationships may exist between the social environment, the development of secure attachments, and vulnerability to depression (Armsden, McCauley, Greenberg, Burke, & Mitchell, 1990; Blatt & Homan, 1992; Gotlib & Hammen, 1992; Ingram, Miranda, & Segal, 1998; Joiner & Coyne, 1999). Early family relationships in which a child's needs for security, affection, nurturance, and responsive, reliable support are not met may lead to the establishment of negativistic beliefs and expectations about the self and relationships with others that, in turn, serve as vulnerability factors for the development of depression (Reinecke & Rogers, 2001; Roberts, Gotlib, & Kassel, 1996). A range of dysfunctional interaction patterns have been found to characterize the home environments of depressed youth (Cole & Rehm, 1986; Reinherz et al., 1989; Sheeber, Hops, Andrews, Alpert, & Davis, 1998; Stark, Humphrey, Crook, & Lewis, 1990). Insofar as depression among youth often is associated with negativistic interactions with family members and with the establishment of an insecure attachment style, clinical interventions may usefully be directed toward developing interaction patterns that are less critical and controlling, more cohesive and supportive, less conflictual, more responsive, less punitive, and more nurturant. Our objective is to develop a more secure attachment between depressed youth and their caregivers, which may serve as a basis for establishing more adaptive beliefs about oneself and others.

Although Theresa's mother was concerned and caring, her relationship with her daughter was characterized by anger, demands, criticism, and episodic, punitive discipline. As noted, Theresa's early home environment was both chaotic and conflicted. She views her father as rejecting and violent—which is consistent with research on depression among adolescents (Baron & MacGillivray, 1989)—and acknowledges maintaining tacit beliefs that she is socially undesirable and that she anticipates being abandoned by others. With this in mind we introduced an "attachment module" during the ninth treatment session.

Working with her mother, we discussed the nature of their relationship, and how transactional links may exist between the quality of their relationship, maladaptive beliefs that each of them may hold, and their mood. Each acknowledged that they would like to improve the quality of their relationship, but felt unsure of how to proceed. We discussed how (based on attachment theory) positive relationships are characterized by nurturance, responsiveness, reliability, and affection. As these qualities did not characterize their current relationship, each was asked to recall a time in their past when these adjectives did apply. Both recalled a time when Theresa was 7–8 years of age, when their relationship was quite close. Theresa and her mother were asked to describe their relationship then in some detail, and to discuss how they felt at the time. With this image in mind, they next discussed how they would like their relationship to be in the future, and how each might work to bring this about. It is, of course, important to note when working with depressed adolescents that their relationship with their parents cannot (and should not) be modeled after childhood relationships. Rather, our goal is to develop a more mature, parent–teen relationship based upon characteristics of nurturance, responsiveness, reliability, and affection. Theresa and her mother found this discussion very helpful, and looked for ways that they might change their behavior toward each other to bring this about. A sense of security in a relationship is based on tacit beliefs about the reliable availability of affection, nurturance, and support; one's acceptability to others; their responsiveness to one's needs; and trust. Difficulties in Theresa's relationship with her mother were longstanding and were based on a wide range of troubling experiences. Changing tacit beliefs about important relationships, then, would take time and persistent effort by both Theresa and her mother. With this in mind, Mrs. G. asked for a referral for counseling for herself so that she might relate to her daughter in a less angry and controlling manner. Both attachment theory and contemporary cognitive models of depression posit that depression stems from maladaptive tacit beliefs or "working models" about the self and one's relationships with others. Theresa acknowledges manifesting negative beliefs in each of these domains. Attachment-based interventions in this module are explicitly designed to address these beliefs and to facilitate the development of a more "secure" relationship between the teenager and caregivers.

Communication and Negotiation

Depressed adolescents frequently experience difficulties communicating with friends and family members. This can take the form of sarcasm, sullen demands, the use of veiled or indirect statements, excessively seeking reassurance from others, arguing, limited interest in others' points of view, and unassertiveness. Over time, this behavior can alienate others, leading to further feelings of isolation. The communication and negotiation module addresses these difficulties by modeling, rehearsing, and practicing specific communication skills. Using psychoeducation, role plays with the therapist, and parent–teenager sessions, the adolescents are encouraged to actively engage others in discussions about their concerns; to directly communicate their thoughts, feelings, and desires; to attend to others' responses; to negotiate with others so that shared goals can be identified; to compromise; to assert themselves (when appropriate); and to express appreciation to others for their efforts and concern.

Relapse Prevention

As noted, depression is often a chronic and recurrent disorder. The majority of adolescents who experience an episode of major depression will experience a recurrence of the disorder, even though they have recovered from the initial episode. Among adults, the probability of experiencing a recurrence of the disorder within 5 years is over 75% (Keller, 1994). Early age of onset and the occurrence of a major depressive episode during adolescence are significant predictors of relapse. With this in mind, prevention of relapse for teenagers who have experienced a depressive episode is a priority.

This is accomplished through the use of a relapse prevention module, scheduled booster sessions during the first 3 months after termination, and the offer of additional "as needed" booster sessions during the following year. The relapse prevention module, like other components of this program, is active, structured, and collaborative. We begin by reviewing with the patient and his or her caregiver(s) the skills they have found to be helpful. Theresa stated that she had found seeking social support and the realistic counterthoughts modules particularly helpful. She observed that the most important skill she had learned was to "keep it all in perspective . . .

don't catastrophize." Theresa reported that the pleasant activities, social activity, problem solving, and identifying maladaptive thoughts modules were also useful. We next discussed how she would apply these skills should she begin to feel depressed once again. We identified a number of potentially problematic situations (including failing a class, arguing with her mother, and breaking up with a boyfriend) and developed plans for managing them. It is important, from this perspective, to note that lapse, relapse, and recurrence are not equivalent. We noted that although she was feeling much better at this time, she should anticipate feeling sad at times in the future (as we all do). This need not mean, however, that the treatment had been ineffective. We discussed how her mood had waxed and waned over the course of treatment, and how, on occasion, she became depressed. Through Socratic discussion she came to see that, by using the techniques and skills she had learned, she was able to reverse this process. In essence, lapses are expected and relapses may be controllable. Theresa's mother participated in this process, and was encouraged to practice these newly learned skills with her daughter should her mood once again begin to "slip."

Follow-Up

Theresa and her mother were asked to complete a battery of objective rating scales at the time she finished treatment and at 3-month intervals during the following year. The results indicate that Theresa was not clinically depressed at the conclusion of therapy, and that she maintained these gains over the course of the follow-up period. Theresa's Clinical Global Assessment Score (CGAS) improved from 50 at the time of her referral for therapy to 72 at termination. Her Affective Disorders Screen (ADS) total score declined from 16 to 4 during this same period. Clinical Global Impression (CGI) severity and improvement ratings completed after 12 weeks of treatment indicated that she was "much improved" and that she was only "mildly ill." One year after termination, Theresa's CGAS score was 65, and CGI ratings suggested that she remained "much improved" and showed "little or no impairment from depressive symptoms."

As important as objective scores were the subjective reports of Theresa and her mother. Mrs. G. reported that her daughter was "happier, more energetic and enthusiastic." She reportedly looks forward to going to school (although she still struggles in math) and is "more receptive to both compliments and constructive feedback. . . . She's in an up mode." As her mother remarked, "She looks real good. . . . She's more expressive and she's breaking out of her shell with friends. . . . I love it, she's revived."

Were Theresa's problems alleviated entirely? Of course not. She continued to experience academic difficulties, remained fearful of failing additional classes, and experienced episodic feelings of dysphoria and pessimism. She continues to live in an impoverished, dangerous neighborhood, and has important questions as to her future and her relationships with others. Theresa is, however, better able to seek assistance from others, and is less likely to avoid stressful situations or to become overwhelmed by day-to-day tasks and challenges.

CONCLUSION

Depression is a complex and often chronic disorder. Although depression during childhood has been recognized as a disorder for barely 30 years, much has been learned about its nature, etiology, course, and treatment. Studies indicate that a number of cognitive, social, and developmental factors are associated with vulnerability for depression. These include maladaptive tacit beliefs or schemas, insecure early attachment, negativistic attributional style, self-focused attention, problem-solving deficits, ruminative style, decreased participation in pleasurable activities, social skills deficits, peer rejection, and stressful life events. Modular CBT is a semi-structured skills-based treatment program based on the assumption that clinical depression stems from the interaction of these risk factors, and that the selection of treatment techniques should be based upon empirically supported formulations of pathological processes. Modular CBT includes general or "required" interventions (which are provided to all patients) in conjunction with optional treatment modules designed to address specific risk factors demonstrated by individual patients. This approach allows treatment to be tailored to the needs of the adolescent and his or her family in a developmentally appropriate manner.

Based on research in cognitive psychotherapy and developmental psychopathology, modular CBT integrates parent and family sessions with individual CBT. As in cognitive therapy with depressed adults, treatment is active, problem-focused, strategic, and collaborative. An emphasis is placed on identifying and rectifying maladaptive beliefs and cognitive processes, developing adaptive coping skills, improving relationships with family and peers, and enhancing the adolescent's ability to think in more flexible, adaptive ways when confronted with problematic situations. Required treatment modules include psychoeducation about depression and the rationale for cognitive therapy, establishing treatment goals, mood and event monitoring, increasing pleasant activities, increasing social activities, rational problem solving, identification of maladaptive thoughts, cognitive restructuring, and relapse prevention. Optional treatment modules include social skills training, relaxation training, communication and negotiation, assertiveness training, establishing a secure attachment, affect regulation, and behavioral parent training.

Modular CBT is a flexible, integrated, developmentally sensitive form of psychotherapy based upon contemporary cognitive diathesis–stress models of depression. As the model attends to the full range of cognitive, social, and behavioral factors associated with risk for depression, and is based upon empirically supported interventions, it may be helpful for some depressed youth. It is worth acknowledging, however, that studies evaluating the effectiveness of modular CBT with depressed adolescents have not been completed (a multisite, longitudinal, placebo-controlled trial comparing CBT alone and in combination with fluoxetine is currently under way). Cognitive therapy has been found effective for reducing depressive symptomatology among both clinically and nonclinically depressed youth. Modular CBT represents an attempt to refine these approaches, and is consistent with the commonly accepted view that treatments should be tailored to the specific need of the child. It shows promise, then, as an approach for treating clinical depression and preventing relapse among youth.

REFERENCES

American Psychiatric Association. (1994). *Diagnostic and statistical manual of mental disorders* (4th ed). Washington, DC: Author.

Angold, A., & Costello, E. (1993). Depressive comorbidity in children and adolescents: Empirical, theoretical, and methodological issues. *American Journal of Psychiatry, 150(12)*, 1779–1791.

Armsden, G., McCauley, E., Greenberg, M., Burke, P., & Mitchell, J. (1990). Parent and peer attachment in early adolescent depression. *Journal of Abnormal Child Clinical Psychology, 18*, 683–697.

Asarnow, J. (1988). Peer status and social competence in child psychiatric inpatients: A comparison of children with depressive, externalizing, and concurrent depressive and externalizing disorders. *Journal of Abnormal Child Psychology, 16*, 151–162.

Asarnow, J., Carlson, G., & Guthrie, D. (1987). Coping strategies, self-perceptions, hopelessness, and perceived family environments in depressed and suicidal children. *Journal of Consulting and Clinical Psychology, 55*, 361–366.

Baron, P., & MacGillivray, R. (1989). Depressive symptoms in adolescents as a function of perceived parental behavior. *Adolescent Research, 4*, 50–62.

Beck, A., Rush, A., Shaw, B., & Emery, G. (1979). *Cognitive therapy for depression.* New York: Guilford Press.

Beck, J. (1995). *Cognitive therapy: Basics and beyond.* New York: Guilford Press.

Birmaher, B., Brent, D. A., Kolko, D., Baugher, M., Bridge, J., Holder, D., Iyengar, S., & Ulloa, R. E. (2000). Clinical outcome after short-term psychotherapy for adolescents with major depressive disorder. *Archives of General Psychiatry, 57*, 29–36.

Birmaher, B., Ryan, N., Williamson, D., Brent, D., Kaufman, J., Dahl, R., Perel, J., & Nelson, B. (1996). Childhood and adolescent depression: A review of the past 10 years. Part 1. *Journal of the American Academy of Child and Adolescent Psychiatry, 35*, 1427–1439.

Blatt, S., & Homan, E. (1992). Parent–child interaction in the etiology of depression. *Clinical Psychology Review, 12,* 47–91.

Brent, D., Holder, D., Kolko, D., Birmaher, B., Baugher, D., Roth, C., Iyengar, S., & Johnson, B. (1997). A clinical psychotherapy trial for adolescent depression comparing cognitive, family, and supportive treatments. *Archives of General Psychiatry, 54,* 877–885.

Brent, D., & Poling, K. (1997). *Cognitive therapy treatment manual for depressed and suicidal youth.* Pittsburgh: Star Center.

Clarke, G., & Lewinsohn, P. (1989). The Coping with Depression Course: A group psychoeducational intervention for unipolar depression. *Behavior Change, 6,* 54–69.

Clarke, G., Lewinsohn, P., & Hops, H. (1990). *Adolescent Coping with Depression Course: Leader's manual for adolescent groups.* Eugene, OR: Castalia.

Cole, D., & Rehm, L. (1986). Family interaction patterns and childhood depression. *Journal of Abnormal Child Psychology, 14,* 297–314.

Coyne, J. (1976). Toward an interactional description of depression. *Psychiatry, 39,* 28–40.

D'Zurilla, T., & Nezu, A. (2001). Problem-solving therapies. In K. Dobson (Ed.), *Handbook of cognitive-behavioral therapies* (2nd ed., pp. 211–245). New York: Guilford Press.

Emslie, G., Rush, A., Weinberg, W., Kowatch, R., Hughes, C., Carmody, T., & Rintelmann, J. (1997). A double-blind, randomized, placebo-controlled trial of fluoxetine in children and adolescents with depression. *Archives of General Psychiatry, 54*(11), 1031–1037.

Essau, C., Conradt, J., & Petermann, F. (1999). Course and outcome of depressive disorders. In C. Essau & F. Petermann (Eds.), *Depressive disorders in children and adolescents: Epidemiology, course and treatment* (pp. 69–103). Northvale, NJ: Aronson.

Essau, C., & Dobson, K. (1999). Epidemiology of depressive disorders. In C. Essau & F. Petermann (Eds.), *Depressive disorders in children and adolescents: Epidemiology, course and treatment* (pp. 69–103). Northvale, NJ: Aronson.

Fremouw, W., Callahan, T., & Kashden, J. (1993). Adolescent suicidal risk: Psychological, problem-solving, and environmental factors. *Suicide and Life-Threatening Behavior, 23,* 46–54.

Gotlib, I., & Hammen, C. (1992). *Psychological aspects of depression: Toward a cognitive-interpersonal integration.* Chichester, UK: Wiley.

Harrington, R., Whittaker, J., Shoebridge, P., & Campbell, F. (1998). Systematic review of efficacy of cognitive behaviour therapies in childhood and adolescent depressive disorder. *British Medical Journal, 316*(7144), 1559–1563.

Hughes, C., Preskorn, S., Weller, E., Weller, R., Hassanein, R., & Tucker, S. (1990). The effect of concomitant disorders in childhood depression on predicting treatment response. *Psychopharmacology Bulletin, 26*(2), 235–238.

Ingram, R., Miranda, J., & Segal, Z. (1998). *Cognitive vulnerability to depression.* New York: Guilford Press.

Joiner, T., & Coyne, J. (Eds.). (1999). *The interactional nature of depression: Advances in interpersonal approaches.* Washington, DC: American Psychological Association.

Kaslow, N., & Thompson, M. (1998). Applying the criteria for empirically supported treatments to studies of psychosocial interventions for child and adolescent depression. *Journal of Clinical Child Psychology, 27,* 146–155.

Kazdin, A., & Weisz, J. (1998). Identifying and developing empirically supported child and adolescent treatments. *Journal of Consulting and Clinical Psychology, 66,* 19–36.

Keller, M. (1994). Depression: A long-term illness. *British Journal of Psychiatry, 165*(Suppl. 26), 9–15.

Keller, M., Beardslee, W., Lavori, P., Wunder, J., Dorer, D., & Samuelson, H. (1988). Course of major depression in non-referred adolescents: A retrospective study. *Journal of Affective Disorders, 15*(3), 235–243.

Kendall, P. (2000). Guiding theory for therapy with children and adolescents. In P. Kendall (Ed.), *Child and adolescent therapy: Cognitive-behavioral procedures* (2nd ed., pp. 3–27). New York: Guilford Press.

Kendall, P., & MacDonald, J. (1993). Cognition in the psychopathology of youth and implications for treatment. In K. Dobson & P. Kendall (Eds.), *Psychopathology and cognition* (pp. 387–430). San Diego: Academic Press.

Kistner, J., Balthazor, M., Risi, S., & Burton, C. (1999). Predicting dysphoria in adolescence from actual and perceived peer acceptance in childhood. *Journal of Clinical Child Psychology, 28,* 94–104.

Lewinsohn, P., Antonuccio, D., Steinmetz-Breckenridge, J., & Teri, L. (1984). *The Coping with Depression Course: A psychoeducational intervention for unipolar depression.* Eugene, OR: Castalia Press.

Lewinsohn, P., & Clarke, G. (1999). Psychosocial treatments for adolescent depression. *Clinical Psychology Review, 19*(3), 329–342.

Lewinsohn, P., Clarke, G., Hops, H., & Andrews, J. (1990). Cognitive-behavioral treatment for depressed adolescents. *Behavior Therapy, 21,* 385–401.

Lewinsohn, P., Hops, H., Roberts, R., Seeley, J., & Andrews, J. (1993). Adolescent psychopathology: I. Prevalence and incidence of depression and other DSM-III-R disorders in high school students. *Journal of Abnormal Psychology, 102*(1), 133–144.

Nezu, A. (1987). A problem-solving formulation of depression: A literature review and proposal of a pluralistic model. *Clinical Psychology Review, 7,* 121–144.

Nolen-Hoeksema, S. (1987). Sex differences in bipolar depression: Evidence and theory. *Psychological Bulletin, 101,* 259–282.

Nolen-Hoeksema, S. (1990). *Sex differences in depression.* Stanford, CA: Stanford University Press.

Panak, W., & Garber, J. (1992). Role of aggression, rejection, and attributions in the prediction of depression in children. *Development and Psychopathology, 4,* 145–165.

Rehm, L., Kaslow, N., & Rabin, A. (1987). Cognitive and behavioral targets in a self-control therapy program for depression. *Journal of Consulting and Clinical Psychology, 55,* 60–67.

Reinecke, M. (1995). Comorbidity of conduct disorder and depression among adolescents: Implications for assessment and treatment. *Cognitive and Behavioral Practice, 2,* 299–326.

Reinecke, M. (2002). Cognitive therapies of depression: A modularized treatment approach. In M. Reinecke & M. Davison (Eds.), *Comparative treatments of depression* (pp. 249–290). New York: Springer.

Reinecke, M., DuBois, D., & Schultz, T. (2001). Social problem-solving, mood, and suicidality among inpatient adolescents. *Cognitive Therapy and Research*, *25* (6), 743–756.

Reinecke, M., & Rogers, G. (2001). Dysfunctional attitudes and attachment style among clinically depressed adults. *Behavioural and Cognitive Psychotherapy*, *29*, 129–141.

Reinecke, M., Ryan, N., & DuBois, D. (1998). Cognitive-behavioral therapy of depression and depressive symptoms during adolescence: A review and meta-analysis. *Journal of the American Academy of Child and Adolescent Psychiatry*, *37* (1), 26–34.

Reinherz, H., Stewart-Berghauer, G., Pakiz, B., Frost, A., Moeykens, B., & Holmes, W. (1989). The relationship of early risk and current mediators to depressive symptomatology in adolescence. *Journal of the American Academy of Child and Adolescent Psychiatry*, *28*, 942–947.

Roberts, J., Gotlib, I., & Kassel, J. (1996). Adult attachment security and symptoms of depression: The mediating roles of dysfunctional attitudes and low self-esteem. *Journal of Personality and Social Psychology*, *70*, 310–320.

Rotheram-Borus, M., Trautman, P., Dopkins, S., & Shrout, P. (1990). Cognitive style and pleasant activities among female adolescent suicide attempters. *Journal of Consulting and Clinical Psychology*, *58*, 554–561.

Sadowski, C., & Kelley, M. (1993). Social problem solving in suicidal adolescents. *Journal of Consulting and Clinical Psychology*, *61*, 121–127.

Sheeber, L., Hops, H., Andrews, J., Alpert, T., & Davis, B. (1998). Interactional processes in families with depressed and non-depressed adolescents: Reinforcement of depressive behavior. *Behavior Research and Therapy*, *36*, 417–427.

Spirito, A., Overholser, J., & Stark, L. (1989). Common problems and coping strategies: II. Findings with adolescent suicide attempters. *Journal of Abnormal Child Psychology*, *17*, 213–221.

Stark, K., Humphrey, L., Crook, K., & Lewis, K. (1990). Perceived family environments of depressed and anxious children: Child's and maternal figure's perspective. *Journal of Abnormal Child Psychology*, *18*, 527–547.

Stark, K., Swearer, S., Kurowski, C., Sommer, D., & Bowen, B. (1996). Targeting the child and the family: A holistic approach to treating child and adolescent depressive disorders. In E. Hibbs & P. Jensen (Eds.), *Psychosocial treatments for child and adolescent disorders: Empirically based strategies for clinical practice* (pp. 207–238). Washington, DC: American Psychological Association.

Tang, T., & DeRubeis, R. (1999). Reconsidering rapid early response in cognitive behavioral therapy for depression. *Clinical Psychology: Science and Practice*, *6* (3), 283–288.

Vernberg, E. (1990). Psychological adjustment and experiences with peers during early adolescence: Reciprocal, incidental, or unidirectional relationships? *Journal of Abnormal Child Psychology*, *18*, 187–198.

SUGGESTED READINGS

Brent, D., & Poling, K. (1997). *Cognitive therapy treatment manual for depressed and suicidal youth*. Pittsburgh: Star Center.

Harrington, R., Wood, A., & Verduyn, C. (1998). Clinically depressed adolescents. In

P. Graham (Ed.), *Cognitive-behaviour therapy for children and families* (pp. 156–193). Cambridge, UK: Cambridge University Press.

Lewinsohn, P., Clarke, G., Rohde, P., Hops, H., & Seeley, J. (1996). A course in coping: A cognitive-behavioral approach to the treatment of adolescent depression. In E. Hibbs & P. Jensen (Eds.), *Psychosocial treatments for child and adolescent disorders: Empirically based strategies for clinical practice* (pp. 109–135). Washington, DC: American Psychological Association.

Spence, S., & Reinecke, M. (in press). Cognitive approaches to understanding, preventing and treating child and adolescent depression. In M. Reinecke & D. Clark (Eds.), *Cognitive therapy across the lifespan: Prospects and challenges.* Cambridge, UK: Cambridge University Press.

Stark, K., Sander, J., Yancy, M., Bronik, M., & Hoke, J. (2000). Treatment of depression in childhood and adolescence. In P. C. Kendall (Ed.), *Child and adolescent therapy: Cognitive-behavioral procedures* (2nd ed., pp. 173–234). New York: Guilford Press.

6

Treatment of Social Anxiety Disorder

ANNE MARIE ALBANO

Once called the "neglected anxiety disorder" (Liebowitz, Gorman, Fyer, & Klein, 1985), social phobia or social anxiety disorder (SAD) is a common and chronic condition characterized by heightened self-consciousness and exaggerated fear of negative evaluation which may be relatively circumscribed or generalized to a variety of social situations and contexts. Although first introduced as a diagnostic category in the third edition of the *Diagnostic and Statistical Manual of Mental Disorders* (DSM-III; American Psychiatric Association, 1980), research and clinical attention to SAD appeared to lag behind that of the other DSM anxiety disorder categories. In part, this initial neglect of SAD may have resulted from a hesitation to "pathologize" what was confused as a variation of a relatively benign personality style or temperament, shyness. However, as clinical scientists turned their attention to understanding the phenomenology and symptoms associated with this disorder in adults, it became apparent that the impairments associated with SAD could involve severe disruption in a number of domains including emotional, social, educational, vocational, and familial functioning (Kessler et al., 1994; Kessler, Foster, Saunders, & Stang, 1995; Kessler & Frank, 1997). Thus, whereas shy individuals may initially appear hesitant to interact or more reserved than their nonshy peers in social contexts, SAD is distinguished from this normally distributed personality trait on a variety of qualitative and quantitative measures of anxiety, distress, and dysfunction (see Beidel & Turner, 1998; Heimberg, Liebowitz, Hope, & Schneier, 1995). Moreover, as research consistently pointed to the onset of this disorder in childhood, attention was turned to the study of social anxiety disorder in youth. The purpose of this chapter is to provide the mental health practitioner with a thorough understanding of the cognitive-behavioral approach to the assessment and treatment of SAD in youth. The chapter begins with an overview of the phenomenology and impact of SAD. Current empirically sound cognitive-behavioral assessment and treatment methods are then presented. The chapter concludes with a detailed case description of an adolescent with social anxiety disorder.

OVERVIEW OF SOCIAL ANXIETY DISORDER

The mental health professional working with children and adolescents will at some point find him- or herself in a quandary when confronted by the referral of a seemingly "normal" child, but with a parent or referral source insisting that "there's something wrong here." A common example is the high-spirited child who may be misperceived as hyperactive but for whom, upon evaluation, all signs indicate a presentation at the higher end of the curve but nevertheless within normal limits. The clinician must then educate the parents and/or referral source about the normative behavior for a child with a given temperament and history, and the distinction between hyperactivity and high activity levels. Concurrently, the clinician must carefully present the information so as not to alienate the parents and/or referral source, but to provide guidance with parenting the high-spirited child and thus encourage appropriate help-seeking behavior if or when necessary in the future.

A different scenario typically occurs in the referral of youth with social anxiety problems. Parents may be prompted by school personnel to bring the child for an evaluation following reports of social isolation, failure to participate in class discussions, or outright refusal to speak in school situations. Alternatively, parents may become concerned when, in contrast to the adolescent's siblings or other adolescents, their teenager "fails" to start tying up the telephone lines, spending hours with friends, or blowing off family functions for parties and other peer gatherings. In such cases the parents may hear for the first time that their son or daughter suffers from an anxiety disorder, one that interferes with the ability to enter and negotiate social and evaluative situations comfortably, and that this problem is not just "a phase" that will spontaneously remit. This diagnosis is particularly difficult when the youth has been consistently viewed as a "good, cooperative, and quiet child" who was "never any trouble." However, it is precisely the nature of the social anxiety disorder, from its earliest stages, that gives the false appearance of a quiet and cooperative child, when in fact the youth is suffering in silence and trying desperately to avoid any undue attention. As such, in these cases the clinician must educate the parents about the difference between being shy on the normal continuum of personality types, and being clinically anxious such that the youth's daily life is impaired and fraught with feelings of distress and anxiety.

Diagnostic Criteria

DSM-IV (American Psychiatric Association, 1994) defines the essential feature of SAD as "a marked and persistent fear of social or performance situations in which embarrassment may occur" (p. 411). In addition, upon exposure to the social situation an individual must invariably experience anxiety, which may take the form of a situationally bound or situationally predisposed panic attack, and must recognize that this anxiety is excessive or unreasonable. The individual with SAD will endure social situations with intense distress and/or escape from or altogether avoid anxiety-provoking situations. Thus, the consequence of the anxiety and resultant avoidance patterns is impairment and interference with the individual's normal routine, social and/or family life, or occupational/academic functioning. When an individual's social anxiety is related to a variety of, or most, social situations, the specifier "generalized" is assigned; otherwise the nongeneralized form of social anxiety refers to circumscribed conditions, such as anxiety in public speaking situations or taking tests.

Four specific provisions, accounting for developmental differences between children and adults, are specified in DSM-IV for assigning the diagnosis to youth (American Psychiatric Association, 1994). First, youth with SAD must show the capacity for age-appropriate social relationships with familiar peers, and the anxiety must occur in peer contexts, not just in the presence of adults. Second, whereas an adult may experience a panic attack when confronted with a challenging social situation, children may express their anxiety through crying, tantrums, freezing, or shrinking away from social situations, especially those involving unfamiliar people. Third, DSM-IV does not require children and adolescents to recognize that their fear in these contexts is unreasonable or excessive. This provision recognizes cognitive-developmental differences between youth and adults, such as the adult's capacity for complex cognitive reasoning, including perspective taking and social comparison skills. These higher-order abstract cognitive skills typically develop throughout the course of adolescence and thus may be arrested due to the social anxiety or not yet fully developed to allow for insight into the nature of the anxiety (see Vasey & Dadds, 2001). Fourth, individuals under the age of 18 must evidence the social anxiety for a minimum of 6 months, allowing for typical and developmentally appropriate transient episodes of social anxiety at critical times of the year (e.g., start of school in the fall, exam periods) or periods of developmental change (e.g., transition from middle school to high school, initiation of romantic relationships).

Associated Features

SAD rarely occurs as a sole diagnosis, as comorbidity with other anxiety disorders, mood disorders, and substance abuse is high (Beidel, 1991; Beidel, Turner, & Morris, 1999; Brady & Kendall, 1992; Wittchen, Stein, & Kessler, 1999). Moreover, epidemiological research indicates that SAD precedes the onset of 85.2% of comorbid substance abuse disorders, 81.6% of mood disorders, and 64.6% of anxiety disorders other than specific phobias (Wittchen et al., 1999). Youth with SAD suffer with higher levels of depressed mood, higher trait anxiety, and lower perceptions of cognitive competence than their nonanxious peers (Albano, Chorpita, & Barlow, 2003). Headaches, stomachaches, and autonomic reactivity in the form of heightened anxiety and panic attacks also accompany the disorder for some youth (Beidel et al., 1999; La Greca, 2001). Youth with SAD report higher levels of loneliness and fewer friends than their same-age peers (Beidel et al., 1999). As such, youth with SAD avoid a wide and generalized range of situations and activities (Hofmann et al., 1999), which may include the ability to attend or stay in school (Kearney, 2001). Thus, the negative impact of social phobia in youth is evident across all domains of functioning.

Etiological Mechanisms

The cognitive-behavioral model understands the etiology of SAD to be a combination of biological and environmental variables, that is, a diathesis–stress model of psychopathology where learning history plays a significant role (see Barlow, 2002). This model incorporates empirical findings from the extant literature, suggesting that biological factors such as genetics and temperament comprise a diathesis for problematic social anxiety (e.g., Hayward, Killen, Kraemer, & Taylor, 1998; Rosenbaum, Biederman, Hirshfeld, Bolduc, & Chaloff, 1991). Furthermore, the model recognizes that the realization of social anxiety symptoms is dependent on other risk and protective factors, including environmental variables such as parental rearing style, observational learning, negative or positive experiences with peers (see Albano et al., 2003) and selective attention to threat-related stimuli (see Kendall, 1992).

Parents are often concerned that they "caused" this anxiety in their child or that, because their child is so different from themselves or their other children, that there could be some "chemical imbalance" in the brain causing this disorder. Regardless of where their concerns may lie, providing the parents and the child or adolescent with an understanding that anxiety is a normal, natural emotion inherent in all human beings (and also animals), and that social anxiety is especially unique to humans, provides the basis for their understanding of the nature of the disorder and how to overcome its deleterious effects. It is important to emphasize to families that normative levels of social anxiety occur in all of us throughout life, in addition to specific periods where we expect to see increases in social anxiety (see the following section on "Onset and Developmental Course"). For some individuals, social anxiety occurs continuously at a high level, at times when it is unnecessary or overly excessive for the situation, which is the case for those who suffer with this anxiety disorder. The reasons for the development of problematic social anxiety are couched in the diathesis–stress/cognitive-behavioral therapy model, in which we emphasize that, for this particular child, a biological vulnerability may exist for more readily experiencing anxiety and that, through a process of oversensitivity to anxiety-provoking cues (via biology, environmental experiences, or cognitive style), the child has learned to react with and anticipate more negative outcomes in social situations than is necessary. Moreover, we discuss with the parents the problem of families becoming drawn into the cycle of anxiety and inadvertently reinforcing escape and avoidance. Certain parental behaviors, reflecting overprotection and overcontrol, have been associated with the maintenance of anxiety disorders (Albano et al., 2003). In fact, studies with anxious children (Barrett, Rapee, Dadds, & Ryan, 1996; Chorpita, Albano, & Barlow, 1996) and adolescents with social phobia (Albano, Logsdon-Conradsen, & Barlow, 1999) demonstrated that parents selectively attend to ambiguous cues in the environment and misinterpret these cues as threatening to their child. The parents then give a verbal message to avoid or escape a situation, rather than engage in constructive problem solving. This process is particularly evident when the parent him- or herself displays high levels of anxiety. It may be that the child's anxiety has "worked on" the parent's natural tendency to protect and comfort, resulting in overprotection. As a result, the parent "takes over" for the child in solving problems and hence prevents the child from learning to cope with various situations through experience and to develop problem-solving and anxiety management skills. In general, we follow a guideline that the more involved the parents are in protecting the child, the more involved they should be in the child or teen's treatment. Depending upon the degree of distress and impairment in the child's life, cognitive-behavioral therapy with or without medication can help the child to master this anxiety and "rein it in" to serve its real, protective function and not overwhelm the individual.

Onset and Developmental Course

Nonclinical levels of social anxiety are present in various forms at all ages, with certain developmental ages associated with increases in social anxiety:

- Prior to age 3, such as when an unfamiliar person is introduced to the toddler.
- Early school age, such as at the start of nursery school or kindergarten and upon meeting new peers in play groups.
- Middle childhood years, during periods of school transitions and during times when teasing becomes a part of the peer-group repertoire.
- Adolescence, when certain developmental tasks are expected such as independent functioning, assertiveness, forming lasting social relationships, initiation of romantic relationships, completion of basic education requirements, and formation of long-term career goals.

It has been noted that social anxiety increases in early to mid-adolescence with the emergence of complex cognitive processes such as perspective taking (Vasey, 1995). This cognitive developmental leap occurs at a time when adolescent peer-group approval becomes extremely important, and exclusion or rejection by peers is felt with exquisite sensitivity for most youth (La Greca, 2001). With regard to the clinical disorder of SAD, epidemiological studies suggest late childhood to early adolescence as the ages for onset of the disorder (between 11.3 and 12.3 years, roughly), although SAD is found and can be diagnosed at any age (see Velting & Albano, 2001). As with other anxiety disorders in youth, SAD runs a chronic and fluctuating course into adulthood (Costello & Angold, 1995; Ferdinand & Verhulst, 1995).

Long-Term Implications

It has been noted that SAD can onset at any age and is associated over time with greater and widespread impairment. Furthermore, it has been suggested that youth with SAD can be hampered in meeting age-related developmental tasks and thus fail to achieve independent functioning. In addition, comorbidity, especially with depression and substance abuse, can complicate the clinical picture by late adolescence. Thus, SAD causes impairment in the individual's social, academic, familial, and occupational functioning and is accompanied by active avoidance of a wide range of everyday situations (Kessler et al., 1995). Among the most notable long-term impairments associated with the condition are failure to complete high school for girls, failure to complete college for both males and females, delayed marriage or entry into unstable marriage, and significant impairment in one's ability to earn a living (Kessler et al., 1995; Kessler & Frank, 1997). It is not unusual for the adolescent with SAD to anticipate that "college or work will be different" than high school with regard to his or her anxiety. However, upon entry into college or the work force, the setting may be different but the challenges are the same, rendering the individual unable to manage the social and evaluative situations that arise in adult life. Hence, dropping out of college or leaving one's job is not uncommon for young adults with SAD, who in many cases return to their parents' home with a greater degree of demoralization and hopelessness. Consequently, in the absence of effective treatment, individuals with SAD can remain dependent upon their families and/or become reliant upon the social welfare system for the long term.

ASSESSMENT

The clinical evaluation of youth suspected of having SAD is critical, especially considering that normal personality variations in sociability and introversion are not clinical syndromes. Thus, while a shy individual may wish to enter cognitive-behavioral therapy (CBT) to learn specific assertiveness skills or deal with other personal goals and issues, it would be inappropriate to automatically assume a diagnosis of social anxiety disorder that could then lead to a treatment regime for SAD, which may include specific CBT protocols or medication. Thus, a multimodal assessment involving multiple informants and both objective and subjective assessments is necessary for accurate diagnosis and treatment planning. This section reviews assessment techniques for use with social anxiety referrals.

Clinical Interview

The structured or semistructured clinical interview is the most widely accepted and reliable method for establishing the presence of DSM diagnoses across the ages (March & Albano, 1998). Valid and standardized clinical interview schedules standardize the diagnostic data collection process, which in turn allows for the quantification of clinical information. Structured diagnostic interviews allow for limited clinical judgment and flexibility on the part of the diagnostician, whereas semistructured interviews provide the clinician with guidelines for adapting inquiries to the age or developmental level of the child, and also allow for some flexibility in probing for clarification and further information as needed. Diagnostic interviews are required in clinical trials to reduce error associated with variance due to method, informant, and interviewer. Also, interviews allow scientists to be confident in outcomes and to compare results across settings using similar methodologies.

The utility of the diagnostic interview in clinical practice lies in providing the clinician with a reliable tool for gathering diagnostic and screening information, identifying and quantifying symptoms and areas of impairment, and defining the targets for therapeutic change. Data gathered from some of the available interviews are quantifiable at both the categorical and dimensional level, and, when provided, the severity level of the diagnostic category can be quantified in one rating. Although structured interviews are the standard for arriving at a reliable and valid diagnosis in clinical trials, practitioners find their use relatively limited due to time constraints, therapist and patient burden, and limitations imposed by third-party payers. Thus, it is recommended that the clinician have at his or her disposal copies of the most widely utilized structured interviews for use when confronted with a differential diagnostic quandary or to use specific diagnostic sections as needed for gathering quantifiable data to track treatment course and outcomes. Such data can be gathered at pre- and posttreatment for charting diagnostic change, guiding posttreatment recommendations, and establishing a record of accountability for the clinician. Critical reviews currently available regarding diagnostic interviews can be found in several publications (e.g., Silverman, 1991; Stallings & March, 1995). What follows is a focus on a specific interview schedule originally developed for the anxiety disorders.

The *Anxiety Disorders Interview Schedule for DSM-IV: Child Version* (ADIS-C; Silverman & Albano, 1996) comprises separate, semistructured interviews for the diagnosis and assessment of children with anxiety disorders along with the range of behavioral and emotional conditions affecting youth ages 7–17. Diagnoses are derived based upon the child and parent reports separately, then combined to form the composite (or working) diagnosis. The ADIS-C interviews were originally developed as a downward extension of the Adult ADIS (DiNardo, O'Brien, Barlow, Waddell, & Blanchard, 1983) due to the low reliability coefficients found for the anxiety diagnoses in existing diagnostic interviews for youth, and because most interviews have historically been less than ideal in their coverage of the anxiety diagnoses (Silverman & Nelles, 1988).

The ADIS-C provides for the differential diagnoses of the DSM anxiety disorders in youth while permitting the clinician to rule out alternative diagnoses. Moreover, these interviews provide quantifiable data concerning symptoms, severity, etiology, course, and a functional analysis to guide treatment planning. Unique to the ADIS are impairment ratings, termed the Clinician Severity Rating (CSR, range = 0–8), which are assigned for each separate diagnosis. A CSR ≥ 4 indicates that all diagnostic criteria are met, including impairment due to the presence of the symptom cluster, and that the disorder is of sufficient intensity to warrant intervention. The disorder (or disorders) with the highest CSR indicates the "worst" condition and can direct the clinician in choosing a treatment protocol and devising the treatment plan. The ADIS has consistently demonstrated good interrater reliability (Silverman & Nelles, 1988; Silverman, Saavedra, & Pina, 2001), retest reliability (Silverman & Eisen, 1992), and sensitivity to treatment effects in studies of youth with anxiety disorders (e.g., Dadds, Heard, & Rapee, 1992; Kendall et al., 1997).

Questionnaire Methods

In contrast to the clinician-administered diagnostic interview, paper-and-pencil self-report scales allow for a relatively time- and cost-efficient means of gathering information from multiple informants (child, parent, teacher). Clinicians are quite attuned to the fact that information gathered from different sources may sometimes be conflicting; however, information gathered from multiple sources is essential to understand the child's presentation across settings, as well as how each person in the youth's environment perceives the child. Diagnoses cannot be derived from such methods; however, dimensional constructs of interest may be identified and tracked throughout the course of treatment. These forms can be administered in the waiting room of the clinic, sent via mail to school personnel (with appropriate permission), or completed in the home and returned to the clinic. Most individual measures take 10–15 minutes to complete, and child measures usually require a second- or third-grade reading level. A wealth of rating scales exist to assess a multitude of constructs in youth (e.g., depression, anger, loneliness, family functioning) with specific scales available for nearly every type of anxiety (e.g., worry, posttraumatic reactions, obsessions). The following is a brief overview of the most common scales used in the assessment of youth with SAD.

The *Multidimensional Anxiety Scale for Children* (MASC; March, Parker, Sullivan, Stallings, & Conners, 1997; March, 1998) is a 39-item self-report rating scale for children 7–17, developed to sample key symptoms of anxious children and adolescents. Only the most relevant symptoms and symptom clusters survived the scale development process, so that the MASC can be seen as representing the population factor structure of anxiety in both children and adolescents. The MASC contains four main factors: physical symptoms (tense/restless and somatic/autonomic subfactors), social anxiety (humiliation/rejection and public performance subfactors), harm avoidance (anxious coping and perfectionism subfactors), and separation/panic anxiety. To a large extent, the empirically derived factor structure of the MASC matches the DSM-IV diagnostic clusters of SAD, separation/panic anxiety, and, averaged across all four factors, generalized anxiety disorder. In addition, the hypothesized division of harm avoidance into perfectionism and approach/avoidance behaviors also received empirical support, which along with gender and age norms allows empirical quantification of distress and impairment. The MASC has shown excellent psychometric properties (e.g., March et al., 1997) and is sensitive to discriminating youth with anxiety disorders from those with depression or no disorder (Dierker et al., 2001).

The *Fear Survey Schedule for Children—Revised* (FSSC-R; Ollendick, 1983) focuses primarily on phobic symptoms, including fear of failure and criticism, fear of the unknown, fear of injury and small animals, fear of danger and death, and medical fears. A parent version of the scale can be administered to assess the parents' perception of their child's number and level of specific fears. The FSSC-R has demonstrated excellent psychometric properties and is widely used across cultures and settings.

The *Social Phobia and Anxiety Inventory for Children* (SPAI-C; Beidel, Turner, & Morris, 1995) is a 26-item inventory most appropriate for children ages 8–14 and assesses anxiety in a variety of social settings. Separate items measure the cognitive, somatic, and behavioral components of social anxiety, thus providing the clinician with an excellent empirically derived measure of the broad construct of social phobia. Items are scored on a 3-point Likert scale, with total scores above 18 indicating a need for a detailed diagnostic evaluation. Beidel and Turner (1998) report excellent psychometric support for the scale, and a parent version of the measure is presently under development.

The *Social Anxiety Scale for Children—Revised* (SASC-R; La Greca, 1998; La Greca & Stone, 1993) comprises 22 items assessing three specific factors: fear of negative evaluation, social avoidance and distress in new situations, and social avoidance and distress in general. The SASC-R is available in a children's version and an adolescent version. Both a 3-point and a 5-point rating format are available, although La Greca (1998) recommends the latter due to better reliability estimates based on this scaling method. The SASC-R has excellent internal consistency and test–retest reliability. Ginsburg, La Greca, and Silverman (1997a, 1997b) evaluated the scale with a sample of children diagnosed with anxiety disorders. Results suggest the SASC-R is a promising instrument for screening children and adolescents to identify socially based anxiety disorders and to evaluate social impairment in youngsters in general. Parent versions are also available for both the child and adolescent versions.

The *School Refusal Assessment Scale* (SRAS; Kearney & Silverman, 1993) is administered to the child and separately to each parent. Instructions are provided for combining the information gained from multiple informants to formulate an accurate picture of the variables motivating and maintaining the school refusal behavior, among which social anxiety often plays a significant role (Kearney, 2001). The child can then be prescribed a specific treatment approach that is proven to effectively treat this type of problem (Kearney, 2001; Kearney & Albano, 2000).

Child self-report measures allow access to private information in a less demanding and stressful manner than direct interviews, yet parent and teacher report forms are also important for accessing a full understanding of the child's presenting issues. Parents and teachers can report on aspects of the child's behavior and attitude that the child fails to report because of limitations in age or cognitive development, social desirability, embarrassment, or oppositional behavior. As noted, parent versions exist for the FSSC-R, SAS-R, and SRAS. Probably the most widely utilized parent and teacher rating scales to assess anxiety within a broader range of childhood problems are the Child Behavior Checklist for parents (CBCL; Achenbach & Edelbrock, 1983) and the corresponding Teacher Report Form (TRF; Achenbach, 1991).

Behavioral Assessment Techniques

Individual Behavioral Avoidance Tests (BATs) are ideographic methods designed by the clinician to assess the behavioral limits of the client when confronted by a phobic stimulus (Barrios & Hartmann, 1997). In the case of SAD, BATs can consist of reading aloud before a small audience, carrying on a conversation with an unfamiliar person, using the telephone, and other situations involving a social or evaluative demand. The BAT can be individually tailored for each client, or standardized for SAD (Albano & Barlow, 1996). Among the parameters to address with the BAT are the following: Can the client even attempt the task? How long can the client stay in the situation? What methods make the situation better or worse for the client? What level of anxiety is reached prior to and during the task? The BAT provides a measure of outcome for evaluating change when administered pre- and posttreatment. Moreover, using thought listing (e.g., "List the thoughts that you had during the speech task"), the therapist can have access to the specific cognitive distortions evident in the mind of the youth with social anxiety.

Family Behavioral Tests (FAM-BATs) provide the therapist with specific information about the ways in which anxiety has infiltrated and may be maintained by the family system. Research indicates that parents of anxious children tend to focus on the threat content of ambiguous situations (Barrett, Rapee, et al., 1996). For example, in a FAM-BAT the parent and child are given the following scenario: "Your child goes out to the playground and approaches a group of kids. They are playing together and start laughing. Some of the children glance over toward your child. What do you think is happening? What should your child do?" Research suggests that parents of anxious children, especially those who themselves are highly anxious (Logsdon-Conradsen, 1998), tend to interpret such situations in a negative way and provide escape or avoidant responses for the children: "Maybe these kids are laughing at my child. They aren't nice kids. Johnny should just go play somewhere else." In comparison, the parent of a nonanxious child may respond: "The kids are having fun. You won't know what they're laughing about until you join in." Family BATs are relatively new to the field of anxiety disorders and used most often in research settings.

The *Fear and Avoidance Hierarchy* (FAH) forms the basis for any exposure-based treatment of anxiety. The FAH lists the "top ten" difficult situations in a graded order according to level of fear and/or avoidance.

These situations are rated by the child and parents on a 0–8 scale (0 = no fear, no avoidance; 8 = extreme fear, always avoids). FAH situations are rated at pretreatment and a blank form is completed every week during treatment. This allows the clinician to track the patient's progress and modify treatment if necessary. Situations from the FAH can be used to design a behavioral test (BAT). Table 6.1 presents a sample FAH for a child with social phobia. Information from the ADIS interviews and questionnaire data are used by the therapist in formulating the FAH, along with further input from the parent and child. The FAH is an easy, ideographic method of tracking treatment progress and providing a measure of long-term follow-up.

TREATMENT

Recent critical reviews support the efficacy of CBT for the range of anxiety disorders in youth (Kazdin & Weisz, 1998; Ollendick & King, 1998), and, indeed, this volume can attest to CBT's wide application across a range of disorders. Nonspecific protocols focused on SAD in addition to separation anxiety and generalized anxiety disorders have proven the efficacy and long-term benefits of CBT through various clinical trials (e.g., Barrett, Dadds, & Rapee, 1996; Kendall, 1994; Kendall & Southam-Gerow, 1996; Mendlowicz et al., 1999; Silverman et al., 1999a, 1999b). Protocols specific to the treatment of SAD in youth have likewise demonstrated excellent efficacy in both small controlled trials and open trials (Albano, Marten, Holt, Heimberg, & Barlow, 1995; Beidel, Turner, & Morris, 2000; Hayward et al., 2000; Spence, Donovan, & Brechman-Toussaint, 2000), with

TABLE 6.1. Sample FAH for Social Phobia

Situation	Fear	Avoidance
1. Answering the telephone at home	4	6
2. Ordering my own food at a restaurant	5	7
3. Taking a test in class	4	4
4. Raising my hand to answer a question	5	8
5. Asking the teacher for help after class	5	8
6. Asking a store clerk to help me find something	5	8
7. Starting a conversation with someone I know	6	7
8. Calling a classmate for missed homework	6	8
9. Starting a conversation with someone I don't know well	7	8
10. Sitting with a group of kids in the cafeteria and eating lunch	8	8

Note. FAH, Fear and Avoidance Hierarchy.

larger controlled studies underway. The remainder of this section is devoted to describing one protocol developed specifically for SAD in adolescents.

Cognitive Behavioral Group Treatment for Adolescent Social Phobia (CBGT-A; Albano et al., 1995) was developed specifically for youth and is based upon the work of Heimberg and colleagues (Heimberg, Dodge, Hope, Kennedy, & Zollo, 1990; Heimberg, Salaman, Holt, & Blendell, 1993) as well as incorporating empirically validated methods for treating shyness in adolescents (see Albano, 1995). Specific components of the program include psychoeducation, skills training (social skills, cognitive restructuring, problem solving), and behavioral exposures (see Table 6.2). The adult CBGT program was adapted to be sensitive to the unique developmental needs and presentation of adolescents with SAD (Albano, 1995; Albano & Barlow, 1996). Specifically, social skills and problem-solving skills training were incorporated into CBGT-A to remediate any skill deficits and provide more practice for the acquisition and refinement of these skills. Although originally designed for 16 group sessions, flexibility in specifying the number of sessions can be determined by the therapist, and roughly 16–20 sessions are needed to allow each group member a sufficient experience in participating in various behavioral exposures. Groups typically consist of both males and females, ages 13–17, with two cotherapists conducting each 2-hour group session. The first four sessions are held within a 2-week period, in order to provide the adolescents with a "jump start" in overcoming their expected and SAD-related resistance to being in a group. Phase I (Sessions 1–8) involves skills training modules. During Phase II (Sessions 9–20) the adolescents engage in behavioral exposures while practicing their anxiety management skills in personally relevant anxiety-provoking situations. These exposures provide the adolescents with a specified, structured experience to practice their skills and confront difficult social situations. As treatment progresses, exposures move from relatively "easy" tasks found on the lower range of each participant's individual hierarchy to more challenging anxiety-provoking tasks. To facilitate generalization beyond the clinic, we have created "Mission Is Possible" tasks, where our group members arrive at the clinic and open a sealed envelope bearing their names. Within is an assignment for them to complete in a public place (taking roughly 30 minutes) and then return to the clinic to process their progress. The group therapists typically accompany the teens but remain at a distance during these *in vivo* exposures. Moreover, we often enlist the help of trainees in psychology, psychiatry, and social work as "confederates" to challenge the youth in these situations. Homework assignments are utilized as a mechanism to foster generalization and maintenance of treatment gains.

At present, parental involvement is minimal and focused on providing education about the disorder and encouraging the parents to coach their adolescents in applying their skills between sessions and after termination.

TABLE 6.2. Session Content for CBGT-A

Session 1	(Parents attend) Ground rules for group Situations causing social anxiety Cognitive-behavioral model of social anxiety Snack time: Therapists share information Overview of treatment program and rationale Monitoring Homework: Monitoring and setting treatment goals
Session 2	(Parents attend) Review self-monitoring Three-component model of anxiety Dissecting social anxiety into three components: Use a common situation Snack time: Therapist's embarrassing moment Expectations for treatment Becoming detectives: Studying the three components Homework: Monitoring and life goals
Session 3	Review of self-monitoring, goals, and model of anxiety Labeling distortions: Introduction to automatic thoughts (ATs) Therapists' role play of ATs Snack time: Guided imagery to the moon Rational responses: Countering ATs Review of session Homework
Session 4	Review of homework Four steps to cognitive restructuring Therapists' role play of cognitive restructuring Snack time: Therapist deals with a problem Steps to problem solving Review Homework
Session 5	Review of homework Therapists model social skills versus "unskilled" Social skills training I: Identifying and improving upon weaknesses Snack time practice: Shaping oral reading skills Social skills training II: Assertiveness Review of session and homework assignment: Preparing a paragraph for next week's snack time
Session 6	Review of homework Social skills training III: Review of skill building steps and focus on perspective taking Group role play: Conversing in the cafeteria Snack time: Reading aloud prepared paragraphs Social skills training IV: More assertiveness Review and homework

(*continued*)

Session 7	Overview and review of skills covered to date: cognitive restructuring, problem solving, social skills Treatment rationale: Simulated exposures Evaluating expectations: "How much better should I be now?" Snack time: Group interaction exercise What to do with your parents: How to access support and be understood Homework
Session 8	(Parents attend) Review of homework Review of expectations: "What should have changed by now?" Treatment rationale: Simulated and between-session exposures Snack time: Informal socializing Role play: Perspective taking—parents and teens switch roles Enlisting support: The coaching team Homework
Sessions 9–14	Review of homework Simulated exposure #1 Snack time: Mini exposures to situations such as taking compliments, giving critical feedback to a friend, etc. Simulated exposure #2 Homework: Individual hierarchy items are assigned for between-session exposure
Session 15 or 19	(Parents attend: Next to last session) Review of monitoring and exposure homework Exposures: Each group member is targeted in an exposure that all parents observe Snack time: Informal socializing Expectations and future plans: Relapse prevention; homework
Sessions 16–20	Review of self-monitoring and exposure homework Final exposures and relapse prevention Snack time: Pizza party Processing of termination and relapse prevention

Note. CBGT-A, Cognitive Behavioral Group Treatment for Adolescent Social Phobia.

Parents are invited to only four sessions, each strategically spaced to provide them with specific information to assist with the progress of the program, but not to become too involved with the adolescent's treatment. The general principle here is that adolescence is a time to develop skills for independent functioning, and taking control of one's social anxiety is a first big step in meeting that specific developmental task. As previously indicated, this idea arises from the finding that parents and family members are often inadvertently drawn into the cycle of anxiety (Albano et al., 1999; Barrett, Rapee, et al., 1996) and that family members may provide reassurance or reinforce escape and avoidance as a way of calming the adolescent or protecting him or her from becoming upset and anxious, rather than focusing the child or teen on problem solving and managing the situation.

Finally, relapse prevention plans are created with each teenager toward the end of the program. These plans involve outlining upcoming proximal and distal social challenges (e.g., confronting a friend, prom night, college interviews) that can be anticipated and worked through using planning sheets for addressing the thoughts, feelings, and behaviors accompanying social anxiety, and a coping plan for managing the situation. Teenagers who have completed the group program are invited back at any time for booster sessions and to participate as confederates in future groups.

CASE EXAMPLE

The following case example is offered to illustrate the presentation of an adolescent with social anxiety disorder and outline the usual course of treatment for this disorder. Names and identifying information are fictitious.

Reason for Referral

During the fall midterm parent–teacher conference, Teresa and Alan Gular were advised by their daughter Lisa's school counselor to seek a clinical consultation with a specialist in adolescent problems due to "persistent shyness and isolation" in the school setting. Although Lisa, at age 15, had been attending high school with no apparent academic difficulties, the school counselor and her teachers had noticed a pattern of withdrawal from any unstructured social activity, such as lunch or free periods, and a complete absence of any effort to participate in class discussions or volunteer a response.

The school personnel were concerned that Lisa was missing out on important social and academic interactions and opportunities, and believed her academic standing could suffer if these patterns persisted. Although her parents were initially reluctant to pursue the referral, upon discussion they agreed that Lisa did isolate and withdraw herself more often than not, even from extended family gatherings and outings. Moreover, in comparison to their older daughter, who was away in her first year of college, Lisa did not bring friends home to "hang out," nor did she share her sister's interests in talking on the phone and going shopping with her girlfriends. Lisa also did not appear to have any interest in dating, as was typical for this age. Although they knew Lisa was their more quiet and shy child, following the school report the Gulars contacted their family physician, who in turn referred them to the NYU Child Study Center's Anxiety and Mood Disorders clinical service.

Background Information

On the basis of the ADIS-IV interviews and questionnaires described earlier, a full picture of Lisa's social anxiety disorder was pieced together, along with its resulting impairment in her life. Lisa was the younger of two girls born to the Gulars. Her older sister, at age 18, was described as a well-rounded young adult, who was "full of life" and had many friends. Lisa's prenatal development and birth were normal and without complications. All developmental milestones were met within normal limits; however, Lisa was described as a "clingy" baby who had difficulty staying with babysitters, even close family members such as her grandmother. Teresa mainly worked from home until Lisa turned 3, at which time the Gulars enrolled her in a small and "nurturing" nursery school. Lisa had much difficulty with separations each morning, and did not become comfortable with being left at the school until some 6 months into the year. For that reason, and because of the Gulars' full-time occupations (Teresa was an accountant; Alan, a stockbroker), Lisa stayed in nursery school throughout the year until she transitioned to kindergarten at a parochial school. This transition was again difficult and characterized by crying, sleep disturbance, clinging, and great difficulty in settling into the school routine.

During her early years, Lisa was described as "generally fearful" with multiple fears including the dark, separation situations, thunderstorms, and small animals. Lisa typically "shrank away" from meeting new people, both adults and children, and consequently the Gulars reportedly often refused invitations for getting together with friends and their families. Lisa preferred solitary activities, such as coloring by herself or reading in her room, but she enjoyed her sister Mary's company up until the time that Mary began having play dates with her peers. Although invited to join in, Lisa more often than not refused to participate in the girls' games and activities. Lisa and her parents reported her having two good friends from kindergarten all the way through the end of eighth grade. One of these girls was described as shy, and the other as just an average kid. Based on questions from the ADIS, Lisa reported having fewer friends than most kids her age, but wished that she could have more. Her parents concurred with her report on this issue. Lisa typically waited for friends to initiate a get-together and rarely did she call someone on the telephone. She preferred to play board games, do crafts, and watch television with her peers, as opposed to going out to movies or other activities. Lisa attended parties as a young child but did not want to host parties as time went on, and, ultimately, with the exception of her two friends, she was no longer invited to parties. Unfortunately, one of the girls moved out of town at the start of high school, but the other, the shy girl, attended high school with Lisa.

Lisa stayed in the same school from kindergarten through eighth grade. Her academic performance was described as "very good," a solid student who was self-directed in completing her homework, studying, and working on her projects. She was "always on time" with her assignments, rarely missed school except when she had the chicken pox or flu, and was described by her teachers as "a perfect student." However, one comment struck the Gulars as telling, although they did not realize it at the time. Lisa's third grade teacher reportedly said: "She is such a delight compared to the rowdy kids in my class . . . so much so that I often forget she is in the classroom." While the parents interpreted this comment as indicative of a polite and well-behaved child, the teacher was likely (without realizing it) identifying the early manifestation of SAD. Over time, teachers interspersed comments into their reports such as "Would like to see Lisa speak up in class" and "She writes so well, if only Lisa would join in the discussions with others." As the demands of academics increased over the years, with a greater emphasis on group projects and oral presentations, Lisa appeared to become more withdrawn. Although she transitioned to a larger parochial high school without complaints, Lisa did not enter with the typical adolescent angst and enthusiasm, nor did she come home from school with stories of the day's events.

Diagnostic questions and inquiries on the ADIS interviews revealed no evidence of any concurrent anxiety disorder; however, subclinical fears of thunderstorms and small animals were noted, probably leftover from earlier fears. The SAD sections of the ADIS were quite telling with regard to the degree of impairment and severity of Lisa's social anxieties. Lisa reported that she felt more anxious than other kids her age in social situations, so much so that she preferred to avoid most of these situations. Moreover, Lisa said that she had had these feelings "for as long as I can remember" and that "it's gotten worse over time." In response to inquiry, Lisa endorsed fears of looking foolish or embarrassing herself, and fears that others would laugh at her or reject her. She preferred solitary activity or small gatherings (one or two friends) to larger groups, and her familiar friends to meeting new people; she was equally uncomfortable with peers of all ages and adults. Lisa's parents concurred with her report.

During the ADIS interview, a list of social situations is presented to the adolescent and separately to the parents. Upon inquiry, Lisa endorsed moderate to severe fear (4 on a 0–8 scale) of most social situations, and also reported she would either avoid or prefer to avoid the situation. As can be seen in Table 6.3, Lisa's parents' ratings were similar to hers for most items, suggesting they had an awareness of her anxiety through observing her avoid situations and activities. Lisa reported that her social anxiety interfered with her life to a "very severe degree" and that she was making decisions about her future based on her social fears. For example, Lisa was reluctant to apply for a summer job because of fear of being rejected or having to deal with people she did not know well. Also, and more poi-

TABLE 6.3. Lisa's and Her Parents' Ratings of Fear and Avoidance for the ADIS-IV Social Situations List

Social situation	Lisa's fear rating[a]	Lisa's avoidance[b]	Parents' fear rating[c]	Parents' avoidance[c]
Answering questions in class	8	Yes	6	Yes
Giving an oral report or reading aloud in front of the class	8	Yes	5	Yes
Asking a teacher a question or for help	6	Yes	2	No
Taking tests	2	No	0	No
Writing on the chalkboard	8	Yes	0	No
Playing with a group of kids	7	Yes	8	Yes
Gym class	5	No	0	No
Walking in the hallways or hanging out by your locker	4	Yes	2	No
Starting or joining in on a conversation	8	Yes	5	No
Using public bathrooms	0	No	0	No
Eating in front of others	7	Yes	3	Yes
Meetings	8	Yes	0	No
Answering or talking on the telephone	6	Yes	7	Yes
Musical or athletic performances	4	Yes	2	No
Inviting a friend to get together	5	No	7	Yes
Speaking to adults	4	No	7	Yes
Talking to persons you don't know well	6	Yes	8	Yes
Attending parties, dances, or school activity nights	4	No	8	Yes
Having your picture taken	0	No	2	No
Dating	3	No	7	Yes
Saying no to something you really don't want to do	6	No	2	Yes
Asking someone to stop doing something you don't like	6	No	2	Yes

Note. ADIS-IV, Anxiety Disorders Interview Schedule for DSM-IV.
[a]Lisa's fear rating: 0–8 scale indicating increasing intensity of fear.
[b]Avoidance question: "Do you try to or would you like to avoid this situation?"
[c]Parents' fear rating and avoidance response are estimates of what they believe Lisa is experiencing.

gnant, Lisa did not think she would apply to college because "it will be just the same as elementary and high school with cliques and social demands."

In addition to the social anxiety, Lisa reported feeling sad more days than not, and feeling blue for most of the day. Although she described a slow and uneven progression of these feelings beginning roughly in sixth grade, with summers being times of relief to some degree but still a low mood, Lisa marked the start of high school as the initiation of a constant and steady depression. In addition to depressed mood, Lisa described a loss of interest in her hobbies and interests (e.g., listening to music), difficulty falling and staying asleep, loss of appetite, lack of energy, and a feeling that things will never get better for her. She reported crying often, but that she did this alone and in her room at night. Lisa denied any clear suicidal ideation or plan; however, she reported, "If these are supposed to be the best years of my life, how bad will it get after high school?" Not surprisingly, the Gulars were unaware of the degree and impact of Lisa's mood disturbance, with the exception of noting her change in appetite and energy.

Diagnostic Formulation and Treatment Recommendations

On the basis of the information obtained, Lisa met criteria for social anxiety disorder at a clinician severity rating (CSR) level of 6 (severely disturbing and disabling). The SAD was exerting a significant impact upon Lisa's ability to access positive reinforcement from her environment, become involved in learning and social tasks, and move forward in her development by meeting and mastering the various tasks of adolescence. So, for example, Lisa had not been able to formulate a self-identity beyond being a "loner," and she was unable to align with a peer group or garner social support from peers. Whereas most adolescents begin to exercise their desire for independence from the family, Lisa made no moves in this direction. Furthermore, she was unable to act upon her desires for dating or exploring romantic relationships, despite the flourishing of teenage romances all around her in school. The severity of her SAD would have been rated higher (CSR of 7 or 8) if Lisa had been compromised in her academic performance or was evidencing school refusal. Also, she did maintain a friendship with the one girl, and occasionally they did things together. Thus, she had the capacity to make and keep friends. But, to add insult to injury, most likely as a consequence of comparing herself to her sister's developmental and social paths, along with looking at same-age peers, Lisa was acutely aware of her limitations and losses. Thus, beginning in sixth grade with a dysthymic disorder, by ninth grade Lisa was in the throes of a full-blown major depressive disorder (MDD). Based on Lisa's and her parents' reports, along with clinical judgment, the MDD was rated as slightly less severe than the SAD and assigned a CSR of 4 (moderately disturbing/

disabling). The comorbidity of SAD and MDD is common in youth who have suffered for the long term with anxiety. Although Lisa may have met criteria for past diagnoses of separation anxiety disorder and specific phobias (e.g., dark, thunderstorms), she was fortunate not to be compromised even more by multiple anxiety diagnoses.

At the NYU Child Study Center, cognitive behavioral group therapy for adolescents with SAD (CBGT-A) was available for Lisa and considered to be the first-line treatment for addressing this condition. However, due to the severity of Lisa's SAD and the comorbid MDD, both individual CBT and pharmacotherapy were also given consideration. There were several options to present to the family in the feedback session described herein. These options were CBGT-A only, CBGT-A plus individual CBT, and either CBGT-A or individual CBT with the addition of pharmacotherapy. The rationales for these options are as follows. First, as noted in this chapter, SAD is highly amenable to treatment through CBT. The opportunity to access CBGT-A and profit from the therapy and social support offered in the group experience could provide Lisa with tools for managing her anxiety. Second, Lisa, although quiet and reserved, provided honest and open answers to the difficult questions posed during intake, indicating a good understanding of the nature of her difficulties and also a level of motivation to change that could facilitate a beneficial response to the psychosocial therapy. However, a third consideration and complicating factor was the comorbidity of the anxiety and depression. Lisa was still functioning well in school, despite these two clinical conditions, and this was a good sign. However, fairly significant symptoms were present for both SAD and MDD, with impairments noted in Lisa's social and familial functioning, along with ongoing vegetative disturbances from these disorders. If the MDD progressed, or even the social anxiety for that matter, a decline could push Lisa into a heightened sense of hopelessness. Also, the potential existed for the combined conditions to act synergistically to prevent Lisa from accessing a beneficial effect from CBGT-A. Thus, individual CBT to focus more specifically on Lisa's depression could be offered to run concurrently with the CBGT-A. In addition, given the nature of these comorbidities and their associated psychosocial and emotional impairments, concurrent treatment with a psychopharmacological agent had also to be considered. Medications, such as the selective serotonin reuptake inhibitors (SSRIs; e.g., fluvoxamine, sertraline, paroxetine, fluoxetine) or a nonspecific serotonin reuptake inhibitor (NSRI; e.g., venlafaxine), may exert broad effects on both the anxiety and depressive symptoms and have a quicker onset than the psychosocial treatment. Clinical psychopharmacological trials of these medications are demonstrating good efficacy in the treatment of SAD in youth (Compton et al., 2001; Mancini, Van Ameringen, Oakman, & Farvolden, 1999; RUPP Anxiety Study Group, 2001), with comparative outcome trials of medications and CBT underway (see Walkup & Ginsburg, 2002). The benefits, risks, and limitations of these treatment options were presented to the Gulars in the diagnostic feedback session.

Feedback Session

Following the diagnostic intake process, the feedback session is conducted and serves several purposes. The clinician meets briefly with the adolescent alone, and then the parents alone, to inquire about any information garnered from the adolescent or parent interviews that should not be shared between parties. This arrangement is set up prior to the start of the diagnostic process to protect the confidentiality of each family member. Our clinicians are careful and clear in outlining the limits of confidentiality as decreed by law and our code of ethical conduct. This brief individual time (approximately 12 minutes total) gives each family member the opportunity to set limits on information to be revealed in the feedback session and also to discuss any pertinent information they may have recalled after leaving the appointment. The family is then brought together and given an agenda for the feedback session. First, the results of the evaluation are presented. Second, questions and any clarification or misunderstanding from the interviews can be addressed. Third, the family's reactions to the findings and comments are solicited and processed. Next, treatment recommendations are offered and the rationale and empirical support for each is outlined. Finally, referrals are provided in addition to offering treatment at our facility, if available.

Lisa and her parents did not set any limits on talking openly about their responses to the intake evaluation. The description of the symptoms and impairment associated with SAD came as no surprise to the Gulars. However, Lisa's parents were caught unaware of the presence of the major depressive disorder, as they had been told that her mood, despite being different from her older sister's, "is typical of adolescents." The Gulars were perplexed by their inability to have recognized the degree of their daughter's distress. However, their guilt was allayed by discussing the difficulty that even trained mental health professionals may have in identifying both SAD and depression in youth. Moreover, it was explained that both these disorders, and most especially SAD, render youth "invisible" as compared to their same-age peers, who may monopolize a teacher's or parent's time with externalizing symptoms. The family was presented with the treatment options outlined earlier, and decided to proceed with CBGT-A as the sole treatment. In consultation with the diagnostician, the family agreed to set observable goals with the assigned therapist and to come to a consensus as to the amount of time that would seem reasonable and safe to let pass with the result of either (1) a reduction of anxiety and mood symptoms, in which case CBGT-A could continue alone, or (2) a rise in anxiety, depression, or the presence of suicidality, in which case medication and/or adjunctive individual treatment would be added to the regime. Lisa signed an agreement to reach out to her parents in the event that she began to experience a decline in her mood or the presence of any suicidal thoughts, and her parents signed this agreement to contact their local emergency room and/or our on-call staff in the event of any problems. The family agreed to begin CBGT-A, and, fortunately, a new adolescent group was to start in 2 weeks. In the meantime, Lisa met with the group therapists once per week to develop her goals for treatment and her individual fear hierarchy, and participated in two individual behavioral tests (giving an impromptu talk; engaging in a conversation with another girl).

Course of Treatment

The first two sessions of CBGT-A involved the adolescents and parents meeting together with the therapists. The group consisted of youth ages 13–16, with three boys and three girls. Lisa was quiet throughout these sessions, which is not unusual for most of the teenagers with SAD. The therapists noted that Lisa was attentive during the groups, that is, she appeared to listen and read from the flip chart as the therapists made notes during the sessions. However, she did not make eye contact with any of the group members or therapists, and kept her head bowed for the most part. Nevertheless, Lisa completed the small, written homework tasks assigned during these early sessions, a good prognostic indicator for her continued participation. Lisa had formulated several short-term goals, including being able to meet new people and invite friends to get together, in addition to wanting to attend school-related social events. These goals are designed with the help of the therapists and should be attainable during the course of the therapy. The Gulars' initial goals for Lisa were to "become more outgoing, learn to relax and enjoy herself, and make more friends." The therapists worked skillfully with the group to alert parents that broad, nonspecific goals would be difficult to achieve. Moreover, Lisa was noted to smile and appear relieved when the therapists assured the youth (in the presence of the parents) that this group was not going to change their personalities and make them into highly outgoing extraverts, but that the goal would be to teach them skills for freeing themselves from anxiety in order to make choices based on likes and dislikes, not fear. Thus, the Gulars revamped their goals to be more specific and obtainable, and consistent with Lisa's.

Cognitive restructuring was initiated with Session 3, and Lisa's homework forms revealed a host of negative, self-defeating thoughts in response to everyday social situations. For example, one entry revealed that one weekend day, upon boarding a train, she recognized a classmate sitting with an empty seat next to her. Rather than sit with the girl, Lisa wrote: "I've never really spoken to her before. I won't know what to say. She probably doesn't want to be bothered." In response to this situation, Lisa exited the train quickly and waited some 15 minutes for the next. Lisa learned that her thoughts raised her anxiety and resulted in a missed opportunity to test out the veracity of these statements. In addition, she reported feeling immediate relief from the anxiety in leaving the train, but then a feeling described as "remorse, sadness, and really feeling like a loser" throughout the remainder of the day. Thus, through the use of the homework diary, where the teens record events that occur along with their corresponding thoughts, anxiety ratings, and behavior, Lisa became aware of the cycle of anxiety and its short- and long-term impact. As the cognitive restructuring continued, Lisa learned to treat her thoughts as hypotheses to be tested, rather than as facts. Thus, she restructured her thoughts as such: "Well, I haven't really spoken to this girl before, but this is an opportunity to do so. If she doesn't talk to me, it could be for any number of reasons, including that she may be shy, too, or maybe she just needs to get to know me better over time."

During the social skills training modules, Lisa worked on improving her eye contact and speaking in a louder voice during conversations. In addition, she had a tendency to "hide" behind her hair by letting it hang in her face, so she was given the response prevention guideline to clip her hair back and away from her face. Lisa began answering questions in the group, first as she was called on by the therapists, and then spontaneously as the sessions progressed. The shaping of this type of behavior is purposeful on the part of the therapists, as they gradually increase the demands for participation as the group progresses in time. This behavior is ecologically valid, as it closely resembles the behavior necessary for participating in class discussions and other academic tasks. Moreover, it was noted that by Session 6 she was beginning to talk to another girl in the group while in the waiting room. Thus, Lisa was seen as making progress in her group participation.

Session 8 involved parents again, and there was a telling interaction between Lisa and her mother (her father could not attend). In the perspective-taking exercise, the adolescents and parents switch roles and work on a social anxiety related situation that has caused them stress or conflict. In this case, Lisa and her mother chose "saying hello to a family friend in a public place." Apparently, Lisa's tendency was to look away or down and minimally whisper a hello when confronted by this situation, such as in a restaurant. During the interaction, while Teresa looked down and failed to respond to the therapist playing the friend, Lisa reached over and pinched her mother on the arm, causing her mother to break from character and yell "ouch!" Lisa and her mother agreed that this was exactly the sequence of events that would occur, yet her mother did not realize that she often pinched her daughter and caused discomfort. Thus, a better understanding of Lisa's anxiety, her mother's frustration, and the underlying conflict that existed in these situations was brought to light. Lisa and her mother agreed to discuss which situations are tough for her, what she could try to do differently, and how her mother could monitor her own impulses and feelings when her daughter struggles with anxiety.

The exposure phase of treatment involved 12 sessions, allowing Lisa the opportunity to be the focus of an exposure four times, but also to be a role player in six other exposures. Exposures involve a prescribed series of steps led by the therapists:

1. The chosen adolescent, in this case Lisa, picks an item from her hierarchy and specifies it clearly: "Having a conversation with someone I know from class." This involves specifying where and when this would occur, and for Lisa this meant speaking to someone in the classroom, before class began.
2. The therapist then lead Lisa in defining clear, observable goals for the exposure: "I will make eye contact for most of the time; I will speak in a clear voice and at a volume that is loud enough to hear; I will ask her two questions."
3. Lisa was then asked to describe any automatic thoughts that she would have in the situation and, with the aid of the other group members, to develop rational responses to these thoughts. For example, for the thought "I won't know what to say," the rationale response of "I'm only responsible for half of the conversation" was found to be very useful by Lisa. After specifying these thoughts and responses, Lisa then chose a rational response to repeat to herself during the exposure.

After a pre-exposure rating was taken on the Subjective Units of Distress Scale (SUDS; from 0–100), the exposure was then conducted for 10 minutes, with additional SUDS ratings taken at 1-minute intervals. Therapists kept track of the SUDS ratings, the time, and whether Lisa was meeting her goals. Figure 6.1 presents Lisa's SUDS ratings over the course of this first exposure. As is typical with youth, Lisa's anticipatory anxiety (pre-rating) was high, but it also escalated at the initiation of the exposure. However, as shown in the figure, with the aid of cognitive restructuring and by staying in the situation that she ordinarily would avoid, her SUDS ratings dropped over the 10-minute exposure. By Lisa's fourth exposure, a much more challenging task, she was evidencing less anticipatory anxiety and a much quicker and dramatic drop in anxiety ratings (Figure 6.2). This was likely due to a number of factors. All teens are assigned the exposure situation practiced in the group as homework to be attempted a minimum of three times prior to the next session. Thus, Lisa had to initiate conversations with familiar peers at least three times during the week, but she was given the guideline not to use her one friend for this homework. Also, Lisa was chosen over time to serve as a role player for other exposures, thus

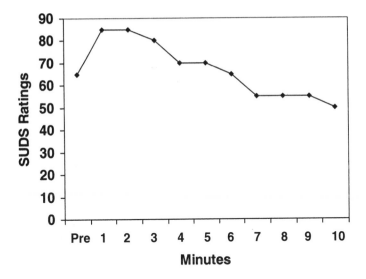

FIGURE 6.1. Lisa's first within-session exposure ratings: Having a conversation with someone I know from class.

gaining more experience in talking to and in front of peers and adults. Finally, as the exposures continued, Lisa was challenged with more difficult situations, as seen in Figure 6.2, giving her the opportunity to improve upon her skills and gather more information to refute her negative predictions and self-defeating thoughts.

Therapists and teens process the results of each exposure, examining whether goals were reached and SUDS decreased, and if not, why. Lisa did at times "get stuck," so that her SUDS did not decrease or a goal was not achieved. At these times she was able to identify negative thoughts "creeping in" during the exposure, such as the thought that "this is not real, just practice, so I won't be able to do this for real at school." These thoughts were challenged by the therapists through cognitive restructuring and by devising behavioral experiments to test these beliefs in the school setting.

Relapse Prevention

CBGT-A involves several relapse prevention strategies including fading of sessions (Sessions 17–20 occur every other week) and the inclusion of parents in the next-to-last session. In addition, we have added the "Mission Is Possible" task, which consists of exposures conducted in local community settings such as bookstores, cafes, and other public places. The following is Lisa's "Mission Is Possible" task.

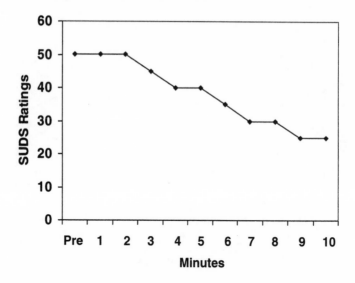

FIGURE 6.2. Lisa's fourth within-session exposure ratings: Initiating a conversation with someone I've never met before.

LISA:

Your mission today, should you decide to accept it (and you'd be avoiding if you didn't!), is to go with us to Borders Bookstore and practice some of your hierarchy items around real people. We would like you to practice a few things *on your own*.

1. We're going to have you continue to practice walking around in front of others like we did last week, only this time you're going to be off on your own instead of with the group of us. Make a note of whether or not people take notice of you and then how they do so. At one point during the exercise, when there are people around you, accidentally (on purpose) *drop a book on the floor* and see how people react.

2. Go to the café in Borders and order something to eat, and then go sit *by yourself* at a table. Take note of how it feels for you to be sitting alone among a group of strangers. By the way, if there are no seats left at the café, there are usually big couches around for people to sit and eat and read. You can go to one of those instead. Just try to be around other customers (non–group members). If you don't have any money on you, see Dr. Albano and she'll give you some.

PLAN TO HEAD BACK TO THE CHILD STUDY CENTER AT 6:30 SO WE CAN DISCUSS HOW THINGS WENT FOR EVERYBODY.

Lisa was successfully engaging in conversations with peers at school and comfortably entering situations that were formerly challenging, such as social events sponsored by the school. Her anxiety continued; however, she reported using her cognitive skills to work through her anxiety in advance and prepare an exposure plan in her mind for the situation. For example, prior to going to a school dance, Lisa, who had never attended a dance before, rehearsed in her mind and also used her group worksheets to outline her goals, examine and challenge her thoughts, and give herself specific structure, such as to plan on staying a minimum of 1 hour, but with the option to stay longer if she wished. Lisa also participated in later groups as a role player for other youth and reported that these experiences helped her to maintain her gains. At the end of treatment, Lisa was reporting the absence of any depressive symptoms and a steady decline in her anxiety. Further evaluation at 6 and 12 months posttreatment revealed no evidence of clinical levels of social anxiety (see Table 6.4). It is interesting to note that both Lisa's and her parents' ratings of her avoidance, on the weekly fear and avoidance hierarchy, were initially higher than the fear ratings, but dropped more dramatically on postevaluation and follow-up. This is a common finding, in that behavioral change will precede the change in emotion or cognition for some youth. Thus, Lisa may still have reported some fear in social situations, but she was pushing herself to enter and master these situations. Her parents noted this pattern by observing what she was doing, as opposed to what she did not do, in her daily life. Lisa's parents concurred with her overall report and were quite pleased with her response to treatment.

CONCLUSION

Social anxiety disorder is a common and often chronic condition warranting serious attention by clinicians and researchers. With onset in late childhood, social anxiety disorder interferes with friendships, academics, and meeting critical developmental tasks. Left untreated, the consequences of social anxiety disorder are far-reaching in adulthood, and result in serious compromises to an individual's ability to live independently and to his or her full potential. Fortunately, the field has advanced such that sensitive and specific assessment tools are available to distinguish social anxiety disorder from other conditions and more benign personality types, such as shyness. Cognitive-behavioral therapy has demonstrated good response for those youth who participate in either individualized treatments or more specialized social anxiety groups. In addition, certain pharmacological agents have proven effective in managing this anxiety disorder, and when used in combination with CBT may prove quite helpful to those youth with

TABLE 6.4. Pre, Post, and Follow-Up Data for Lisa

Measure	Pretreatment	Posttreatment	6-month follow-up	12-month follow-up
ADIS diagnoses (Composite of teen and parent report)	Social phobia CSR = 6 Major depression CSR = 4	Social phobia = 4 MDD = 2	Social phobia = 2 MDD = Full remission	Social phobia = Full remission MDD = Full remission
Mean Fear Score for 10-item FAH—Lisa's report	7.0	4.5	3.0	3.0
Mean Avoidance Score for FAH—Lisa's report	7.5	3.5	2.5	1.0
Mean Fear Score for 10-item FAH—parents' report	6.0	4.0	2.0	2.0
Mean Avoidance Score for 10-item FAH—parents' report	8.0	4.0	2.0	0.0

Note. ADIS, Anxiety Disorders Interview Schedule; CSR, Clinician Severity Rating; MDD, major depressive disorder; FAH, Fear and Avoidance Hierarchy.

serious disabilities and complex clinical pictures that would be resistant to CBT alone. Overall, the advances in the treatments of social anxiety disorder, as evidenced by the case description of Lisa, give hope to many youth who suffer in silence for the potential to master this anxiety and lead a full and productive life.

REFERENCES

Achenbach, T. M. (1991). *Manual for the Child Behavior Checklist 4–18 and 1991 Profile*. Burlington: Department of Psychiatry, University of Vermont.

Achenbach, T. M., & Edelbrock, C. (1983). *Manual for the Child Behavior Checklist and Revised Child Behavior Profile*. Burlington: Department of Psychiatry, University of Vermont.

Albano, A. M. (1995). Treatment of social anxiety in adolescents. *Cognitive and Behavioral Practice, 2*, 271–298.

Albano, A. M., & Barlow, D. H. (1996). Breaking the vicious cycle: Cognitive behavioral group treatment for socially anxious youth. In E. D. Hibbs & P. S. Jensen (Eds.), *Psychosocial treatments for child and adolescent disorders: Empirically based strategies for clinical practice* (pp. 43–62). Washington, DC: American Psychological Association.

Albano, A. M., Chorpita, B. F., & Barlow, D. H. (2003). Anxiety disorders. In E. J. Mash & R. A. Barkley (Eds.), *Child psychopathology* (2nd ed., pp. 279–329). New York: Guilford Press.

Albano, A. M., Logsdon-Conradsen, S., & Barlow, D. H. (1999, March). *Verbal interactions of social phobic adolescents and their parents: Evidence for the FEAR effect.* In M. Patterson & S. Tracey (Chairs), Social phobia in youth. Symposium presented at the Anxiety Disorders Association of America, San Diego, CA.

Albano, A. M., Marten, P. A., Holt, C. S., Heimberg, R. G., & Barlow, D. H. (1995). Cognitive-behavioral group treatment for social phobia in adolescents: A preliminary study. *Journal of Nervous and Mental Disease, 183,* 685–692.

American Psychiatric Association. (1980). *Diagnostic and statistical manual of mental disorders* (3rd ed.). Washington, DC: Author.

American Psychiatric Association. (1994). *Diagnostic and statistical manual of mental disorders* (4th ed.). Washington, DC: Author.

Barlow, D. H. (2002). *Anxiety and its disorders* (2nd ed.). New York: Guilford Press.

Barrett, P., Dadds, M., & Rapee, R. (1996). Family treatment of childhood anxiety: A controlled trial. *Journal of Consulting and Clinical Psychology, 64,* 333–342.

Barrett, P., Rapee, R., Dadds, M., & Ryan, A. (1996). Family enhancement of cognitive style in anxious and aggressive children. *Journal of Abnormal Child Psychology, 24,* 187–203.

Barrios, B. A., & Hartmann, D. P. (1997). Fears and anxieties. In E. J. Mash & L. G. Terdal (Eds.), *Behavioral assessment of childhood disorders* (2nd ed., pp. 249–337). New York: Guilford Press.

Beidel, D. C. (1991). Social phobia and overanxious disorder in school-age children. *Journal of the American Academy of Child and Adolescent Psychiatry, 30,* 545–552.

Beidel, D. C., & Turner, S. M. (1998). *Shy children, phobic adults: Nature and treatment of social phobia.* Washington, DC: American Psychological Association.

Beidel, D. C., Turner, S. M., & Morris, T. L. (1995). A new inventory to assess childhood social anxiety and phobia: The Social Phobia and Anxiety Inventory for Children. *Psychological Assessment, 7,* 73–79.

Beidel, D. C., Turner, S. M., & Morris, T. L. (1999). Psychopathology of childhood social phobia. *Journal of the American Academy of Child and Adolescent Psychiatry, 38,* 643–650.

Beidel, D. C., Turner, S. M., & Morris, T. L. (2000). Behavioral treatment of childhood social phobia. *Journal of Consulting and Clinical Psychology, 68,* 1072–1080.

Brady, E., & Kendall, P. C. (1992). Comorbidity of anxiety and depression in children and adolescents. *Psychological Bulletin, 111,* 244–255.

Chorpita, B. F., Albano, A. M., & Barlow, D. H. (1996). Cognitive processing in children: Relation to anxiety and family influences. *Journal of Clinical Child Psychology, 25,* 170–176.

Compton, S. N., Grant, P. J., Chrisman, A. K., Gammon, P. J., Brown, V. L., & March, J. S. (2001). Sertraline in children and adolescents with social anxiety disorder: An open trial. *Journal of the American Academy of Child and Adolescent Psychiatry, 40,* 564–571.

Costello, E. J., & Angold, A. (1995). Epidemiology in anxiety disorders in children and adolescents. In J. S. March (Ed.), *Anxiety disorders in children and adolescents* (pp. 109–124). New York: Guilford Press.

Dadds, M. R., Heard, P. M., Rapee, R. M. (1992). The role of family intervention in the treatment of child anxiety disorders: Some preliminary findings. *Behaviour Change, 9,* 171–177.

Dierker, L., Albano, A. M., Clarke, G. N., Heimberg, R. G., Kendall, P. C., Merikangas, K. R., Lewinsohn, P. M., Offord, D. R., Kessler, R., & Kupfer, D. J. (2001). Screening for anxiety and depression in early adolescence. *Journal of the American Academy of Child and Adolescent Psychiatry, 40,* 929–936.

DiNardo, P. A., O'Brien, G. T., Barlow, D. H., Waddell, M. T., & Blanchard, E. B. (1983). Reliability of the DMS-III anxiety disorder categories using a new structured interview. *Archives of General Psychiatry, 40,* 1070–1074.

Ferdinand, R. F., & Verhulst, F. C. (1995). Psychopathology from adolescence into young adulthood: An 8-year follow-up study. *American Journal of Psychiatry, 152,* 586–594.

Ginsberg, G., La Greca, A. M., & Silverman, W. K. (1997a, November). *Social anxiety among children with anxiety disorders: Relation with social functioning.* Paper presented at the annual meeting of the Association for the Advancement of Behavior Therapy, Miami Beach, FL.

Ginsberg, G., La Greca, A. M., & Silverman, W. K. (1997b, November). *The Social Anxiety Scale for Adolescents (SAS-A): Utility for youth with anxiety disorders.* Paper presented at the annual meeting of the Association for the Advancement of Behavior Therapy, Miami Beach, FL.

Hayward, C., Killen, J., Kraemer, H., & Taylor, C. (1998). Linking self-reported childhood behavioral inhibition to adolescent social phobia. *Journal of the American Academy of Child and Adolescent Psychiatry, 37,* 1308–1316.

Hayward, C., Varady, S., Albano, A. M., Thieneman, M., Henderson, L., & Schatzberg, A. F. (2000). Cognitive behavioral group therapy for female socially phobic adolescents: Results of a pilot study. *Journal of the American Academy of Child and Adolescent Psychiatry, 39,* 721–726.

Heimberg, R. G., Dodge, C. S., Hope, D. A., Kennedy, C. R., & Zollo, L. J. (1990). Cognitive behavioral group treatment for social phobia: Comparison with a credible placebo control. *Cognitive Therapy and Research, 14,* 1–23.

Heimberg, R. G., Liebowitz, M., Hope, D. A., & Schneier, F. R. (Eds.) (1995). *Social phobia: Diagnosis, assessment, and treatment.* New York: Guilford Press.

Heimberg, R. G., Salaman, D. G., Holt, C. S., & Blendell, K. A. (1993). Cognitive-behavioral group treatment for social phobia: Effectiveness at five-year follow-up. *Cognitive Therapy and Research, 17,* 325–339.

Hofmann, S., Albano, A. M., Heimberg, R. G., Tracey, S., Chorpita, B. F., & Barlow, D. H. (1999). Subtypes of social phobia in adolescents. *Depression and Anxiety, 9,* 8–15.

Kazdin, A. E., & Weisz, J. R. (1998). Identifying and developing empirically supported child and adolescent treatments. *Journal of Consulting and Clinical Psychology, 66,* 19–36.

Kearney, C. A. (2001). *School refusal behavior.* Washington, DC: American Psychological Association.

Kearney, C. A., & Albano, A. M. (2000). *When children refuse school: A therapist's manual.* San Antonio, TX: Psychological Corporation.

Kearney, C. A., & Silverman, W. K. (1993). Measuring the function of school refusal behavior: The School Refusal Assessment Scale. *Journal of Clinical Child Psychology, 22*, 85–96.

Kendall, P. C. (1992). Childhood coping: Avoiding a lifetime of anxiety. *Behaviour Change, 9*, 229–237.

Kendall, P. C. (1994). Treating anxiety disorders in children: Results of a randomized clinical trial. *Journal of Consulting and Clinical Psychology, 62*, 100–110.

Kendall, P. C., Flannery-Schroeder, E., Panicelli-Mindel, S. M., Southam-Gerow, M. A., Henin, A., & Warman, M. (1997). Therapy for youths with anxiety disorders: A second randomized clinical trial. *Journal of Consulting and Clinical Psychology, 65*, 366–380.

Kendall, P. C., & Southam-Gerow, M. A. (1996). Long-term follow-up of a cognitive behavioral therapy for anxiety disordered youth. *Journal of Consulting and Clinical Psychology, 64*, 724–730.

Kessler, R. C., Foster, C. L., Saunders, W. B., & Stang, P. E. (1995). Social consequences of psychiatric disorders: I. Educational attainment. *American Journal of Psychiatry, 152*, 1026–1032.

Kessler, R. C., & Frank, R. G. (1997). The impact of psychiatric disorders on work loss days. *Psychological Medicine, 27*, 861–873.

Kessler, R. C., McGonagle, K., Zhao, S., Nelson, C. B., Hughes, M., Eshleman, S., Wittchen, H. U., & Kendler, K. S. (1994). Lifetime and 12-month prevalence of DSM-III-R psychiatric disorders in the United States. *Archives of General Psychiatry, 51*, 8–19.

LaGreca, A. M. (1998). *Social anxiety scales for children and adolescents: Manual and instructions for the SASC, SASC-R, SAS-A and parent versions of the scales.* Unpublished manuscript available from the author. University of Miami, Coral Gables, FL.

La Greca, A. M. (2001). Friends or foes? Peer influences on anxiety among children and adolescents. In W. K. Silverman & P. Treffers (Eds.), *Anxiety disorders in children and adolescents* (pp. 159–186). New York: Cambridge University Press.

La Greca, A. M., & Stone, W. L. (1993). Social Anxiety Scale for Children—Revised: Factor structure and concurrent validity. *Journal of Clinical Child Psychology, 22*, 17–27.

Liebowitz, M. R., Gorman, J. M., Fyer, A. J., & Klein, D. F. (1985). Social phobia: Review of a neglected anxiety disorder. *Archives of General Psychiatry, 42*, 729–735.

Logsdon-Conradson, S. (1998). *Family interaction patterns in adolescents with social phobia.* Unpublished doctoral dissertation, University of Louisville, Louisville, KY.

Mancini, C., Van Ameringen, M., Oakman, J., & Farvolden, P. (1999). Serotonergic agents in the treatment of social phobia in children and adolescents: A case series. *Depression and Anxiety, 10*, 33–39.

March, J. (1998). *Manual for the Multidimensional Anxiety Scale for Children (MASC).* Toronto: MultiHealth Systems.

March, J. S., & Albano, A. M. (1998). Advances in the assessment of pediatric anxiety disorders. *Advances in Clinical Child Psychology, 20*, 213–241.

March, J. S., Parker, J. D. A., Sullivan, K., Stallings, P., & Conners, K. (1997). The Multidimensional Anxiety Scale for Children (MASC): Factor structure, reliability, and validity. *Journal of the American Academy of Child and Adolescent Psychiatry, 36,* 554–565.

Mendlowitz, S. L., Manassis, K., Bradley, S., Scapillato, D., Miezitis, S., & Shaw, B. F. (1999). Cognitive-behavioral group treatments in childhood anxiety disorders: The role of parental involvement. *Journal of the American Academy of Child and Adolescent Psychiatry, 38,* 1223–1229.

Ollendick, T. H. (1983). Reliability and validity of the revised Fear Survey Schedule for Children (FSSC-R). *Behaviour Research and Therapy, 21,* 395–399.

Ollendick, T. H., & King, N. J. (1998). Empirically supported treatments for children with phobic and anxiety disorders. *Journal of Clinical Child Psychology, 27,* 156–167.

Rosenbaum, J. F., Biederman, J., Hirshfeld, D. R., Bolduc, E. A., & Chaloff, J. (1991). Behavioral inhibition in children: A possible precursor to panic disorder or social phobia. *Journal of Clinical Psychiatry, 52,* 5–9.

RUPP Anxiety Study Group (2001). Fluvoxamine for the treatment of anxiety disorders in children and adolescents. *New England Journal of Medicine, 344,* 1279–1285.

Silverman, W. K. (1991). Diagnostic reliability of anxiety disorders in children using structured interviews. [Special issue: Assessment of childhood anxiety disorders.] *Journal of Anxiety Disorders, 5,* 105–124.

Silverman, W. K., & Albano, A. M. (1996). *The Anxiety Disorders Interview Schedule for DSM-IV—Child and parent versions.* San Antonio, TX: Graywind Publications (division of The Psychological Corp.).

Silverman, W. K., & Eisen, A. R. (1992). Age differences in the reliability of parent and child reports of child anxious symptomatology using a structured interview. *Journal of the American Academy of Child and Adolescent Psychiatry, 31,* 117–124.

Silverman, W. K., Kurtines, W. M., Ginsburg, G. S., Weems, C. F., Lumpkin, P., White, C., & Hicks, D. (1999a). Treating anxiety disorders in children with group cognitive-behavioral therapy: A randomized clinical trial. *Journal of Consulting and Clinical Psychology, 67,* 995–1003.

Silverman, W. K., Kurtines, W. M., Ginsburg, G. S., Weems, C. F., Rabian, B., & Serafini, L. T. (1999b) Contingency management, self-control, and education support in the treatment of childhood phobic disorders: A randomized clinical trial. *Journal of Consulting and Clinical Psychology, 67,* 675–687.

Silverman, W. K., & Nelles, W. B. (1988). The Anxiety Disorders Interview Schedule for Children. *Journal of the American Academy of Child and Adolescent Psychiatry, 27,* 772–778.

Silverman, W. K., Saavedra, L. M., & Pina, A. A. (2001). Test–retest reliability of anxiety symptoms and diagnoses with the Anxiety Disorders Interview Schedule for DSM-IV: Child and parent versions. *Journal of the American Academy of Child and Adolescent Psychiatry, 40,* 937–944.

Spence, S. H., Donovan, C., & Brechman-Toussaint, M. (2000). The treatment of childhood social phobia: The effectiveness of a social skills training-based, cognitive-behavioural intervention, with and without parental involvement. *Journal of Child Psychology and Psychiatry, 41,* 713–726.

Stallings, P., & March, J. S. (1995). Assessment. In J. S. March (Ed.), *Anxiety disorders in children and adolescents* (pp. 125–147). New York: Guilford Press.

Vasey, M. W. (1995). Social anxiety disorders. In A. R. Eisen, C. A. Kearney, & C. A. Schaefer (Eds.), *Clinical handbook of anxiety disorders in children and adolescents* (pp. 131–168). Northvale, NJ: Jason Aronson.

Vasey, M. W., & Dadds, M. R. (Eds.). (2001). *The developmental psychopathology of anxiety.* New York: Oxford University Press.

Velting, O. N., & Albano, A. M. (2001). Current trends in the understanding and treatment of social phobia in youth. *The Journal of Child Psychology and Psychiatry and Allied Disciplines, 42,* 127–140.

Walkup, J., & Ginsburg, G. (Guest Eds.). (2002). Anxiety disorders in children and adolescents. *International Review of Psychiatry.*

Wittchen, H. U., Stein, M., & Kessler, R. (1999). Social fears and social phobia in a community sample of adolescents and young adults: Prevalence, risk factors, and comorbidity. *Psychological Medicine, 29,* 309–323.

SUGGESTED READINGS

Albano, A. M. (1995). Treatment of social anxiety in adolescents. *Cognitive and Behavioral Practice, 2,* 271–298.

Beidel, D. C., & Turner, S. M. (1998). *Shy children, phobic adults: Nature and treatment of social phobia.* Washington, DC: American Psychological Association.

Hofmann, S. G., & DiBartolo, P. M. (Eds.). (2001). *Social phobia and social anxiety: An integration.* New York: Plenum Press.

Velting, O. N., & Albano, A. M. (2001). Current trends in the understanding and treatment of social phobia in youth. *Journal of Child Psychology and Psychiatry, 42,* 127–140.

7

Treatment of Obsessive– Compulsive Disorder

MARTIN E. FRANKLIN
MOIRA RYNN
EDNA B. FOA
JOHN S. MARCH

Pediatric obsessive–compulsive disorder (OCD) has been the subject of increased scientific investigation and mass media attention alike in the last 10 years. Once believed to be extremely rare, the disorder is now thought to affect about 1 in 200 children and adolescents in the United States (Flament et al., 1988; Valleni-Basille et al., 1994). The efficacy of cognitive-behavioral therapy (CBT) involving exposure and ritual prevention (EX/RP) and pharmacotherapy with serotonin reuptake inhibitors (SRIs) is now well established for adult OCD (for reviews, see Franklin & Foa, 1998; Pigott & Seay, 1998), yet fewer data are available regarding treatment of pediatric OCD. Similarity in clinical presentation between pediatric and adult OCD (Swedo, Rapoport, Leonard, Lenane, & Chelsow, 1989) suggests that effective treatment for adults may also be helpful for children and adolescents, but controlled outcome trials involving younger samples must be conducted before strong conclusions can be drawn. Generally speaking, the pharmacotherapy treatment outcome literature for pediatric OCD is more advanced than is the CBT literature, although several controlled trials of CBT are currently under way.

In this chapter we review briefly the extant literature on pediatric OCD treatment, then present clinical case material designed to illustrate how to conduct CBT for children and adolescents. We have chosen to include material from several different OCD patients, as age of the child in treatment and OCD subtype require so much tailoring that a single case

162

may not do justice to the varied clinical problems likely to be encountered by therapists treating pediatric OCD. Case material presented is derived from composite cases, a method that provides additional protections against breach of confidentiality and allows for more in-depth discussion of clinical issues than would typically be seen in a single case.

THEORETICAL FOUNDATIONS

As is often the case in pediatric psychology and psychiatry, the theoretical conceptualization and hence the rationale for treatment for pediatric OCD is built largely upon research conducted with adults. When developmental differences between adults and children, such as ability to introspect, are taken into account, there appears to be a great deal of formal similarity in OCD presentations across the developmental spectrum, which further justifies the extrapolation. Thus, Mowrer's (1939, 1960) two-factor theory, which posits that obsessions give rise to anxiety and compulsions and other avoidance behaviors reduce and thereby maintain it, is thought to be applicable to pediatric as well as adult OCD. A behavioral rationale for exposure and ritual prevention follows logically from this conceptualization of the disorder: If rituals can be successfully blocked, their negative reinforcing properties will be reduced and the obsessional symptoms necessarily will be decreased.

The same dissatisfaction with two-factor theory as an explanation for the etiology of obsessions that led to cognitive theories of adult OCD is also now evident with respect to causal factors in pediatric OCD. Recent studies have indicated that cognitive factors thought to be involved in adult disorders are also present in pediatric clinical samples suffering from those disorders (e.g., elevated probability and cost ratings for social situations in social anxiety disorder; Rheingold, Herbert, & Franklin, 2002), yet no research has been done in OCD to establish that cognitive factors thought to be of relevance in adult OCD—such as elevated sense of responsibility, thought suppression, and thought–action fusion (e.g., Clark, 1999; Salkovskis, 1996)—are also present in younger sufferers. Nevertheless, most modern conceptualizations of OCD and the effects of exposure-based treatments emphasize the importance of changing erroneous beliefs (e.g., Foa & Kozak, 1985, 1986); treatments derived from these information-processing approaches are consistent with the use of informal cognitive procedures to augment exposure. The specific relevance of these conceptualizations and associated treatment methods to very young children with OCD remains to be seen. Biological studies, such as those conducted by Baxter and colleagues (e.g., 1992) with adult OCD, have yet to be attempted with younger samples. The interrelationship between biological and cognitive-behavioral accounts of OCD will undoubtedly be an area of careful study in the next decade, and, ideally, will provide us with greater knowledge of the disorder that will facilitate both treatment and prevention efforts.

TREATMENT OUTCOME IN PEDIATRIC OBSESSIVE–COMPULSIVE DISORDER

In keeping with the logic described earlier with respect to theoretical conceptualizations of adult and pediatric OCD, researchers have conducted several "age-downward extension" treatment studies in pediatric OCD that adjust the treatments of established efficacy in adults for developmental differences. Three controlled studies with children and adolescents have evaluated the efficacy of clomipramine (CMI; DeVeaugh-Geiss et al., 1992; Flament et al., 1985; Leonard et al., 1989), a tricyclic antidepressant that inhibits serotonin reuptake but also affects other neurotransmitter systems (e.g., DeVeaugh-Geiss, Landau, & Katz, 1989). In the largest of these pediatric CMI studies, DeVeaugh-Geiss and colleagues (1992) found a mean 37% reduction on the Children's Yale–Brown Obsessive Compulsive Scale (CY-BOCS) for CMI versus 8% for placebo in a pediatric OCD sample, which is remarkably consistent with findings from the multicenter adult CMI study (DeVeaugh-Geiss et al., 1989). Thus, CMI is superior to placebo, produces partial symptom reduction on average, and yields similar results in adults and children.

Despite evidence for the efficacy of CMI, the *selective* SRIs (SSRIs; fluoxetine, fluvoxamine, sertraline, and paroxetine) are more typically used as a first-line treatment of pediatric OCD in clinical practice. This is likely due to their generally more favorable side-effect profile in comparison to that of CMI (March, Frances, Kahn, & Carpenter, 1997). Several SSRIs have been found effective for children and adolescents with OCD in controlled studies. Fluoxetine was found superior to placebo in a double-blind, placebo-controlled, crossover study (Riddle et al., 1992). In the largest pediatric OCD placebo-controlled study conducted to date, sertraline was also found superior to placebo (March et al., 1998). Two other recently completed multicenter studies suggest that fluoxetine (Geller et al., 2001) and fluvoxamine (Riddle et al., 2001) are also superior to placebo for pediatric OCD. Notably, no study has directly compared the efficacy of one SRI versus another using a pediatric OCD sample, nor are such studies common in the adult literature. On the whole, it appears that CMI and the SSRIs are effective treatments for pediatric OCD, with no clear superiority of a particular compound (March et al., 1998).

The short-term efficacy of SRIs relative to placebo having been established, several caveats about pharmacotherapy for pediatric OCD need to be underscored. Mean CY-BOCS reductions from the controlled studies described earlier range from 31% to 44%, suggesting that most patients have residual OCD symptoms following treatment, and approximately one-third of pediatric OCD patients fail to respond at all to a particular SRI (DeVeaugh-Geiss et al., 1992). Relapse following CMI withdrawal was almost universal in a small pediatric OCD sample, indicating that maintenance treatment is necessary (Leonard et al., 1991); the rate of relapse upon SSRI discontinuation has yet to be established in children. Thus, pharmacotherapy appears to be far from a completely or universally effective form of treatment for pediatric OCD, and the need to develop alternative or augmentative treatments remains apparent.

As mentioned earlier, the CBT literature in pediatric OCD is less well developed than the pharmacotherapy literature. The literature is comprised primarily of case studies, small open trials largely involving samples that were receiving concomitant pharmacotherapy with SRIs, and one direct randomized comparison with pharmacotherapy. March, Mulle, and Herbel (1994) found a mean posttreatment CY-BOCS reduction of 50% in 15 children and adolescents following a CBT program that included psychoeducation, cognitive training, EX/RP, and anxiety management training (AMT); all but one child received concurrent pharmacotherapy with an SRI. In a second examination of this protocol, 14 children and adolescents treated with CBT involving EX/RP evidenced a mean 67% and 62% CY-BOCS reduction at posttreatment and at follow-up, respectively (Franklin et al., 1998). In the largest of the published open trials involving CBT for juvenile OCD, Wever and Rey (1997) reported a mean posttreatment CY-BOCS reduction of 68% in 57 children and adolescents who received CBT and concomitant pharmacotherapy. DeHaan and colleagues (deHaan, Hoogduin, Buitelaar, & Keijsers, 1998) randomly assigned pediatric patients to treatment with CBT or CMI, and found that CBT was superior to CMI in reducing OCD symptoms as measured by the CY-BOCS. Collectively these findings are encouraging, yet much more empirical research is needed before definitive conclusions can be drawn about the relative and combined efficacy of CBT and pharmacotherapy for pediatric OCD. In the interim, clinical decision making regarding CBT for children and adolescents is guided by the few studies mentioned earlier, case study data (for a review, see March, 1995), and expert consensus (March, Parker, Sullivan, Stalling, & Conners, 1997), as well as the extensive adult EX/RP treatment outcome literature. Notably, controlled studies are currently under way that will examine the relative efficacy of CBT, sertraline, and their combination (Pediatric OCD Collaborative Study Group, 2001), and the relative efficacy of CBT versus a psychosocial control condition.

In speaking with children and their parents about the treatment alternatives currently available for pediatric OCD, we typically share with them findings from the controlled and uncontrolled studies reviewed earlier so that they are well informed prior to making a treatment decision. We describe to the family what we do know from this literature, while at the same time openly discussing what we do not know. In addition we discuss what we have learned in the clinical setting about these treatments, and try to help each family arrive at a decision about clinical services that matches their needs and their child's readiness to work on the OCD. We emphasize that CBT will take a considerable amount of effort on the part of the patient and the family, and by definition require the ability to tolerate anxiety in the short run in order to reduce anxiety in the long run. Children who are adamantly opposed to experiencing any anxiety in the treatment context or taking any risks of their feared consequences occurring may not be good candidates for CBT, as acceptance of these conditions is an essential part of doing CBT.

COGNITIVE-BEHAVIORAL THERAPY PROTOCOL

The CBT program that we typically employ was published as a book by March and Mulle in 1998 (see Table 7.1 for visit summary). In the context of the randomized controlled outcome study we are currently conducting, this program has been adapted for research purposes to include 14 sessions over 12 weeks in Phase I. Phase II consists of four monthly follow-up sessions for patients who responded to EX/RP or to combination treatment (Pediatric OCD Collaborative Study Group, 2001). Typically we treat children and adolescents using this protocol with this visit schedule; however, in some cases we adapt the treatment from its once-weekly format to a daily intensive regimen, depending in large part on the particulars of the case. For example, weekly treatment may be more easily accommodated by busy families during the school year, whereas parents from out of the region seeking expert help may prefer a more intensive schedule. Clinical factors also come into play: A child with extremely severe OCD might be better served by frequent visits, especially if between-session compliance with EX/RP proves to be less than optimal. Preliminary evidence suggests that the visit schedule was not associated with outcome in pediatric OCD (Franklin et al., 1998) and adult OCD (Abramowitz, Foa, & Franklin, 2003), but this awaits confirmation in controlled trials involving random assignment.

As shown in Table 7.1, the CBT protocol consists of 14 visits over 12 weeks that involve (1) psychoeducation, (2) cognitive training, (3) mapping OCD, (4) exposure and response prevention, and (5) relapse prevention. Except for Weeks 1 and 2, when patients come to treatment twice weekly, all visits are administered as once-weekly sessions of 1 hour each. In addition to these in-person visits, a brief telephone contact is conducted after

TABLE 7.1. CBT Treatment Protocol

Visit number	Goals
Week 1 and 2	Psychoeducation Cognitive training
Week 1	Mapping OCD Cognitive training
Weeks 3–12	Exposure and ritual prevention
Weeks 11–12	Relapse prevention
Visits 1, 7, and 11	Parent sessions

each of the weekly sessions in which the therapist provides encouragement and answers questions about homework assignments. E-mail is also a reasonable substitute for telephone contacts for patients who prefer this method; we have often used e-mail to create and to provide feedback for imaginal exposures to feared disasters. Each in-person session includes a statement of goals, review of the previous week, provision of new information, therapist-assisted practice (when appropriate), homework for the coming week, and monitoring procedures.

Parents were directly involved in Sessions 1, 7, and 11, with the first session devoted to psychoeducation and explaining the treatment process to the family and the latter two devoted to guiding the family about how to assist the child with homework assignments and with reinforcing efforts to combat OCD. Parents are also invited into the other sessions, usually at the end of the session, in order to keep them up to speed regarding progress and the week's assignments. In some cases, extensive family involvement in rituals and/or the developmental level of the child require that family members play a more central role in treatment. The CBT protocol provides sufficient flexibility to accommodate variations in family involvement dictated by the OCD symptom picture and by the developmental stage of the child. In one notably exceptional case, a highly motivated teenager who initiated treatment herself after seeing the newspaper ad for the program wished to involve her parents minimally in her treatment. She felt strongly that this approach would be best given the many interpersonal conflicts that were ongoing in the home. Her parents agreed that this was indeed the case, and would dutifully drive her to and from sessions while remaining "out of her business." Decisions about when and how to involve parents are made in clinical supervision, where factors such as the child's ability to discuss his or her symptoms directly with the therapist, the extent to which obsessional content and/or rituals involves parents, and likelihood of successful completion of exposure homeworks and self-monitoring tasks are all taken into consideration.

CASE EXAMPLES

We now present material from several pediatric OCD composite cases treated with CBT at our respective centers. We begin with a discussion of assessment, as adequate CBT requires a thorough assessment of obsessions, compulsions, comorbidity, functional impairment, and family strengths and difficulties. Assessment also presents a golden opportunity for psychoeducation, as does the creation of treatment hierarchies; we describe several examples of each in the assessment section. Following this section we describe early CBT sessions involving EX/RP; these sessions set the stage for later success on more difficult hierarchy items and are thus critical to CBT's long-term effectiveness. Moving up the EX/RP hierarchy is described next; these sessions often require reconceptualization of the case in the wake of new information about the patient's OCD symptoms and overall functioning, and we present several such examples in this section. The next section describes reaching the top of the treatment hierarchy, which often involves managing the patient's and the family's anxiety about confronting the most difficult items. In the next section, relapse prevention and wrapping up, we describe the process of preparing the patient to be his or her own therapist if and when symptoms arise in the future. We have also included a section on booster sessions, as many patients remain in occasional contact with their CBT provider long after core CBT has been completed. We have also chosen to include a final section on the role of cognitive techniques in CBT involving EX/RP, as we have encountered some misunderstanding about this issue in our professional encounters and because using cognitive techniques in pediatric OCD poses some particular challenges to the therapist.

Pretreatment Assessment

An adequate assessment of pediatric OCD should include a comprehensive evaluation of current and past OCD symptoms, current OCD symptom severity and associated functional impairment, and a survey of comorbid psychopathology. In addition, the strengths of the child and family should be evaluated, as well as their knowledge of OCD and its treatment. There are many self-report and clinician-administered instruments available for these purposes. We typically mail several relevant self-report questionnaires (e.g., Children's Depression Inventory [CDI]; Kovacs et al., 1985; Multidimensional Anxiety Scale for Children [MASC]; March, Parker, Sullivan, Stallings, & Conners, 1997; March & Sullivan, 1999) prior to the intake visit, then review these completed materials prior to meeting with the child. If it is apparent from these materials that comorbid depression or other anxiety problems besides OCD are prominent, we discuss these as well in the intake. The Anxiety Disorders Interview Schedule for Children (ADIS-C; Albano & Silverman, 1996; Silverman, 1991) is a semistructured interview that can be used to examine comorbid problems in greater detail. We use the ADIS in our current collaborative study examining the relative efficacy of CBT, sertraline, combined treatment, and pill placebo (Pediatric OCD Collaborative Study Group, 2001). For patients with highly unusual OCD symptoms, such as fear of losing their essence by discarding trash, or with extremely fixed beliefs about the veracity of their OCD fears, it is important to carefully survey positive and negative symptoms of thought disorder rather than assume that such presentations are necessarily psychotic symptoms.

For surveying history of OCD symptoms and current symptom severity we use the Children's Yale–Brown Obsessive Compulsive Scale checklist and severity scale (Scahill et al., 1997). One decision to make prior to assessment with the CY-BOCS is whether to interview the child with or without the parent present. We typically conduct a conjoint interview, directing questions to the child but soliciting parental feedback as well. Sometimes discrepancies between the parent and child arise when conducting a conjoint CY-BOCS, but this information can be invaluable in conceptualizing the case and ought to be courted rather than thwarted. We tell families upfront that it is often the case that parents become accurate observers of compulsions and functional impairments whereas the patient him- or herself usually has more knowledge about internal stimuli such as the frequency and intensity of obsessions, and that both reports help us arrive at the most comprehensive picture of the child's functioning. We do this specifically to minimize the common arguments over which report is "right." If it is clear that a patient is reluctant to discuss certain symptoms with a parent present (e.g., sexual obsessions), the therapist can skip that item on the CY-BOCS checklist and save some time at the end of the interview to revisit these potentially sensitive issues alone with the patient.

Prior to administering the CY-BOCS, the therapist should explain the concepts of obsessions and compulsions, using examples if the child and/or parent have difficulty grasping the concepts. Because children often feel as if they are the only ones suffering in this way, we make a point to tell them about the prevalence, nature, and treatment of OCD, which may increase their willingness to disclose their specific symptoms. It is also important to observe the child's behavior carefully during the intake and to inquire if certain behaviors (e.g., unusual movements, vocalizations) might be compulsions designed to neutralize obsessions or to reduce distress. Tic disorders are commonly comorbid with OCD, and it also is important to try to make a differential diagnosis as compulsions and tics would be targeted by different treatment procedures. Surveying common obsessions with a checklist instead of asking the child to disclose the fears tends to help with this problem, as does encouragement on the part of the therapist (e.g., "Lots of the kids I see have a hard time talking about these kinds of fears"). We have found that flexibility in the manner of disclosing the obsession is warranted. Thus, for example, we allow the child to write down the fears, or nod as the therapist describes examples of similar fears, in order to help the child share his or her OCD problems. In this way we can convey to the child and family that we recognize the difficulty associated with disclosure.

Pediatric OCD patients' medical histories should also be surveyed, with particular attention to the presence of recurrent Strep infection. At this point experts agree that the base rate of pediatric autoimmune neuropsychiatric disorders associated with streptococcal infections (PANDAS) given OCD is currently unknown and that the diagnosis cannot be assigned retrospectively at this juncture (Leonard et al., 1999; Swedo et al., 1998). Current research diagnostic criteria for PANDAS require at least two prospectively documented episodes of exacerbations in OCD and tic symptoms associated with streptococcal infection. Unfortunately, an unambiguous retrospective diagnosis of PANDAS is next to impossible in a clinically referred population of youth with OCD (March, unpublished data). Clinically, children who have unambiguous cases of PANDAS should be referred for appropriate treatment of their group A β-hemolytic streptococcal (GABHS) infection. Once treated for strep, the clinician should then also consider CBT and/or SSRI pharmacotherapy strategies. Many parents of children and adolescents with OCD have already heard of PANDAS and are very interested in determining whether their child suffers from this condition. Thus, awareness of this phenomenon on the part of the diagnostic and treatment team is likely to enhance the family's confidence in the facility in which treatment may be provided.

Brief descriptions of our core assessments follow.

Children's Yale–Brown Obsessive–Compulsive Scale (CY-BOCS)

The primary instrument for assessing OCD is the CY-BOCS, which assesses obsessions and compulsions separately on time consumed, distress, interference, degree of resistance, and control (Goodman, Price, Rasmussen, Mazure, Delgado, et al., 1989; Goodman, Price, Rasmussen, Mazure, Fleischmann, et al., 1989). We use the pediatric version (Scahill et al., 1997) of the CY-BOCS symptom checklist and symptom scale to inventory past and present OCD symptoms, initial severity, total OCD severity, relative preponderance of obsessions and compulsions, and degree of insight. The CY-BOCS is a clinician-rated instrument merging data from clinical observation and parent and child report.

Anxiety Disorders Interview Schedule for Children (ADIS-C)

The child and adolescent ADIS is a semi-structured interview for assessing DSM-IV anxiety disorders in youth that shows excellent psychometric properties for internalizing conditions relative to other available instruments, such as the Diagnostic Interview Schedule for Children (DISC) (Silverman, 1991). The ADIS utilizes an interviewer–observer format, thereby allowing the clinician to draw information from the interview and from clinical observations. Scores are derived regarding (1) specific diagnoses and (2) level of diagnosis-related interference.

OCD Impact Scale (OCIS)

We also obtain child and parent versions of the OCD Impact Scale, which shows preliminary evidence favoring psychometric adequacy and sensitivity to change (Jaffer & Piacentini, 2001; Piacentini, Jaffer, Liebowitz, & Gitow, 1992), for use in analyses of functional impairment from OCD. This instrument enables us to estimate whether the CY-BOCS improvements result in normalization as assessed by functional impairment.

Multidimensional Anxiety Scale for Children (MASC)

The MASC has four factors and six subfactors: physical anxiety (tense/restless, somatic/autonomic), harm avoidance (perfectionism, anxious coping), social anxiety (humiliation/rejection, performance anxiety), and separation anxiety. It is in use in a variety of NIMH-funded treatment outcome studies. The MASC shows test–retest reliability in clinical (ICC > .92) and school samples (ICC > .85); convergent/divergent validity is similarly superior (March et al., 1997; March & Sullivan, 1999). There is also the MASC OC Screener, a 20-item questionnaire that surveys OCD symptoms frequently reported by children and adolescents.

Children's Depression Inventory (CDI)

The CDI (Kovacs, 1985) is a 27-item self-report scale that measures cognitive, affective, behavioral, and interpersonal symptoms of depression. Each item consists of three statements, of which the child is asked to select the one statement that best describes his or her current functioning. Items are scored from 0 to 2; therefore, scores on the CDI can range from 0 to 54. The CDI shows adequate reliability and validity (Kovacs, 1985). This scale is useful to assess for symptoms of depression, which assists in tailoring the treatment plan.

Setting Up Cognitive-Behavioral Therapy: Sessions 1–4

Once key information about the child and his or her OCD has been gathered, psychoeducation and treatment planning may commence. In our protocol the initial parent session involves a detailed discussion of OCD as a neurobehavioral disorder. We describe the areas of the brain that may be implicated in the pathophysiology of OCD, the serotonin hypothesis, and the positron-emission tomography (PET) scan studies suggesting that behavioral changes after EX/RP may affect these areas of the brain (Baxter et al., 1992). For one young child who found this particularly interesting, we drew brains in the initial session and tried to replicate Baxter's PET scans in drawings, emphasizing during this exercise that the rest of her brain seemed just fine and that with some treatment the "brain hiccough" may be greatly reduced. We endeavor to help the family view OCD as a medical illness rather than as a series of habits that the child/adolescent could stop if he or she tried hard enough. The former view promotes the externalizing of OCD and fosters a more collaborative spirit. It is also important in this first session to explain how the treatment process follows logically from our understanding of the disorder, and that successful CBT will ultimately, but not immediately, require elimination of all rituals and other avoidance behaviors.

With the goal of developing a shared vocabulary with which to promote understanding of core treatment concepts, the therapist should take the time to find out about the patient's interests and hobbies early on in the treatment. Sometimes this discussion must seem odd to parents who want the therapist to begin immediately working on their child's symptoms, but patience in these early sessions pays off later, when the therapist can use the patient's day-to-day experiences to drive home core concepts. For instance, one patient of ours was a fanatic football fan who would talk about his favorite team at any given opportunity. Quickly recognizing an "in," the therapist was able to make use of the child's keen interest in the sport to foster a common vocabulary that allowed the patient to quickly master the core principles of EX/RP while at the same time having fun in the sessions. The patient and the therapist cast OCD as a division-leading football team that was known for its aggressive defensive strategies. The early CBT sessions were cast as "film sessions" in which the therapist (the coach) and the patient (the starting quarterback) dissected OCD's strategies in order to create a proper game plan in the face of OCD's fairly consistent tendencies. This shifting of the discussion promoted the patient's active engagement in the treatment, which is an essential element of successful CBT. It is also important to recognize that even though psychoeducation is formally presented in these early sessions, this education can take place throughout treatment. The therapist should take advantage of opportunities to point out flaws in OCD's logic, and reinforce the child for mastering key concepts and for designing exposure and ritual prevention strategies on his or her own based on the child's understanding of these concepts.

In Sessions 2–4 the therapist meets with the patient and develops a treatment hierarchy. The hierarchy is often created in the form of a "map" in which OCD themes, their interconnections, and their relative severity are documented. One patient's OCD map included an island for thoughts of harming friends intentionally, a nearby island for thoughts of harming him-self, and the largest and most intimidating island for thoughts of harming his father intentionally. Based on this mapping technique, the patient and therapist were able to recognize that the best "battle plan" would be to take the small islands first, which would promote increased confidence about taking the largest island. Islands are usually colored to reflect how successful the child is in resisting OCD related to a particular theme, a term described elsewhere as the "transition zone." With a very young child more concrete examples might be needed. For instance, the therapist asked the child to move a small bulldozer across a tabletop to reflect how often it was that OCD was able to "get its way" across situations involving contamina-tion and urges to wash at home, at school, and at her grandmother's house. The child's moving of the bulldozer to varying points on the table conveyed to the therapist that resisting urges to wash was most challenging at home, followed by at her grandmother's, and then at school. The toy bulldozer was used throughout treatment so that the child could convey progress in the treatment and play with an interesting toy at the same time. Once the hierarchy is completed, it is imperative to convey to the child/adolescent that the treatment will progress at the pace he or she feel is manageable, while at the same time helping the child to recognize that inordinate delays in moving up the hierarchy will slow the much-desired reduction of obses-sional frequency/distress.

As listed in Table 7.1, cognitive training is also an element of our treat-ment. The purpose of this training, or learning to "talk back to OCD," is to encourage the child/adolescent to remain in feared situations without ritualizing in order to promote habituation and a change in core OCD be-liefs. Thus, when faced with obsessions about contamination and associ-ated urges to ritualize, a child might begin to say "You're not the boss of me" in order to encourage him- or herself to stay in the fear-provoking situ-ation. Accordingly, the purpose of the positive self-talk is not to reduce short-term anxiety during exposure but to strengthen the child's ability to stay in the feared situation long enough for short-term and long-term habit-uation. Self-talk can also be used to introduce humor into the exposure ex-ercises, which is another distancing strategy that if used properly may help younger patients move forward with exposures. For example, after exten-sive discussions in session, a child with fears of losing his soul to the devil created a poem to remind himself to stay with exposures when devil fears arose: "What I once feared will become a bore; the devil is just a meta-phor." For this particular child, the poem served both as positive self-talk and as an exposure in and of itself, as he previously feared writing or saying the word "devil" and saying definitively that he did not believe in a devil, which he feared would leave his soul more vulnerable to acquisition.

One potential risk of the positive self-talk may arise if the child does not understand this function of cognitive training. If not, he or she may be vulnerable to using these self-statements in a ritualized fashion, that is, to reduce obsessional distress during exposure, which may compromise outcome and actually prolong the difficulties. For instance, one patient began to repeat over and over to herself, "Nothing bad will happen to me or my loved ones," while conducting exposures to situations in which these fears arose. This neutralizing of obsessions was successful in keeping her from becoming anxious, yet did not allow her to fully test her OCD's hypothesis that harm thoughts that were not neutralized in some way would come true. The therapist designed a series of exposures with the patient to eliminate the neutralizing phrases; as is typical, the patient's anxiety increased significantly once these phrases were dropped, but it eventually reduced over time in the session, which weakened the fear considerably. Thus, the therapist should teach the child/adolescent this purpose of positive self-talk and should pay particular attention to make sure that cognitive training is not producing what essentially would amount to new mental rituals. Because some children cannot tolerate the distress associated with exposure, positive self-talk and other anxiety management strategies such as relaxation exercises and deep breathing may be necessary at first to help these children engage in exposures. These techniques should be faded later as the child experiences successes, such as within- and between-sessions habituation and changes in core OCD beliefs.

The first practice exposure conducted during Session 4 should be chosen in collaboration with the child and should come from the bottom end of the hierarchy. There is often considerable pressure to move quickly to the most obvious and impairing targets, yet this pressure should be resisted as the purpose of the trial exposure is to demonstrate procedures and to promote optimism regarding the possibility of success. One child with checking fears was having great difficulty leaving his house for fear that a light would be left on, a sink would be left running, or a window or door left unlocked. The checking rituals were designed to reduce the chance that disastrous consequences (e.g., fire, flood, burglary) would ensue. Notably, the therapist encouraged the child to choose a much easier trial exposure, namely, refraining from checking his bookbag. This item was rated rather low on the fear hierarchy but nevertheless would allow the therapist to model how to conduct exposure and would virtually guarantee a successful outcome. The child was able to refrain from ritualizing in the trial exposure session; his anxiety habituated within just a few minutes; and he reported that the bookbag exposures gave him no trouble whatsoever in the week between Sessions 4 and 5. Having completed this exercise successfully, the therapist could review its outcome and use it as an example of how the more difficult exposures would be conducted. Parents anxious to see their child's dysfunction reduced immediately need to be coached at this point in praising the child for this success regardless of whether other items await confrontation. One exasperated parent asked the therapist after Session 4, "Why are you working on touching the chair in your office when she can't even go near a public bathroom?" The therapist replied, "Because she can't even go near a public bathroom," and went on to discuss the importance of conducting hierarchy-driven exposures at a pace that the child could manage without being overwhelmed.

Moving Up the Hierarchy

Assuming that the child successfully completed the trial exposure as homework, the next session (Session 5) involves selecting another exposure exercise to be conducted. The child with the checking fears returned to report excellent progress in that realm and chose to work in Session 5 on turning off sinks and leaving the room without checking, as this was slightly more difficult than the bookbag but much easier than leaving the house without checking the locks or the appliances. Thus, the *in vivo* exposure for Session 5 involved using sinks throughout the building, turning them off quickly and without excessive tightening (another method used by the patient to reduce likelihood of a flood), and leaving the room without looking back. The therapist inquired whether there was an auditory check taking place, as he noticed that the patient stopped talking to the therapist immediately after turning off the sink but resumed discourse in the hallway outside the various bathrooms. The patient acknowledged this subtle form of ritual of which he had previously been unaware, and subsequent exposures were designed to block this automatic ritual by conversing loudly throughout the exposure. After doing this exposure in about 10 different bathrooms the patient was led back to the therapist's office, where they discussed the feared and realistic consequences of the exposure:

THERAPIST: So, as we're sitting in my office now how likely does it seem that the unit is being flooded with water from one of these sinks that we worked on?

PATIENT: Pretty unlikely—I'm pretty sure we turned them all off.

THERAPIST: But the problem is that your OCD usually doesn't like "pretty sure"—it will only rest if it's 100% guaranteed, right?

PATIENT: Yeah, it says you never can be too sure.

THERAPIST: And what we're trying to prove is that even if you don't have an absolute guarantee the bad stuff your OCD bugs you about doesn't happen anyway.

PATIENT: But it's hard to believe that when you're checking.

THERAPIST: Exactly—there's even been some research suggesting that checking may actually make people less sure of themselves.

PATIENT: And you think I'll be more sure of myself if I don't check?

THERAPIST: I do, which is why we should continue to hang out here for awhile until your anxiety goes down. The lower your anxiety gets, the easier it will be for you to see that you don't need to check in order to feel better, or for the sinks to be off for that matter.

PATIENT: It would be funny if we left one on though, wouldn't it?

THERAPIST: Sounds like your OCD has got you wondering a little bit about how safe this was to do.

PATIENT: Maybe a little bit; I'm like a 3 on the Fear Thermometer now.

THERAPIST: Which isn't a 10 but isn't a 1 yet either, which means you're still a little anxious.

PATIENT: Yeah, I am.

THERAPIST: Well let's see what happens to your anxiety if we sit here for a while longer.

(*The patient and the therapist continued in this fashion until session's end, at which point the therapist prepared the patient to leave the building without doing any checking for his feared disasters.*)

THERAPIST: Well I'm going to walk you out now, and I want to prepare you for the possibility that your OCD might make one final attempt to get you to check while you walk past the bathrooms we just worked in.

PATIENT: Yeah that's what it does at home usually—I can check the sink, but every time I go past the bathroom I feel like I should check again because I'm already there.

THERAPIST: So we know it's going to act up a little bit—what do you need to do?

PATIENT: I need to walk past, not look under the doors for water, not listen for sounds of the sink overflowing, and just leave.

THERAPIST: Exactly, just leave. Can you leave at a regular pace or do you need to sprint down the hall?

PATIENT: I think I can leave regular, but if it starts getting on me I should pick up the pace a little bit.

THERAPIST: Right, and keep your eyes looking upward so your OCD doesn't get you checking for surf in the corridor.

PATIENT: I didn't bring my board anyway.

THERAPIST: Well let's go then, ready?

PATIENT: Ready.

THERAPIST: You did a nice job today on this stuff—good work.

PATIENT: Thanks.

As demonstrated in the preceding exchange, the therapist discusses probability theory with the patient in addition to habituation. The therapist should provide emotional support and aid the patient in examining the likelihood of the occurrence of feared outcomes without providing guarantees of safety or excessive reassurance. The therapist also tried to introduce levity into the discussion, which the patient responded to positively. If the patient feels as if he or she is being laughed at, however, the relationship can be undermined and the therapy compromised, so such attempts should be made cautiously and with a good working knowledge of the patient's style. Another point illustrated in the preceding exchange is that both patient and therapist are referring to OCD as if it were a third person in the room, a process known as externalizing (March & Mulle, 1998). With younger children this can take the form of giving OCD a nickname to be used during the treatment, so as to further reinforce the notion that the child is not to blame for these unusual fears and compulsions, but, rather, the OCD is to blame. Some therapists may worry that externalizing might cause the child to feel powerless in the face of a fearsome opponent, and indeed this possibility needs to be considered by the therapist as the dialogue about OCD continues.

In a case involving more unusual content, the progression up the hierarchy moves similarly. For example, in a case we have presented in detail elsewhere (Franklin et al., 2001), a patient in CBT was combating fears that he might turn into another person if he inadvertently bumped into someone. Moving up the hierarchy in that case involved first determining the parameters of the fear—for example, is it worse to turn into a boy than a girl?—then simply stepping up the list in light of the patient's willingness to tolerate anxiety and refrain from rituals. Confrontation of these fears began with the therapist asking George to shake hands with him, which George was able to do with only mild anxiety. Next, he was introduced to other staff members and asked to shake hands with them as well. The next step, confronted in subsequent sessions, was to bump into people. As with the handshaking exposures, these exercises began with the therapist and then progressed quickly to bumping into other staff members. The fear of bumping into random strangers outside the office was greater than what he had accomplished already, and these exposures were planned for subsequent sessions. All the while the therapist and George discussed whether he had indeed turned into anyone else and whether his essence was being lost by doing repeated exposures; OCD's logic was thereby attacked systematically. George was later instructed to begin bumping into strangers in crowded places, starting with the hospital cafeteria, progressing to a local store, and finally in a crowded shopping area and city street. The OCD's logic weakened by discussion and by the disconfirming evidence, the bumping exposures were soon ceased and other areas of concern were addressed.

As with adults, imaginal exposure is often a useful adjunct to *in vivo* exposure for patients with feared consequences. Conducting imaginal exposure with very young children can be challenging, however, as the task of narrating a story with eyes closed and incorporating all of the desired anxiety-evoking elements can prove to be daunting, and children may become discouraged from doing so. One way we have found to conduct imaginal exposure with young children is to do "story writing" exercises; many of the patients who like creative writing take well to this method. We also conduct demonstrations in the office designed to disconfirm fears that images that are not neutralized are more likely to come true. For example, a 6-year-old patient with many intrusive images of harm befalling herself, her family, and the planet was having difficulty refraining from neutralizing and reassurance seeking when confronted with these images, and imaginal exposure appeared to be called for. The therapist and the patient worked on this problem as follows:

THERAPIST: OK, Kristin, remember we said today we'd try to work on the scary pictures that come into your head?

PATIENT: How are we going to do that?

THERAPIST: Well, first I want to show you a trick. Last time you were here you said that "Tummy Tickle" (OCD) tells you that if you have one of those scary pictures in your head and you didn't tell Mommy that maybe it would happen and it would be your fault?

PATIENT: I still think that.

THERAPIST: Well let's see if we can mess with it a bit. First I want you to look at that soda bottle on my desk. See it there?

PATIENT: Yeah, I see it.

THERAPIST: Well I want you to get a good picture of it in your head, and then close your eyes and imagine it in your head. Can you do that?

PATIENT: Yeah.

THERAPIST: OK, good. Now I want you to move the soda bottle in your head from one side of the desk to the other.

PATIENT: Do I need to move the real one too?

THERAPIST: No, just the one in your head.

PATIENT: OK, I did it.

THERAPIST: Great, now make it grow wings and fly across the room like a butterfly.

PATIENT: What color should the wings be?

THERAPIST: Whatever color you like.

PATIENT: OK, it's flying now.

THERAPIST: Can you make it smile?

PATIENT: It doesn't have a face.

THERAPIST: OK, give it a face and make it smile.

PATIENT: It's smiling now.

THERAPIST: Can you see it really clearly now?

PATIENT: Yes, I can see its bright blue wings and its big happy teeth.

THERAPIST: Great, now open your eyes. Where's the soda bottle now?

PATIENT: (*Laughs.*) It's still on your desk, silly!

THERAPIST: I thought it was flying around the room like a smiling butterfly?

PATIENT: No, that's just the one in my head.

THERAPIST: So even if you see something really clearly in your head it doesn't mean that it's real, right?

PATIENT: Right.

THERAPIST: Let's go back to it now—close your eyes, and give the soda bottle back its mouth.

PATIENT: OK.

THERAPIST: Can you make it bite my hand?

PATIENT: That wouldn't be very nice.

THERAPIST: Well how about a little bite.

PATIENT: OK, I guess so.

THERAPIST: Did it bite me?

PATIENT: Yup, right on the finger.

THERAPIST: Which finger?

PATIENT: The little finger.

THERAPIST: Why don't you have it bite me on the thumb now, OK?

PATIENT: OK.

THERAPIST: OK, now open your eyes again. Do you see any teeth marks?

PATIENT: No.

THERAPIST: How come?

PATIENT: Because it was only pretend.

THERAPIST: And what does this say about the scary pictures that come into your head, like the one you had today while driving in with your parents?

PATIENT: Well, maybe they're pretend too, and I don't have to make them go away any more.

THERAPIST: I think that's right, but what do you say we find that out?

The therapist conducted this experiment for several reasons. First, the therapist wanted to ascertain whether the child was able to conjure up and then hold images in her mind, which she apparently could do. Next, he wanted to help the patient recognize that having and manipulating vivid images in her mind did not have any consequences in reality. He first used a pleasant image to demonstrate this point, then moved to a slightly more fearful one to further demonstrate that even if the valence of the image changed that the external consequences did not. Having demonstrated this successfully to the child, the next step in the session involved her picking an image that bothered her at least a little bit, and conducting the same exercise. The child mentioned that before the session, when she drove with her parents over the bridge into the city, she had a vivid and scary image of a large flood in the city. In the wake of this image, she asked her parents repeatedly to check if the city was in fact flooding and to reassure her that cities ordinarily do not flood without warning. Stepping now from the more neutral stimuli in the preceding sample dialogue to this image of the city flooding, the therapist and the child stared out at the city and then attempted to start such a flood by imagining the entire city under water. The child was able to imagine the scene clearly and had previously been concerned about thought–action fusion and troubled by an exaggerated sense of responsibility to prevent bad outcomes such as floods (Salkovskis, 1985). Thus, the process of holding the flooded city image in her mind served as an imaginal exposure designed to promote within- and between-session habituation to the image. In addition, it serves as a "behavioral experiment" in that the failure to flood the city despite having vivid images of such a scene in her mind helped to weaken her belief that an un-neutralized image would cause the feared outcome.

Confronting the Most Difficult Items

Building upon past successes, the gradual ascent up the treatment hierarchy must culminate with the confrontation of the most difficult thoughts and situations. We advise that such items be addressed in Sessions 10–12 of our 14-session protocol, as saving the worst item for the last session may not allow the patient enough time to work with the therapist to overcome the fear. We also advise that ritual prevention success and exposure to lower level items should be taken into account when deciding when to confront these highest items: If a patient is still washing regularly in response to touching office doorknobs, it may not be prudent to advance to bathroom-related stimuli until the patient can successfully refrain from such ritualizing. When confronting the most difficult items, it is imperative to remind the child how much progress he or she has made in the treatment, and that confronting the harder items works just like confronting the easier ones: Stay in the situation, show your OCD who's boss, and refrain from rituals and avoidance so that your body's alarm system can shut itself off. Explaining and helping the child manage strong physiological sensations of anxiety is often more relevant at the very top of the hierarchy, so advance preparation for what to expect can be useful. Although, for obvious reasons, we steer clear of guaranteeing patients that their feared outcomes will not come to pass, we also let our patients know that we would not allow them to do exposures that we thought were objectively dangerous and that we would not do ourselves. This point should not be construed as reassurance giving, but instead viewed as encouragement to confront the most difficult items. Nonfearful modeling also comes into play when doing these kinds of exposures: A child who watches the therapist touch a public toilet seat and then contaminate his hair without exhibiting any reaction will learn how the therapist wants the exposure done but also witnesses that not everyone responds to such exercises with extreme fear. Parental reinforcement of the child's efforts to confront the most difficult items may also improve follow-through with homework assignments pertaining to these items, and this point should be emphasized with the family.

Relapse Prevention and Wrapping Up

Sessions 12–14 in our protocol emphasize continuing to confront fears that have yet to be reduced, and thus in vivo exposures are usually included in these later sessions. In addition, for patients who have made progress in CBT, we also begin to emphasize the maintenance of treatment gains. For one of our patients who made considerable progress in treatment, the child with the checking fears described earlier, there was little left to conquer on the hierarchy but much left to do in terms of helping the child realize that he could maintain his gains over the long run without weekly sessions. In his case we made up "OCD quizzes" to test his knowledge of key concepts and his ability to generalize, and again, to interject some humor into the treatment process. Glenn was taught the difference between lapses and relapses in accord with discussions from the treatment of other disorders (e.g., Marlatt & Gordon, 1985), and was asked to describe how he would respond if his fears of disasters and related checking urges crept back in. The therapist and the patient also generated a list of identifiable stressors that might exacerbate his currently subclinical symptoms, and Glenn was advised that the time to work hardest on OCD in the future (e.g., devising exposures, self-monitoring) was when the symptoms were more prevalent and distressing. Session 14 is usually devoted to further discussion of relapse prevention, a review of progress, an exposure if needed, and a small celebration of treatment completion. This final session is also an opportunity to convey to the parents that the family has learned how to conduct EX/RP for OCD and that they should continue to work collaboratively to address residual symptoms or to deal with new themes as they arise. The therapist should do everything possible to enhance the patient's and the family's confidence that they can handle lingering or new symptoms effectively, as the complete remission of all OCD is apparently quite rare.

Staying in Touch: Booster Sessions

In the context of our randomized controlled trial, patients receive 14 sessions of CBT conducted over approximately 12 weeks during the acute phase, followed by four booster sessions conducted over 4 months for patients who responded to CBT. In the clinical setting we try to work out a similar schedule that allows for continuing contact while at the same time giving increasing responsibility for EX/RP to the child. Usually booster sessions are reviews of the past few weeks of OCD symptoms, discussion of the patient's plan to deal with these symptoms, survey of any new themes that might have developed and discussion of how to combat these new issues, and also a more general discussion of stressors and accomplishments over the same period of time. One adolescent patient with contamination fears and washing rituals who had responded extremely well to CBT began to notice in follow-up that she had increased contamination concern immediately following normative washing, such as after going to the bathroom or working with her mother in the garden with bare hands:

PATIENT: Right after I wash regularly now I notice that I'm more scared to touch things.

THERAPIST: Is the wash a ritualized one?

PATIENT: No, I've actually found that I can wash faster than most of my friends do, and I don't make sure I get soap on every spot the way I used to.

THERAPIST: Nevertheless you're finding yourself more anxious after these handwashes.

PATIENT: Yeah, like I've got the germs off now and I better be careful.

THERAPIST: This is actually a pretty common thing that happens, and we'll need to work on it.

PATIENT: How?

THERAPIST: Well, do you remember during the treatment when we talked about reexposure after doing a ritual?

PATIENT: Yeah, you told me that if I gave in and did what OCD wanted that I should try right then to recontaminate myself and try not to wash.

THERAPIST: Right, this way OCD wouldn't get its way and you'd be able to show it who's in charge.

PATIENT: But that was after rituals—these aren't really rituals, are they?

THERAPIST: No, they're what most people would do after getting lots of soil on their hands or after going to the bathroom, but I think your OCD is trying to sneak back into the picture by telling you that now that you're decontaminated that you should try to maintain that.

PATIENT: So I should probably touch something contaminated right after washing to let the OCD know that I'm not going to fall for it, right?

THERAPIST: Right. Now we need to decide what thing to touch. Based on how we did this before, how would you arrive at a decision about this?

PATIENT: Probably based on how much things bother me.

THERAPIST: Right—there's no sense recontaminating with something that doesn't feel contaminated.

PATIENT: I had been using the bottom of my shoes but that's no problem now.

THERAPIST: Well let's think about this—is there anything in your house that feels even a little bit yucky?

PATIENT: Not that I can think of.

THERAPIST: How about outside your house?

PATIENT: Well touching a public toilet seat or handle is still a little gross.

THERAPIST: But your OCD doesn't tell you it will make you sick any more?

PATIENT: It tries to, but I don't listen and therefore it stopped saying much.

THERAPIST: But it still says a little bit about it. Given that, how do you think you can do the recontamination exercises successfully?

PATIENT: I suppose I could touch something to the toilet handle and then use that to contaminate myself after a regular handwash.

THERAPIST: What kind of thing should it be?

PATIENT: Something that I have with me a lot, that doesn't get washed, and that won't fall apart.

THERAPIST: Do you have anything like that?

PATIENT: How about my necklace? I never take it off so it'll be with me anywhere I go.

THERAPIST: I think that's a great idea! Now how would you do this?

PATIENT: I'll have to touch it to a public toilet handle and then put it back on, then make sure I touch it right after I wash my hands.

THERAPIST: After ritualized handwashes?

PATIENT: (*Smiles.*) No, after any handwashes.

THERAPIST: Good. I'd suggest that you use it any time you're feeling decontaminated—reload with toilet handle germs and really show your OCD who's boss.

PATIENT: So I'll basically be walking around all day with a toilet handle around my neck, just in case. Sorta like that poem about the sailor with the dead bird that he had to wear because he killed it.

THERAPIST: (*Laughs.*) Yeah, it is a bit of an albatross, but hopefully one that helps keep your OCD from getting the best of you.

HOW "COGNITIVE" IS COGNITIVE-BEHAVIORAL THERAPY FOR PEDIATRIC OBSESSIVE–COMPULSIVE DISORDER?

The role of cognitive theory and interventions in CBT involving EX/RP has traditionally been given short shrift in writings about this form of treatment, which may contribute to growing confusion about their relevance in this context. Most OCD theorists, including those in our own group (e.g., Foa & Kozak, 1985, 1986), have stated unequivocally that cognitive change is essential to good outcome: Successfully treated OCD patients should be more willing to accept low risks and be less dependent on guarantees of safety. Thus, if a treatment is thought to be "cognitive" in that cognitive change is of interest, then our treatment approach would fit this description (Kozak, 1999). The question then becomes a more practical one: What is the best way to achieve these desired cognitive changes? In that regard our CBT involving EX/RP can also be cast as a "cognitive" treatment, at least in part, in that we use cognitive methods as part of our therapeutic repertoire. For example, we educate patients about the perils of thought suppression, discuss mistaken OCD beliefs, consider probability theory, and discuss the meaning of anxiety reduction for the patient's previously untested hypotheses. As is demonstrated earlier, exposure exercises involve confrontation of the feared thoughts and situations, but discussion before, during, and after exposure is included in order to facilitate both behavioral and cognitive change. As we have stated elsewhere, cognitive methods are used in this context to anticipate and accompany exposure rather than to replace it (Foa, Franklin, & Kozak, 1998). Tests of "pure" behavioral and cognitive methods have yet to be conducted in children and adolescents, and although their outcomes would be of interest theoretically, they would not address important unanswered questions about how best to blend behavioral and cognitive methods to maximize short- and long-term treatment outcome.

REFERENCES

Abramowitz, J. S., Foa, E. B., & Franklin, M. E. (2003). Cognitive behavior therapy for obsessive compulsive disorder: Effectiveness of twice weekly versus intensive treatment sessions. *Journal of Consulting and Clinical Psychology, 71*(2).

Albano, A. M., & Silverman, W. K. (1996). *Anxiety Disorders Interview Schedule for DSM-IV: Child version.* San Antonio, TX: Psychological Corporation.

Baxter, L. J., Schwartz, J. M., Bergaman, K. S., Szuba, M. P., Guze, B. H., Mazziotta, J. C., Alazraki, A., Selin, C. E., Ferng, H. K., & Munford, P. (1992). Caudate glucose metabolic rate changes with both drug and behavior therapy for obsessive compulsive disorder. *Archives of General Psychiatry, 49,* 681–689.

Clark, D. A. (1999). Cognitive behavioral treatment of obsessive compulsive disorder: A commentary. *Cognitive and Behavioral Practice, 6,* 408–415.

deHaan, E., Hoogduin, K. A. L., Buitelaar, J. K., & Keijsers, G. P. J. (1998). Behavior therapy versus clomipramine for the treatment of obsessive–compulsive disorder in children and adolescents. *Journal of the American Academy of Child and Adolescent Psychiatry, 37,* 1022–1029.

DeVeaugh-Geiss, J., Landau, P., & Katz, R. (1989). Treatment of OCD with clomipramine. *Psychiatric Annals, 19,* 97–101.

DeVeaugh-Geiss, J., Moroz, G., Biederman, J., Cantwell, D., Fontaine, R., Greist, J. H., Reichler, R., Katz, R., & Landau, P. (1992). Clomipramine hydrochloride in childhood and adolescent obsessive–compulsive disorder: A multi-center trial. *Journal of the American Academy of Child and Adolescent Psychiatry, 31,* 45–49.

Flament, M. F., Rapoport, J. L., Berg, C., Sceery, W., Kilts, C., Mellstrom, B., & Linnoila, M. (1985). Clomipramine treatment of childhood obsessive–compulsive disorder. *Archives of General Psychiatry, 42,* 977–988.

Flament, M. F., Whitaker, A., Rapoport, J. L., Sceery, W., Kilts, C., Mellstrom, B., & Linnoila, M. (1988). Obsessive–compulsive disorder in adolescence: An epidemiological study. *Journal of the American Academy of Child and Adolescent Psychiatry, 27,* 764–771.

Foa, E. B., Franklin, M. E., & Kozak, M. J. (1998). Psychosocial treatments for obsessive compulsive disorder: Literature review. In R. P. Swinson, M. M. Antony, S. Rachman, & M. A. Richter (Eds.), *Obsessive–compulsive disorder: Theory, research, and treatment* (pp. 258–276). New York: Guilford Press.

Foa, E. B., & Kozak, M. J. (1985). Treatment of anxiety disorders: Implications for psychopathology. In A. H. Tuma & J. D. Maser (Eds.), *Anxiety and the anxiety disorders* (pp. 421–452). Hillsdale, NJ: Erlbaum.

Foa, E. B., & Kozak, M. J. (1986). Emotional processing of fear: Exposure to corrective information. *Psychological Bulletin, 99,* 20–35.

Franklin, M. E., & Foa, E. B. (1998). Cognitive-behavioral treatments for obsessive compulsive disorder. In P. E. Nathan & J. M. Gorman (Eds.), *A guide to treatments that work* (pp. 339–357). New York: Oxford University Press.

Franklin, M. E., Kozak, M. J., Cashman, L. A., Coles, M. E., Rheingold, A. A., & Foa, E. B. (1998). Cognitive-behavioral treatment of pediatric obsessive–compulsive disorder: An open clinical trial. *Journal of the American Academy of Child and Adolescent Psychiatry, 37,* 412–419.

Franklin, M. E., Tolin, D. F., March, J. S., & Foa, E. B. (2001). Intensive cognitive-behavior therapy for pediatric OCD: A case example. *Cognitive and Behavioral Practice, 8,* 297–304.

Geller, D. A., Hoog, S. L., Heilgenstein, J. H., Ricardi, R. K., Tamura, R., Kluszynski, S., & Jacobson, J. G. (2001). Fluoxetine treatment for obsessive compulsive disorder in children and adolescents: A placebo-controlled clinical trial. *Journal of the American Academy of Child and Adolescent Psychiatry, 40,* 773–779.

Goodman, W. K., Price, L. H., Rasmussen, S. A., Mazure, C., Delgado, P., Heninger, G. R., & Charney, D. S. (1989). The Yale–Brown Obsessive Compulsive Scale: II. Validity. *Archives of General Psychiatry, 46,* 1012–1016.

Goodman, W. K., Price, L. H., Rasmussen, S. A., Mazure, C., Fleischmann, R. L., Hill, C. L., Heninger, G. R., & Charney, D. S. (1989). The Yale–Brown Obsessive Compulsive Scale: I. Development, use, and reliability. *Archives of General Psychiatry, 46,* 1006–1011.

Jaffer, M., & Piacentini, J. (2001, July). The Child OCD Impact Scale (COIS): Clinical applications. In D. McKay (Chair), *Childhood OCD: Bringing research into the clinic.* Paper presented at the World Congress of Behavioral and Cognitive Therapies, Vancouver, BC.

Kovacs, M. (1985). The Children's Depression Inventory (CDI). *Psychopharmacology Bulletin, 21,* 995–998.

Kozak, M. J. (1999). Evaluating treatment efficacy for obsessive–compulsive disorder: Caveat practitioner. *Cognitive and Behavioral Practice, 6,* 422–426.

Leonard, H. L., Swedo, S. E., Garvey, M., Beer, D., Perlmutter, S., Lougee, L., Karitani, M., & Dubbert, B. (1999). Post-infectious and other forms of obsessive–compulsive disorder. *Child and Adolescent Psychiatry Clinics of North America, 8,* 497–511.

Leonard, H. L., Swedo, S. E., Lenane, M. C., Rettew, D. C., Cheslow, D. L., Hamburger, S. D., & Rapoport, J. L. (1991). A double-blind desipramine substitution during long-term clomipramine treatment in children and adolescents with obsessive–compulsive disorder. *Archives of General Psychiatry, 48,* 922–927.

Leonard, H. L., Swedo, S. E., Rapoport, J. L., Koby, E., Lenane, M. C., Cheslow, D. L., & Hamburger, S. D. (1989). Treatment of obsessive–compulsive disorder with clomipramine and desipramine in children and adolescents: A double-blind crossover comparison. *Archives of General Psychiatry, 46,* 1088–1092.

March, J. S. (1995). Cognitive-behavioral psychotherapy for children and adolescents with OCD: A review and recommendations for treatment. *Journal of the American Academy of Child and Adolescent Psychiatry, 34,* 7–18.

March, J. S., Biederman, J., Wolkow, R., Safferman, A., Mardekian, J., Cook, E. H., Cutler, N. R., Dominguez, R., Ferguson, J., Muller, B., Riesenberg, R., Rosenthal, M., Sallee, F. R., & Wagner, K. D. (1998). Sertraline in children and adolescents with obsessive–compulsive disorder: A multicenter randomized controlled trial. *Journal of American Medical Association 280,* 1752–1756.

March, J., Frances, A., Kahn, D., & Carpenter, D. (1997). Expert consensus guidelines: Treatment of obsessive–compulsive disorder. *Journal of Clinical Psychiatry, 58,* 1–72.

March, J. S., & Mulle, K. (1998). *OCD in children and adolescents: A cognitive-behavioral treatment manual.* New York: Guilford Press.

March, J. S., Mulle, K., & Herbel, B. (1994). Behavioral psychotherapy for children and adolescents with obsessive–compulsive disorder: An open trial of a new protocol-driven treatment package. *Journal of the American Academy of Child and Adolescent Psychiatry, 33,* 333–341.

March, J., Parker, J., Sullivan, K., Stallings, P., & Conners, K. (1997). The Multidimensional Anxiety Scale for Children (MASC): Factor structure, reliability and validity. *Journal of the American Academy of Child and Adolescent Psychiatry, 36,* 554–565.

March, J. S., & Sullivan, K. (1999). Test–retest reliability of the Multidimensional Anxiety Scale for Children. *Journal of Anxiety Disorders, 13,* 349–358.

Marlatt, G. A., & Gordon, J. R. (Eds.). (1985). *Relapse prevention.* New York: Guilford Press.

Mowrer, O. H. (1939). A stimulus–response analysis of anxiety and its role as a reinforcing agent. *Psychological Review, 46,* 553–565.

Mowrer, O. H. (1960). *Learning theory and behavior.* New York: Wiley.

Pediatric OCD Collaborative Study Group (2001, July). Recent developments in the treatment of pediatric obsessive compulsive disorder. In S. Taylor (Chair), *New developments in treating obsessive compulsive disorder: Behavior therapy and beyond.* Paper presented at the World Congress of Behavioral and Cognitive Therapies, Vancouver, BC.

Piacentini, J., Jaffer, M., Liebowitz, M., & Gitow, A. (1992, November). *Systematic assessment of impairment in youngsters with obsessive–compulsive disorder: The OCD impact scale.* Poster presented at the annual meeting of the Association for the Advancement of Behavior Therapy, Boston, MA.

Pigott, T. A., & Seay, S. (1998). Biological treatments for obsessive–compulsive disorder: Literature review. In R. P. Swinson, M. M. Antony, S. Rachman, & M. A. Richter (Eds.), *Obsessive–compulsive disorder: Theory, research and treatment* (pp. 298–326). New York: Guilford Press.

Rheingold, A. A., Herbert, J. D., & Franklin, M. E. (2002). *Cognitive bias in adolescents with social anxiety disorder.* Manuscript submitted for publication.

Riddle, M., Reeve, E., Yaryura-Tobias, J., Yang, H., Claghorn, J., Gaffney, G., Greist, J., Holland, D., McConville, B., Pigott, T., & Walkup, J. (2001). Fluvoxamine for children and adolescents with obsessive compulsive disorder: A randomized, controlled, multicenter trial. *Journal of the American Academy of Child and Adolescent Psychiatry, 40,* 222–229.

Riddle, M. A., Scahill, L., King, R. A., Hardin, M. T., Anderson, G. M., Ort, S. I., Smith, J. C., Leckman, J. F., & Cohen, D. J. (1992). Double-blind, crossover trial of fluoxetine and placebo in children and adolescents with obsessive–compulsive disorder. *Journal of the American Academy of Child and Adolescent Psychiatry, 31,* 1062–1069.

Salkovskis, P. M. (1996). Cognitive-behavioural approaches to the understanding of obsessional problems. In R. Rapee (Ed.), *Current controversies in the anxiety disorders* (pp. 103–133). New York: Guilford Press.

Scahill, L., Riddle, M. A., McSwiggin-Hardin, M., Ort, S. I., King, R. A., Goodman,

W. K., Cicchetti, D., & Leckman, J. F. (1997). Children's Yale–Brown Obsessive–Compulsive Scale: Reliability and validity. *Journal of the American Academy of Child and Adolescent Psychiatry, 36,* 844–852.

Silverman, W. K. (1991). Diagnostic reliability of anxiety disorders in children using structured interviews. [Special issue: Assessment of childhood anxiety disorders]. *Journal of Anxiety Disorders, 5,* 105–124.

Swedo, S. E., Leonard, H. L., Garvey, M., Mittleman, B., Allen, A. J., Perlmutter, S., Dow, S., Zamkoff, J., Dubbert, B., & Lougee, L. (1998). Pediatric autoimmune neuropsychiatric disorders associated with streptococcal infections: Clinical description of the first 50 cases. *American Journal of Psychiatry, 155,* 264–271.

Swedo, S. E., Rapoport, J. L., Leonard, H., Lenane, M., & Cheslow, D. (1989). Obsessive–compulsive disorder in children and adolescents: Clinical phenomenology of 70 consecutive cases. *Archives of General Psychiatry, 46,* 335–341.

Valleni-Basille, L. A., Garrison, C. Z., Jackson, K. L., Waller, J. L., McKeown, R. E., Addy, C. L., & Cuffe, S. P. (1994). Frequency of obsessive–compulsive disorder in a community sample of young adolescents. *Journal of the American Academy of Child and Adolescent Psychiatry, 33,* 782–791.

Wever, C., & Rey, J. M. (1997). Juvenile obsessive–compulsive disorder. *Australian and New Zealand Journal of Psychiatry, 31,* 105–113.

SUGGESTED READINGS

Kendall, P., Chu, B., Pimentel, S., & Choudhury, M. (2000). Treating anxiety disorders in youth. In P. Kendall (Ed.), *Child and adolescent therapy: Cognitive-behavioral procedures* (2nd ed., pp. 235–287). New York: Guilford Press.

March, J., & Mulle, K. (1996). Banishing OCD: Cognitive-behavioral psychotherapy for obsessive–compulsive disorders. In E. Hibbs & P. Jensen (Eds.), *Psychosocial treatments for child and adolescent disorders: Empirically-based strategies for clinical practice* (pp. 83–102). Washington, DC: American Psychological Association.

March, J., & Mulle, K. (1998). *OCD in children and adolescents: A cognitive-behavioral treatment manual.* New York: Guilford Press.

Shafran, R. (1998). Childhood obsessive–compulsive disorder. In P. Graham (Ed.), *Cognitive-behaviour therapy for children and families* (pp. 45–73). Cambridge, UK: Cambridge University Press.

8

Strategies to Modify Low Self-Esteem in Adolescents

STEPHEN SHIRK
REBECCA BURWELL
SUSAN HARTER

Concerns about poor self-image and low self-esteem are common among the problems presented by parents of clinic-referred adolescents. Although problems with self-esteem are not recognized as a disorder or syndrome, self-related difficulties in the form of low self-worth, unstable self-image, high self-criticism, and distorted self-evaluations are among the diagnostic or associated features of a wide range of disorders. Low self-esteem is identified most commonly with depressive disorders and is included among the defining features of both dysthymic disorder and major depressive disorder (DSM-IV; American Psychiatric Association, 1994). However, low self-esteem is an associated feature of attention-deficit/hyperactivity disorder, oppositional defiant disorder, social phobia, and bulimia nervosa (see, e.g., American Psychiatric Association, 1994).

Research indicates that low self-esteem is found among adolescents with learning disabilities (Boetsch, Green, & Pennington, 1996), particularly among girls (Heath & Ross, 2000), and is associated with maladaptive academic achievement strategies among non-learning-disabled teens (Aunola, Stattin, & Nurmi, 2000). Low self-esteem also has been found among maltreated older children (Vondra, Barnett, & Cicchetti, 1989) and among children of alcoholic parents (Rodney & Mupier, 1999). Furthermore, low self-esteem has emerged as a predictor of adolescent substance abuse (Unger, Kipke, Simon, Montgomery, & Johnson, 1997), and is common among adolescents with eating disorders (Silverstone, 1990), even among those who do not endorse other depressive symptoms (van der

189

Ham, van-Strien, & van Engeland, 1998). As these findings indicate, low self-esteem, though not a specific disorder, is associated with a range of clinical problems.

Nevertheless, low self-esteem has not been a prominent target for intervention among cognitive-behavioral therapists (cf. Kendall, 1991). This is surprising in light of developmental formulations of the self as a cognitive-affective representation that is constructed through cognitive processes (Harter, 1999; Leahy & Shirk, 1985). Instead, most cognitive-behavioral research and treatment has focused on self-schemas, that is, cognitive structures that influence attention to and recall of self-relevant information (Leahy, 1985). For example, among depressed youth, self-schemas are assumed to be characterized by overgeneralization ("Since I'm bad at math, I'm a lousy student"), all-or-none thinking ("I'm totally stupid"), and dysfunctional attitudes ("If I fail at one thing, I'm a loser"). Negative self-schema, assessed in terms of memory for negative self-descriptors, has been demonstrated among 8- to 16-year-old clinically depressed youth (Zupan, Hammen, & Jaenicke, 1987). Furthermore, there is growing evidence that the content of self-schemas varies by type of disorder; for example, the self-schema of depressed individuals includes contents pertaining to failure and loss, whereas the contents of anxious individuals reflect social threat (Westra & Kuiper, 1997). Thus, one might reasonably assume that low self-esteem, like other cognitive contents, could result from schematic processing biases or cognitive distortions, and thus represents an important target for cognitive-behavioral intervention.

There may be other reasons why self-esteem has not been a prominent target for cognitive-behavioral therapy (CBT). A major issue for cognitive-behavioral clinicians concerns the *function* of psychological constructs. For many, self-esteem is viewed, at best, as a consequence or marker of other pathogenic processes that are responsible for maladjustment. In essence, low self-esteem is typically viewed as a symptom of, rather than a cause of, emotional or behavioral disorders. However, recent research indicates that self-esteem plays a more important functional role in adjustment than once believed.

First, there is evidence that self-esteem is not only a predictor of various outcomes, but that it also functions as a mediator and/or moderator for various clinical problems. As a moderator, level of self-esteem has been shown to impact the relationship between body dissatisfaction and disordered eating, such that young women with low self-esteem are more likely than those with high self-esteem to develop disordered eating patterns (Twamley & Davis, 1999). In addition, level of self-esteem was found to be an important moderator of treatment response for women with eating disorders (van der Ham et al., 1998). Harter (1986) has demonstrated that self-esteem mediates the relationship between children's perceived social support and competence and their academic motivation. Similarly, research by Juvonen, Nishina, and Graham (2000) reveals that, in addition to loneliness and depression, self-esteem mediates the relationship between perceived peer harassment and school outcomes (including GPA and attendance). Self-esteem appears to be closely linked to peer relationships in adolescence, and findings by Kahle, Kulka, and Klingel (1980) indicate that self-esteem is a better predictor of subsequent interpersonal problems than vice versa. Thus, self-esteem does not appear to be a mere correlate or consequence of other functional pathogenic processes. Rather, self-esteem may be integrally involved in the etiology and maintenance of various forms of child and adolescent psychopathology.

A second important issue concerns whether it is possible to change self-esteem through psychotherapy. Although self-esteem may play a functional role in adaptive behavior, it may not be responsive to therapeutic interventions. Early meta-analytic results supported this perspective. Few child treatment studies ($N = 3$) have targeted self-esteem, and those that did produced virtually no effect (mean effect size = .08) (Casey & Berman, 1985). However, in their recent meta-analysis of interventions for self-esteem, Haney and Durlak (1998) uncovered significantly more studies that included self-esteem as an outcome ($N = 116$), and found substantially larger treatment effects (mean effect size = .47) than reported earlier. This moderate effect size suggests that self-esteem can be improved through treatment. Furthermore, treatments that specifically targeted self-esteem produced significantly larger effects than those that merely included a measure of self-esteem but focused on another treatment target, such as social skills (Haney & Durlak, 1998). Consistent with other results in the child treatment literature (Weisz, Donenberg, Han, & Kauneckis, 1995), findings suggest that treatments that focus on a specific target tend to produce more beneficial effects than treatments that attempt to affect an associated target indirectly. From a clinical standpoint, it appears that changes in self-esteem can be attained through improving adolescents' skills and relationships, but treatment strategies that directly target self-esteem may yield additional benefits.

A third issue concerns the degree to which changes in self-esteem will translate into improvements in adaptive functioning. Typically, low self-esteem is one of many problems presented at intake. Is there any evidence that modifying self-esteem contributes to general improvements in adjustment?

One might expect to see limited broadband benefits from specific self-esteem interventions. However, in comparing treatments that focused on self-esteem with those that had a different focus, Haney and Durlak (1998) found that the former set of treatments produced larger effects on collateral problems than the latter. This was true for children with both externalizing and mixed problems, but not for children with internalizing problems, for which both approaches were equally effective (Haney &

Durlak, 1998). For example, among children with externalizing problems, self-esteem–focused treatments had approximately twice the impact on collateral behavior problems compared to treatments without a self-esteem focus (effect size = .66 vs. 34). A similar but more pronounced difference was found for academic outcomes (Haney & Durlak, 1998). Although the causal connection between changes in self-esteem and changes in collateral problems remains ambiguous, these results demonstrate that targeted changes in self-esteem are associated with positive changes in other areas of functioning.

In summary, recent findings indicate that self-esteem plays a functional role in adjustment and can be changed through treatment, especially through treatments that target it for change. Improvements in self-esteem also are linked with other positive outcomes. A critical question, then, is what types of cognitive strategies might be used to modify low self-esteem?

COGNITIVE STRATEGIES TO MODIFY LOW SELF-ESTEEM

One of the limitations of meta-analysis is its inability to identify treatment components or processes associated with positive outcomes. In part, this problem is most apparent when a range of treatment strategies are used across reviewed studies. As a result, meaningful aggregation of treatments often is precluded (Haney & Durlak, 1998). But to a large extent, identification of effective strategies in meta-analyses is constrained by the evaluation of broad treatment packages, rather than specific treatment processes in most outcome studies (Shirk & Russell, 1996).

In an effort to identify promising cognitive interventions, a subset of treatment studies that utilized cognitive procedures was more closely examined. Treatments that included cognitive or cognitive-behavioral terms in the title and that were included in the original meta-analysis by Haney and Durlak (1998) were reviewed. A review of articles produced 12 outcome studies that met the foregoing criteria.[1] All but one study was available for review and a second study that focused on career counseling was excluded, thereby resulting in 10 reviewed articles.[2]

Only three of the studies were designed as self-esteem or self-concept interventions; the remaining seven included a measure of self-esteem along with other outcome measures. Targeted problems in these studies included self-control problems, anxiety, achievement issues, and, most frequently, depressive symptoms. Like most outcome studies, the majority of treat-

---

[1]Evaluations of rational-emotive therapy were not included in this review. Only cognitive or cognitive-behavioral treatments were examined.

[2]These 10 articles are indicated by asterisks in the reference list.

ments involved multiprocedural packages (Shirk, 1999); four studies evaluated a specific treatment procedure such as cognitive restructuring.

Among the four studies that evaluated a specific procedure, assertiveness training, attribution restructuring, and social reinforcement of positive self-referent statements yielded significant improvements in self-esteem. It is noteworthy that two of these studies directly targeted *cognitive* processes hypothesized to be associated with self-esteem, and both produced significant positive changes. A fourth study that examined cognitive restructuring failed to produce significant changes in self-esteem, but the intervention was part of a primary prevention program and many students did not report low self-esteem at the start of intervention.

A number of cognitive or cognitive-behavioral strategies were evaluated in studies that did not specifically target self-esteem. Social problem-solving, self-instructional, and relaxation training were all shown to be associated with reductions in targeted emotional or behavioral problems. Despite improvements in targeted problems, these common cognitive-behavioral strategies did not produce improvements in self-esteem relative to control conditions.

An exception to this pattern was multicomponent treatment packages for depression. Among three treatments targeting depressive symptoms (which includes low self-esteem), all yielded significant improvements in self-esteem over time, and two produced moderate to large treatment effects relative to controls. All three treatments (Kahn, Kehle, Jenson, & Clark, 1990; Reynolds & Coates, 1986; Stark, Reynolds, & Kaslow, 1987) involved multiple components such as practice in goal setting, problem solving, scheduling pleasurable activities, self-reinforcement, and self-monitoring. Consequently, it is difficult to identify a set of specific treatment processes that account for change in self-esteem. It is noteworthy, however, that all three treatments included procedures that targeted *self-evaluative processes* such as the accuracy of self-evaluations and distortions in self-standards. Although far from conclusive, this pattern suggests that these treatments actually targeted self-esteem to some degree and that cognitive strategies aimed at restructuring self-evaluative processes had a beneficial impact on self-esteem. For example, Stark et al. (1987) concluded that it is likely that improvements in self-esteem were related to the development of realistic self-standards.

Overall, then, the results of this focused review suggest that cognitive treatments that target specific self-evaluative processes show significant promise for improving low self-esteem. A number of treatments that included common cognitive-behavioral strategies, but did not specifically target self-evaluative processes, failed to change self-esteem. The only exception to this pattern was one study that improved self-esteem through assertiveness training. The foregoing conclusion, however, is offered with considerable caution. Procedures aimed at altering self-evaluative processes often were embedded in multicomponent treatment packages, and consequently the specific procedures that were responsible for change remain unclear.

COGNITIVE-BEHAVIORAL FORMULATIONS
FOR LOW SELF-ESTEEM

One interesting finding to emerge from the meta-analysis by Haney and Durlak (1998) was that treatments based on prior self-esteem research produced larger treatment gains than those based on general therapy models (e.g., rational-emotive therapy) or based on investigator-generated hypotheses. This finding appears to be consistent with the notion that the design of treatments should be closely linked to research on developmental psychopathology (Persons, 1989; Shirk & Russell, 1996). As Shirk and Russell (1996) have proposed, intervention strategies should be based on empirically grounded formulations of pathogenic process. That is, selection of specific treatment procedures for a particular case should follow from an assessment of pathogenic processes that contribute to manifest problems. Like most clinical problems, low self-esteem can be reached through different pathways or different processes (Harter, 1999).

According to the case formulation approach (Shirk, 2000), treatment planning involves answering a series of questions. First, what are the manifest problems in this case? Second, what pathogenic mechanisms have been shown to be associated with these problems? Answers to the second question require a review of evidence from developmental psychopathology. Third, is there evidence that one or more of these pathogenic mechanisms is present in this specific case? Answers to the third question will define, in part, specific targets for treatment. Fourth, what treatment procedures have been shown to alter the identified pathogenic process? Ironically, despite substantial developments in child and adolescent therapy research, answers to the last question are still elusive largely because research has not focused on specific treatment processes for specific pathogenic mechanisms (Shirk & Russell, 1996). Nevertheless, identification of specific pathogenic mechanisms in a particular case provides a useful starting point for the selection of potentially effective interventions. To this end, a set of empirically grounded, cognitive formulations for low self-esteem are presented.

Unrealistic Self-Standards

One pathogenic mechanism linked with low self-esteem is unrealistic standards for self-evaluation. Perhaps the best-known example involves perfectionistic expectations for the self. Research indicates that maladaptive perfectionism and socially prescribed perfectionism (i.e., the belief that others expect perfection) are negatively correlated with self-esteem (Flett, Hewitt, & DeRosa, 1996; Rice, Ashby, & Slaney, 1998).

Unrealistic expectations for the self have been conceptualized as dysfunctional attitudes (Weissman, 1980), and have been shown to cluster into two types, perfectionistic and socially dependent. Perfectionistic dysfunctional attitudes involve rigid adherence to extreme performance standards as a means of achieving a sense of acceptability and worthiness (e.g., "If I fail partly, it's as bad as being a complete failure"). Socially dependent attitudes involve excessive reliance on others' approval for self-worth (e.g., "I am nothing if a person I love does not love me"). Not surprisingly, endorsement of these rigid and excessive attitudes has been shown to be associated with low self-esteem (Kuiper & Dance, 1994; Roberts, Gotlib, & Kassel, 1996).

It is interesting to note that ideal standards for the self (ideal self-image) have been shown to increase with age and developmental level, reflecting both increasing cognitive abstraction and internalization of societal norms (Glick & Zigler, 1985). One cost of this process, however, is accompanying declines in real self-image (Leahy, 1985). That is, as higher standards are incorporated into the ideal self-image and applied to the real self-image, increasingly negative self-evaluations appear to follow (Leahy, 1981). It is not clear that ideal self-images are inherently unrealistic; however, *idealized* expectations for the self are likely to be difficult to attain. Such extreme contingencies for self-acceptance may represent an important target for cognitive restructuring.

Inaccurate Self-Evaluations

Closely linked to the first formulation is the problem of inaccurate self-evaluations. From a developmental perspective, inaccuracies in self-evaluation are to be expected among young children (Harter, 1988a). In fact, young children, especially in the preschool and early elementary school years, typically *overrate* their abilities (Harter, 1988a; Ruble, Boggiano, Feldman, & Loebl, 1980). Harter (1988a) has proposed that children at this age fail to differentiate what they are really like from what they wish they were like. By middle childhood, however, increasing accuracy and realism begin to characterize children's self-evaluations. Also, it is during this period that children begin to link domain-specific evaluations to global evaluations of the self such as self-esteem (Harter, 1986).

Despite the developmental trend toward increasing accuracy, some groups of children and adolescents show inaccurate self-evaluations. For example, both maltreated and conduct-disordered children have been found to report exaggerated (overly positive) self-evaluations (Hughes, Cavell, & Grossman, 1997; Vondra et al., 1989). It is not clear if this pattern reflects a developmental delay in self-evaluation or a defensive strategy for masking underlying feelings of inferiority. In contrast, research with depressed children (Kendall, Stark, & Adam, 1990) has indicated that self-evaluations are negatively distorted relative to external standards.

Inaccurate self-evaluations, especially negatively valenced evaluations, could result from a number of maladaptive cognitive processes. First, such problems could stem from the selective use of social comparison information. Adolescents often compare their characteristics to those of peers and may selectively attend to reference groups that deflate their self-esteem. For example, Matthews and Siegel (1983) have found that children differ in their choice of comparison targets especially in the absence of well-defined criteria for performance. Some children (e.g., those with strong achievement strivings) compare themselves only to top performers on a task. Similar processes are likely to be operative in adolescents' evaluations of their physical appearance, a characteristic closely tied to self-esteem (Harter, 1999).

Adolescents may also show information-processing biases in their evaluations of information that are important to self-esteem. Harter (1986, 1999) has demonstrated that perceptions of competence and social support are closely linked to level of self-worth, and that adolescents vary in their relative weighting of these two sources of information. Moreover, perceptions of competence or support can be subject to cognitive bias. For example, Shirk, Van Horn, and Leber (1997) demonstrated that dysphoric teens perceive videotaped, supportive interactions as less responsive, helpful, and authentic than do nondysphoric peers. This research indicated that differences in perceptions of supportive interactions could be attributed to schematic processing biases. Adolescents with these processing biases also showed lowered self-esteem.

Alternatively, inaccurate self-evaluations could be closely tied to unrealistic self-standards. That is, despite clear feedback or performance criteria some teens may harbor unrealistic, internal standards that result in distorted evaluations of the self. Unrealistic self-contingencies could contribute to biased recall of self-relevant information such that flaws or minor "failures" become highly salient and easily retrieved.

Another cognitive process that can undermine self-evaluative accuracy is a biased explanatory style (Nolen-Hoeksema, Girgus, & Seligman, 1986). According to the reformulated learned helplessness model (Abramson, Seligman, & Teasdale, 1978), the tendency to attribute negative events to stable, internal causes produces a defined cluster of helplessness characteristics, including lowered self-esteem. Research with children and adolescents has revealed consistent associations between depressive symptoms, including low self-esteem, and a biased explanatory style (cf. Robinson, Garber, & Hilsman, 1995)

In summary, a number of cognitive processes, including unrealistic self-standards, biased social information processing, selective recall of self-relevant information, and a biased explanatory style could contribute to negatively distorted self-evaluations. As such, these processes represent potential targets for cognitive-behavioral interventions.

Undifferentiated Self-Structure

With development children and adolescents increasingly differentiate aspects or domains of self-evaluation, including evaluations of the self that are linked to specific relational contexts (Harter, 1999; Leahy & Shirk, 1985). In this connection, one structural feature of the self that has received considerable attention is level of self-complexity, or the number of self-aspects an individual uses for organizing information and their degree of distinctiveness (Linville, 1985). Low levels of self-complexity in adolescence have been shown to be related to low global self-worth and to elevated levels of both internalizing and externalizing behaviors (Evans, 1994). Linville (1985) has proposed that low levels of complexity render individuals vulnerable to affective lability and sharp shifts in self-evaluation. In brief, limited differentiation provides the conditions for spreading evaluative coloring of self-appraisals. With few self-aspects, positive or negative feedback in one domain carries greater implications for global self-esteem than in a highly differentiated system. Consistent with this hypothesis, Linville (1985, 1987) has demonstrated that individuals with less complex cognitive representations of the self are more vulnerable to extreme swings in affect and self-evaluation after failure or success experiences than those with greater complexity. Thus, it is possible that adolescents who present with low self-esteem may show poorly differentiated self-concepts, and have placed *all their self-evaluative eggs in one large cognitive basket* (Linville, 1985). Differentiation of the self may represent an important step in improving self-esteem and protecting adolescents from the negative impact of stressful events. In fact, Linville (1987) has shown that high self-complexity functions as a buffer against stress-related illness and depression.

A related issue involves the degree to which adolescents evaluate the *importance* of different aspects or domains of the self. Harter (1999) has shown that domains of the self that are important to adolescents have a significantly larger impact on global self-worth than those that are less important. Thus, an adolescent might differentiate multiple aspects of the self, but really only view one or a few as important. Such overvaluing of single aspects of the self can increase vulnerability to low self-esteem. In essence, negative events or feedback in important domains are not offset by positive evaluations of other aspects of the self because they are regarded as unimportant. Perhaps the best example of this phenomenon is in the area of physical appearance or body image where weight gain, a minor blemish, or a perceived slight can undermine self-esteem among teens who overvalue this aspect of self. One aim of intervention, then, is to help the adolescent to recognize or to develop other important self-aspects.

Inauthentic or False Self

False self—the suppression or hiding of one's authentic self and of one's thoughts, feelings, and beliefs—represents another important pathogenic mechanism associated with low self-esteem. False self is a particularly salient issue during adolescence, a time when awareness of the self is magnified, and when teens are attempting to distinguish between their multiple selves in different relationships in order to define their "true" self (Harter, 1999). False-self behavior in the form of suppressing or hiding one's true thoughts, feelings, and beliefs is associated with low global self-worth in adolescence (Harter, Marold, Whitesell, & Cobbs, 1996) and may interfere with the development of mutual peer relations that are critical to identity development (Harter, 1999).

The emergence of false-self behavior appears to have strong interpersonal roots. Research reveals an association between false self and adolescents' perceptions of low, and primarily conditional, support from others. In modeling relations among self-related constructs, Harter et al. (1996) found that the association between perceptions of contingent support and the presentation of false self operated through hopelessness about pleasing others. It is important to note that such hopelessness may, in fact, be realistic for some adolescents. False-self behavior may be particularly challenging for adolescent girls as they begin to identify with cultural proscriptions involving the expression of thoughts and beliefs by women. Loss of "voice" is linked with low self-esteem (Harter et al., 1996) and may contribute to the emergence of gender differences in depressive symptoms during adolescence. Recent findings indicate that loss of voice is related to gender identity such that feminine girls, particularly in public contexts, show the lowest level of voice.

Taken together, these findings suggest that false-self behavior is embedded in both social and cultural processes. Consequently, efforts to alter false-self behavior may need to address not only the cognitive underpinnings of this problem but the contextual factors that maintain it.

Summary

According to the case formulation approach, the selection of treatment strategies is guided by the identification of pathogenic processes for a set of manifest problems (Persons, 1989). It is our proposal that this process should be informed by empirical evidence on associations between pathogenic mechanisms and specific clinical problems. In the case of low self-esteem, four cognitive-behavioral formulations of pathogenic process have been presented, including unrealistic self-standards, inaccurate self-evaluation, undifferentiated self-structure, and inauthentic or false-self behavior, along with supporting evidence for each. Although by no means exhaustive, these cognitive-behavioral formulations provide a starting point for assessment in specific cases and, ultimately, for the selection of treatment strategies.

By no means do we wish to convey that low self-esteem is solely the result of maladaptive cognitive processes. There is far too much evidence to indicate that family processes such as high parental criticism (Kernis, Brown, & Brody, 2000), traumatic life events such as sexual abuse (Bolger, Patterson, & Kupersmidt, 1998), and other life circumstances can have a corrosive impact on self-esteem. Thus, a caveat is in order: Self-esteem is not simply a function of internal processes. In many cases, deleterious processes in the social environment take their toll on youngsters' self-esteem. However, such deleterious experiences are processed through a cognitive filter; consequently, cognitive processes can amplify or ameliorate the impact of negative events.

In the following section, two case reports will be presented in order to illustrate a cognitive-behavioral case formulation approach to the treatment of low self-esteem in adolescence. Although both teens presented with low self-esteem, their treatments were guided by different cognitive-behavioral formulations.

CASE EXAMPLES

Chris

Chris, a 16-year-old high school junior, was referred for psychotherapy following an emotional episode during which he expressed a wish to kill himself. Over the previous 2 years, Chris, who was an outstanding student/athlete has shown signs of social withdrawal and self-deprecating thinking. There had been no overt suicide attempts, but suicidal ideation was prominent in his thinking.

Initial Assessment

Following interviews with Chris and his mother, it was learned that Chris was near the top of his class academically, well integrated socially, and a starter for the basketball team. His mother noted that he was a "model son" but was perplexed by his demands to be "perfect." For example, when Chris failed to achieve the highest grade on a physics exam, he did not permit himself to see his close friends for over a week; instead, he spent time sequestered in his room studying. Asked about family expectations for Chris, his mother noted that she and her husband would be happy with a solid B average. Chris, in fact, acknowledged that the pressure he felt did not come from his parents.

On the Youth Self-Report (YSR), Chris showed clinically significant elevations on several of the internalizing narrow bands, including anxiety/depression (Internalizing $T = 72$). However, the most prominent feature in his presentation was self-criticism. He set extremely high standards for himself and was sharply self-punitive when he failed to attain them. On several occasions he had slapped himself on the face following what he perceived to be academic "failure" (not getting an A). Not surprisingly, he reported low global self-worth (nearly two standard deviations below the normative mean) on the Self-Perception Profile for Adolescents (Harter, 1988b). His self-esteem was clearly vulnerable. Acknowledged achievements brought limited feelings of satisfaction, and were often discounted, whereas perceived failure resulted in sustained self-reproach.

Family history was noteworthy in that Chris had been adopted as an infant. His biological mother, a teenager, had attempted to raise him but, given her limited resources including little family support, found the task overwhelming and relinquished custody of Chris. Chris had been informed of his adoption at an early age, but given the "closed" nature of the adoption he had no contact with his birth mother. In interview, he reported no desire to search for her, and expressed a strong sense of "belonging" in his adoptive family.

Case Formulation and Treatment Plan

The most prominent features in Chris's presentation were his high self-standards, strong self-critical tendencies, and depressed mood that appeared to follow from self-punitive thinking. Chris's low self-esteem appeared to be a function of *unrealistic self-standards* and his tendency to utilize *self-punishment* as his primary method of self-regulation. Consequently, the aims of treatment were to modify Chris's standards for self-evaluation and to help him develop alternatives to self-punishment for coping with disappointments. In brief, self-evaluative processes were directly targeted. Chris seemed motivated for treatment and expressed a strong desire to find relief from what he called his "internal pressure." Our initial alliance was forged around the mutual goal of finding a "relief valve" for this pressure.

Course of Treatment

Early in treatment, Chris and I (SRS) explored his goals and expectations for himself. Consistent with the initial interview, his academic performance expectations were extremely high and somewhat at odds with his long-term goals, namely, to attend a state university and become an architect. Neither goal required the high level of performance Chris demanded of himself.

One of the first interventions, a series of homework assignments, required Chris to seek information about college requirements and the academic criteria for admission to a program in architecture. The aim was to provide both realistic information and to highlight the incongruity between his perfectionistic standards and his realistic goals. Chris met with his high school guidance counselor, and his parents arranged a visit to a local architectural firm. Despite feedback about what would be "realistically" required to attain his goals, little change in his self-expectations resulted from these "psychoeducational" interventions.

In an effort to alter his self-punitive tendencies, I asked Chris to keep a log of his "inner pressure," noting any occasion when he acted punitively toward himself. He was an active recorder of his moods and thoughts, which typically included references to his "stupidity" and "worthlessness." At this point, I began to challenge the connection between his high expectations and his harsh self-criticism through a series of role plays aimed at introducing a new perspective on his situation. After linking his tendency to punish himself for failing to meet his performance standards, I asked Chris if he held the same standards for his friends, and, more importantly, if he would treat them so harshly if they failed to perform perfectly. Not surprisingly, Chris was far more forgiving of his friends and certainly did not expect them to be perfect. We focused on this "double standard" for several sessions. During this time, I role played one of his friends. In a typical scenario, I would express disappointment with my performance. It was Chris's task to demonstrate how he would console or encourage his friend. Chris had little difficulty being supportive in the role plays and he had no trouble generating alternative strategies for dealing with disappointment that he *consistently* failed to use with himself. It was easy to see why Chris had a broad network of friends. In relation to *others* he was empathic and supportive, but in relation to himself, he was a harsh taskmaster.

Chris's difficulty with self-punishment did not fit a deficit model; instead, he had the skills in his repertoire but failed to utilize them with himself. Thus, the aim of therapy came to be defined as "teaching Chris to be a friend to himself." In an effort to transfer the skills and attitudes that Chris clearly demonstrated in relation to others, we recorded the calming and encouraging statements he used with friends (e.g., "Don't take it so hard; there'll be another test"; "So this one didn't go so well—think about everything else you have going for you"). In session, we continued the role plays, but this time Chris was asked to recall episodes of disappointment and to practice the self-calming statements.

Unfortunately, Chris continued to struggle with perfectionism and self-criticism. Although he appeared to have the "skills" needed to be less self-critical, the recalcitrant nature of this cognitive pattern appeared to be embedded in deeper assumptions about the self and others. A recurrent theme in Chris's thinking was a close link between "failure" (lack of perfection) and interpersonal rejection. For example, Chris made numerous comments that his interpersonal security was tied to outstanding performance across multiple domains (e.g., "They'll laugh at me if I make a mistake"; "I don't measure up so I have to show I'm better than them"; "No one wants to hang around a loser"). These expectations had all the hallmarks of cognitive distortions. First, they were overgeneralized and unqualified; second, they were inconsistent with what I had learned about Chris's family and friends. Chris's low self-esteem was linked to unrealistic self-standards, and the roots of these standards appeared to go far beyond his current life circumstances.

Given evidence that Chris's schematic expectation (imperfection = rejection) was not based on current interpersonal experiences, we began a "developmental analysis" of the origins of his belief. After noting this cognitive pattern, I assured Chris that he must have good grounds for holding such a belief, and that our new task was to discover how he came to believe in it. Chris was willing to search for the origins of his belief, still motivated to find some relief for his "internal pressure." He initially focused on the anxiety he experienced when he changed schools at age 13. Not surprisingly, the theme of this memory revolved around anticipated rejection by teachers and classmates. However, as we continued to focus on the possible origins of his expectations of rejection, our conversations quickly turned to his adoption.

Chris and his parents knew relatively little about the circumstances of his relinquishment, yet Chris was adamant that he had played a role in the process. As we explored the possibilities, he alluded to being "too difficult" and to "being a burden." Eventually, with a great outpouring of emotion, he simply said, "Something must have been wrong with me." This core assumption, undoubtedly constructed during childhood to make sense of his early experience, found expression in his current schematic belief that "others will reject me (or I must reject myself), if I am not perfect."

The final phase of treatment involved gentle challenges to Chris's core assumption about his relinquishment. Much of this work centered around consideration of alternative reasons for his placement, noting that each was as plausible as the "theory" Chris had constructed. His adoptive mother participated in several sessions to counter Chris's claim that he was a difficult or burdensome baby. A marked shift occurred in his emotion expression. For the first time, Chris directed his anger not at himself, but toward his birth mother, whom he regarded as "weak." In a later session I noted that he was now turning his harshness in another direction, and although I was pleased to see him direct it away from himself, we needed to recall that his perception of his birth mother as weak also was only a theory. Although Chris initially reacted by directing anger toward me, this intervention appeared to open the door for a process of grieving his early loss. The strength of the emotions expressed during the ensuing sessions provided strong testimony for the tight link between core schemas and intense emotions. Although this phase of therapy had been guided by an analysis of cognitive assumptions, it was evident that schema transformation involved the experience and expression of associated emotion. In many ways this final phase of treatment is consistent with recent findings on change processes in cognitive therapy; specifically, that depth of emotional experiencing in cognitive therapy is predictive of symptomatic change (Castonguay, Goldfried, Wiser, Raue, & Hayes, 1996).

Treatment Outcome

It was evident that Chris had attained significant distance from his maladaptive assumption linking perfection with acceptance. Maternal report indicated increased involvement in social activities and an emerging interest in romantic relationships. The intensity of his achievement concerns and his drive for perfection were clearly in better balance with other age-appropriate interests. More directly, Chris no longer showed the self-punitive cognitive pattern following "perceived failure" (not getting the top grade), even though his achievement standards remained relatively, though not excessively, high. It appeared that attaining some perspective on, and processing emotions related to, his maladaptive core assumptions enabled him to use adaptive coping skills already in his repertoire. Perhaps of greatest relevance, at time of termination Chris reported feeling "less internal pressure" and, not surprisingly, his report of global self-worth on the SPP showed a noteworthy jump in a positive direction to within a half a standard deviation of the normative mean. Consistent with this shift, his Internalizing T score dropped into the non-clinical range ($T = 58$).

Russ

Russ is a 14-year-old high school freshman who was referred by his parents following an academic year described by his mother as "catastrophic." Russ was in a gifted and talented program during elementary school and had performed consistently above grade level. He was described as a youngster with great curiosity and a unique talent for writing and performing in plays. During the preceding year, Russ had "shut down" academically, failed to complete numerous assignments, and had lost interest in play writing. Neither Russ nor his parents reported any significant life events that might account for this marked change in academic functioning. Because of Russ's intellectual strengths he passed eighth grade by performing well on tests with relatively little effort.

Initial Assessment

Given the sharp decline in motivation, Russ was interviewed for symptoms of depression. Although he acknowledged loss of interest in school and play writing, he remained invested in family activities (skiing and hiking) and in attending concerts with friends. He noted that it was difficult to get up on school days but he did not report sleep problems or being tired on weekends or over vacations. Russ further acknowledged that he felt down and "kind of empty" a lot of the time, especially during the last 6 months. However, overall level of depressive symptoms on the Child Depression Inventory (CDI) was only slightly elevated, with a score of 11. Russ appeared to meet criteria for dysthymic disorder based on the constellation and duration of symptoms and evidence of functional impairment (school) derived from the interview. His CDI score suggested that, at present, he was mildly depressed or what might be better termed dysphoric. Closer examination of his CDI profile indicated that two clusters accounted for his slightly elevated score, low self-worth (critical of and disappointed with himself, with suicidal ideation), and low energy and interest (bored and tired easily).

In interview Russ was at a loss to explain the change in his mood and academic functioning. He did mention that he felt like he was "in a slump" and that he simply needed to push himself a little harder. At one point he mentioned with more than a hint of anger that his "parents were really bent about his [play] writing." When pressed to elaborate, Russ simply said, "They really get off on the awards." He also noted that he felt increasingly distant from his friends at school, whom he described as "jocks" or "preps" who spent most of their time flirting or talking about shopping. In contrast to school, he felt "connected" to teens in a youth group he belonged to and noted that he could talk about anything with them. The problem was that he rarely saw these friends because they resided in a different school district. He noted that when he was with them he felt a "whole different energy."

A collateral interview with his parents suggested that they were very perplexed about the change in Russ. In fact, they were very concerned about his loss of interest in play writing and acting. His mother noted that he had won several competitions for his scripts and was quite distressed because he currently showed no interest in writing or trying out for school plays. She ended the initial interview by stating, "I just don't want to see him throw his life away."

Case Formulation and Treatment Plan

Based on the initial assessment, three sets of problems were evident in Russ's presentation. First, his motivation for academic achievement had dropped sharply, and was so low that it was distressing to both Russ and his parents. Second, he often felt bored and uninterested in activities that once had been engaging, although the scope of this problem appeared to be limited to schoolwork and play writing. There was some evidence that he was beginning to disengage with school friends as well. Third, he was critical of and disappointed with himself, both markers of problems with self-esteem.

From a cognitive-behavioral perspective, the first two problems could be addressed with familiar, empirically supported strategies. In order to address the decline in academic motivation, a contingency contract could be negotiated to increase incentives for homework completion. Similarly, in order to offset Russ's low energy and boredom, scheduling pleasurable activities and increasing physical exercise could be prescribed. In fact, these strategies were employed but were secondary to other cognitive strategies that followed from an emerging case formulation.

As Persons (1989) has observed, a good case formulation ties together the patient's problems so that presenting problems do not appear as a "random collection of difficulties" (pp. 37–38). Of course, one way of tying Russ's problems together would be to attribute them to a depressive disorder. This approach, however, would represent only the first step in understanding his problems. From a case formulation perspective, it is necessary to develop hypotheses about the underlying pathogenic mechanisms that account for the constellation of symptoms.

In Russ's case, there were a number of indicators that problematic cognitions about the self were contributing to his difficulties. First, it was noteworthy that Russ described his emotional distress as emptiness rather than sadness. Corresponding to this affective experience, he described himself as "playing a role" and "feeling fake" in relation to his friends at school. In sharp contrast to these experiences, he felt "connected," "alive," and "comfortable with himself" with his friends in the youth group. As he noted in an early session, with these kids "I can be who I really am," and an important part of Russ involved his intellectual curiosity and interest in religious and philosophical issues. Thus, there appeared to be a close connection between his emotions and his experience of self.

Complicating the picture were cognitions related to his play writing. He commented that he "felt like he was going through the motions of writing," and even though he could still produce material, none of it seemed to feel like his own. Although his parents strongly supported his play writing and had sent him to summer workshops, his recent attempts at writing some "weird dark stuff" had been discouraged by his parents. As Russ noted, "They only respond when I stay in the mainstream; then they love it." In brief, it appeared that intrinsic interest in an activity had been undermined by increasing performance expectations, and by Russ's wish to meet them. Although he did not share this aspect of himself with his school friends for fear they would see him as a "nerd," he had performed several of his plays with his friends in the youth group.

Thus, a core cognitive dilemma for Russ involved the presentation of his "true self" in different relational contexts. With his classmates he felt like he was fake, but fearful that exposure of his true self would result in rejection. With his parents, one of his core self-attributes, as a playwright, felt like it had been co-opted in the service of parental pride and admiration. In many ways, then, Russ's problems appeared to fit the *inauthentic or false-self formulation*. Although adolescence is the period during which awareness of false-self behaviors becomes particularly acute (Harter, 1999), for Russ such awareness appeared to be tightly connected with his academic difficulties and loss of interest. Furthermore, as demonstrated by developmental research, adolescents with the highest levels of false-self issues report the lowest levels of self-worth and dysphoric affect (Harter et al., 1996). Therefore, in addition to interventions aimed at boosting energy and motivation for schoolwork, the cognitive focus of therapy revolved around assumptions pertaining to Russ's true self.

Course of Treatment

Russ and I (SRS) agreed that our treatment goal would be to help him out of his "rut" of boredom and low energy. I told him that "getting back on track" might involve "finding a new track" rather than returning to the same old way of doing things. After prescribing an exercise program (Russ was an avid biker) and scheduling pleasurable activities, we turned to taking care of old business. The first task involved helping Russ complete a project that he had failed to finish during the previous academic year. Although his parents agreed to reward him with concert tickets when he finished, Russ and I focused on self-control strategies (e.g., setting aside gradually increasing amounts of time for work, and building self-reinforcement plans for incremental completion of the project). This approach was in contrast to a maladaptive pattern of procrastination identified by Russ. In addition, the focus on *self-control* appeared to be consistent with the developmental press toward increasing autonomy and self-direction that is typical at Russ's age. Russ felt good about this approach, and was pleased to be "rid of a burden" after he completed the project over the first 6 weeks of therapy. He also felt this approach would make it easier to deal with burdensome homework during the coming school year.

Also during the early phase of treatment, I began to have Russ monitor and record his moods, including both "feeling down" and "feeling empty" each day. Overall, he reported that his moods had already improved slightly, but there were still times when he felt distressed. The following week Russ began to record the contexts for his moods as well as the *inner dialogue* that covaried with them. Given his interest in drama, I suggested that he might be "playing out a script he might want to rewrite."

It was during this phase of treatment that Russ's problematic cognitive schemas became most evident. These schemas were structured as "if . . . then" contingencies for interpersonal acceptance (Baldwin & Sinclair, 1996). For example, "If I show my friends at school I like musicals, they'll think I'm strange"; "My parents ignore my writing if I try something weird"; "I just act like I'm into sports and stuff so the other kids don't ignore me." On the other hand, meeting these interpersonal expectations was taking a toll. Russ felt like he was "being fake" or "artificial," and his suppression of what Harter (1999) has called "voice," that is, his true thoughts, feelings, interests, and opinions, appeared to leave him feeling "empty" and at times "irritated." In terms of self-esteem, Russ was angry and disappointed with himself for falling into this false-self pattern.

It was noteworthy that Russ observed that these feelings were not part of his experience with his youth group. In that context he felt free of the contingencies he experienced with his school friends and parents. Here he could be "intellectual," into "all kinds of music," and be "accepted for the real me." Not surprisingly, he felt alive and energized with this set of friends.

At this point in treatment (the tenth session), our work began to focus on "bringing all of Russ onto stage." The first strategy was to increase Russ's contact with the members of his youth group, who appeared to support aspects of himself that he valued. In session we began a close examination of aspects he exposed or hid in different contexts. Russ then rank ordered aspects of himself from the easiest to the most difficult to reveal in different settings. This activity was aimed, in part, at addressing the "either/or" quality of his thinking about true and false self. We also recorded his expectations of what might happen if he showed more of his true self in these settings. This work centered on clarifying his "if . . . then" contingencies for acceptance.

Our work then moved in two directions. First, it was not clear that Russ's contingencies for acceptance were marked by distortion or, given the premium on conformity in suburban high school culture, were actually right on the mark. Consequently, we worked on identifying contexts within the school in which it might be possible for him to begin to show more of his true self. This strategy served two functions: First, it allowed Russ to test his assumptions under conditions where they might be disconfirmed, and, second, it provided a relatively safe exposure trial. Russ could gradually present more of himself to kids with whom he did not have long-standing connections. He then could decide if he wanted to take the same risks with teens he had known for a long time, or if he wanted to establish new friendships. In this connection, we simultaneously began to reevaluate his desire to be accepted by the "popular kids."

With the goal of finding a supportive peer group, Russ identified the debate club and theater group as two contexts to practice "being himself." Fortunately, he was surprised to find that teens in the debate club actually valued his sharp wit and intellectual strength. One aspect of self thus found a new context for expression. Russ was equally pleased to find that the group not only included smart kids, but attractive girls (one of his concerns about showing his intelligence was that he would repel potential dates). In turn, he began to feel less "phony." He reported that he was not struggling to get up in the morning to go to school and that he had new friends to "hang with" at lunch.

Russ's treatment illustrates an important aspect of cognitive therapy. Although his difficulties could be understood in cognitive terms, treatment involved both uncovering and reworking of cognitive schemas that undermined self-esteem *and* the identification and use of social contexts that could support aspects of the self that had been hidden. In essence, we often use social contexts to test maladaptive cognitions, but at other times we need to find contexts that are consistent with patient cognitions as well.

Treatment Outcome

Russ's treatment was reduced to periodic monitoring after 23 sessions. He reported fewer episodes of feeling tired and empty, and his CDI score dropped to 5, or slightly below the normative mean. From a behavioral perspective, Russ no longer struggled to complete his school assignments. Thus, the functional impairment that led to referral was substantially altered. With regard to self-esteem, Russ reported less anger at himself for being "fake" and greater comfort with his expressed self. This latter development was captured in a session when Russ reported that one of his friends had dropped by while he was listening to folk music. He noted that most of his friends thought folk to be "pathetic," and that he would have shut off the music in the past. This time he let it play because it was "a part of him" that he "didn't want to hide." In essence, his dependence on social approval appeared to be diminished, and his capacity to validate his own voice had grown stronger.

Russ had not returned to play writing at the end of regular sessions. In part, it seemed that this activity represented the final frontier of contingent self-worth. That is, with both parents and at least a subset of his peers, Russ's play writing had been a vehicle for recognition, admiration, and acceptance, yet with other classmates it carried a different meaning—it made him different, and potentially vulnerable to exclusion. However, as an indicator of change in this area, Russ ventured back to drama by trying out for and getting a part in a class play. Not only did he rediscover the positive emotions connected with drama, he found a group who supported this aspect of himself.

CONCLUSIONS

Although self-esteem has not been a prime target for cognitive therapists, it is clear that problematic cognitions about the self are part of a number of disorders and associated with a range of clinical problems. Furthermore, there is growing evidence that self-esteem has a functional role in emotional and behavioral adjustment, that it can be modified through treatment, and that changes in self-esteem can impact other aspects of adaptive functioning. Our review of the literature also suggests that modification of self-esteem is most promising when self-evaluative processes are directly targeted for change.

As in the treatment of most disorders, a "one size fits all" approach to treating low self-esteem in adolescence is unlikely to be most effective. Instead, the choice of specific strategies depends on the formulation of pathogenic processes contributing to low self-esteem. To this end, we identified four empirically supported formulations for low self-esteem, including unrealistic self-standards, inaccurate self-evaluation, undifferentiated self-structure, and inauthentic or false-self behavior. Assessment of these processes in a particular case provides the framework for selecting specific cognitive strategies for low self-esteem.

In our case reports, we illustrated treatments based on two of the prototypical self-esteem formulations. Although both treatments involved well-known cognitive procedures such as thought monitoring, uncovering and challenging interpersonal assumptions, and the development of self-control strategies, variations in implementation of these procedures followed from different case formulations. Kurt Lewin once commented that there is nothing as practical as a good theory. Similarly, we would propose that there is nothing as clinically useful as an empirically supported case formulation. Such formulations not only provide order to diverse presenting problems, they provide a compass for guiding the course of therapy.

REFERENCES

*Indicates studies included in the analysis of effect sizes for cognitive procedures on self-esteem.

Abramson, L. Y., Seligman, M. E., & Teasdale, J. D. (1978). Learned helplessness in humans: Critique and reformulation. *Journal of Abnormal Psychology, 87*(1), 49–74.

American Psychiatric Association (1994). *Diagnostic and statistical manual of mental disorders* (4th ed.). Washington, DC: Author.

Aunola, K., Stattin, H., & Nurmi, J. E. (2000). Adolescents' achievement strategies, school adjustment, and externalizing and internalizing problem behaviors. *Journal of Youth and Adolescence, 29*(3), 289–306.

*Baker, S. B., Thomas, R. N., & Munson, W. W. (1983). Effects of cognitive restructuring and structured group discussion as primary prevention strategies. *School Counselor, 31,* 26–33.

Baldwin, M. W., & Sinclair, L. (1996). Self-esteem and "if . . . then" contingencies of interpersonal acceptance. *Journal of Personality and Social Psychology, 71*(6), 1130–1141.

Boetsch, E. A., Green, P. A., & Pennington, B. F. (1996). Psychosocial correlates of dyslexia across the lifespan. *Development and Psychopathology, 8*(3), 539–562.

Bolger, K. E., Patterson, C. J., & Kupersmidt, J. B. (1998) Peer relationships and self-esteem among children who have been maltreated. *Child Development, 69*(4), 1171–1197.

Casey, R., & Berman, J. (1985). The outcome of psychotherapy with children. *Psychological Bulletin, 98,* 388–400.

Castonguay, L., Goldfried, M., Wiser, S., Raue, P., & Hayes, A. (1996). Predicting the effect of cognitive therapy for depression: A study of unique and common factors. *Journal of Consulting and Clinical Psychology, 64,* 497–504.

*Elias, M. J. (1983). Improving the coping skills of emotionally-disturbed boys through television based social problem-solving. *American Journal of Orthopsychiatry, 53,* 61–72.

Evans, D. (1994). Self complexity and its relation to development, symptomatology, and self-perception in adolescence. *Child Psychiatry and Human Development, 24,* 173–182.

Flett, G. L., Hewitt, P. L., & DeRosa, T. (1996). Dimensions of perfectionism, psychosocial adjustment, and social skills. *Personality and Individual Differences, 20*(2), 143–150.

Glick, M., & Zigler, E. (1985). Self-image: A cognitive-developmental approach. In R. Leahy (Ed.), *The development of the self* (pp. 1–55). New York: Academic Press.

Haney, P., & Durlak, J. (1998). Changing self-esteem in children and adolescents: A meta-analytic review. *Journal of Clinical Child Psychology, 27,* 423–433.

Harter, S. (1986). Processes underlying the construction, maintenance, and enhancement of self-concept in children. In J. Suls & A. Greenwald (Eds.), *Psychological perspectives on the self* (Vol. 3, pp. 137–181). Hillsdale, NJ: Erlbaum.

Harter, S. (1988a). Development and dynamic changes in the nature of the self-concept. In S. Shirk (Ed.), *Cognitive development and child psychotherapy* (pp. 119–160). New York: Plenum Press.

Harter, S. (1988b). *Self-Perception Profile for Adolescents.* Unpublished manual. University of Denver.

Harter, S. (1999). *The construction of the self: A developmental perspective.* New York: Guilford Press.

Harter, S., Marold, D. B., Whitesell, N. R., & Cobbs, G. (1996). A model of the effects of parent and peer support on adolescent false self behavior. *Child Development, 67,* 360–374.

Heath, N. L., & Ross, S. (2000). Prevalence and expression of depressive symptomatology in students with and without learning disabilities. *Learning Disability Quarterly, 23*(1), 24–36.

Hughes, J., Cavell, T., & Grossman, P. (1997). A positive view of self: Risk or protection for aggressive children? *Development and Psychopathology, 9,* 75–94.

Juvonen, J., Nishina, A., & Graham, S. (2000). Peer harassment, psychological adjustment, and school functioning in early adolescence. *Journal of Educational Psychology, 92*(2), 349–359.

Kahle, L., Kulka, R., & Klingel, D. (1980). Low adolescent self-esteem leads to multiple interpersonal problems. *Journal of Personality and Social Psychology, 39,* 496–502.

*Kahn, J., Kehle, T., Jenson, W., & Clark, E. (1990). Comparison of cognitive-behavioral, relaxation, and self-modeling interventions for depression among middle school students. *School Psychology Review, 19,* 196–211.

Kendall, P. (Ed.). (1991). *Child and adolescent therapy: Cognitive-behavioral procedures.* New York: Guilford Press.

*Kendall, P., & Braswell, L. (1982). Cognitive-behavioral self-control therapy for children: A components analysis. *Journal of Consulting and Clinical Psychology, 50,* 672–689.

Kendall, P., Stark, K., & Adam, T. (1990). Cognitive deficit or cognitive distortion in childhood depression. *Journal of Abnormal Child Psychology, 18,* 255–270.

Kernis, M. H., Brown, A. C., & Brody, G. H. (2000). Fragile self-esteem in children and its associations with perceived patterns of parent–child communication. *Journal of Personality, 68*(2), 225–252.

Kuiper N. A., & Dance, K. A. (1994). Dysfunctional attitudes, role stress evaluations, and psychological well-being. *Journal of Research in Personality, 28*(2), 245–262.

Leahy, R. (1981). Parental practices and the development of moral judgment and self-image disparity during adolescence. *Developmental Psychology, 17,* 580–594.

Leahy, R. (1985). The costs of development: Clinical implications. In R. Leahy (Ed.), *The development of the self* (pp. 267–294). New York: Academic Press.

Leahy, R., & Shirk, S. (1985). Social cognition and the development of the self. In R. Leahy (Ed.), *The development of the self* (pp. 123–150). New York: Academic Press.

Linville, P. (1985). Self complexity and affective extremity: Don't put all your eggs in one cognitive basket. *Social Cognition, 3,* 94–120.

Linville, P. (1987). Self complexity as a cognitive buffer against stress-related illness and depression. *Journal of Personality and Social Psychology, 52,* 663–676.

Matthews, K., & Siegel, J. (1983). Type A behaviors by children, social comparison, and standards for self-evaluation. *Developmental Psychology, 19,* 135–140.

Nolen-Hoeksema, S., Girgus, J. S., & Seligman, M. E. (1986). Learned helplessness in children: A longitudinal study of depression, achievement, and explanatory style. *Journal of Personality and Social Psychology, 51*(2), 435–442.

Persons, J. (1989). *Cognitive therapy in practice: A case formulation approach.* New York: Norton.

*Phillips, R. H. (1984). Increasing positive self-referent statements to improve self-esteem in low-income elementary school children. *Journal of School Psychology, 22,* 155–163.

*Reynolds, W., & Coates, K. (1986). A comparison of cognitive-behavioral therapy and relaxation training for the treatment of depression in adolescence. *Journal of Consulting and Clinical Psychology, 54,* 653–660.

Rice, K. G., Ashby, J. S., & Slaney, R. B. (1998). Self-esteem as a moderator between perfectionism and depression: A structural equation analysis. *Journal of Counseling Psychology, 45*(3), 304–314.

Roberts, J. E., Gotlib, I. H., & Kassel, J. D. (1996). Adult attachment security and symptoms of depression: The mediating roles of dysfunctional attitudes and low self-esteem. *Journal of Personality and Social Psychology, 70*(2), 310–320.

Robinson, N., Garber, J., & Hilsman, R. (1995). Cognitions and stress: Direct and moderating effects on depressive versus externalizing symptoms during the junior high transition. *Journal of Abnormal Psychology, 104,* 453–563.

Rodney, H. E., & Mupier, R. (1999). The impact of parental alcoholism on self-esteem and depression among African-American adolescents. *Journal of Child and Adolescent Substance Abuse, 8*(3), 55–71.

Ruble, D., Boggiano, A., Feldman, N., & Loebl, J. (1980) Developmental analysis of the role of social comparison in self-evaluation. *Developmental Psychology, 16,* 105–115.

Shirk, S. (1999). Integrated child psychotherapy: Treatment ingredients in search of a recipe. In S. Russ & T. Ollendick (Eds.), *Handbook of psychotherapies with children and families* (pp. 369–384). New York: Kluwer Academic/Plenum Press.

Shirk, S. (2000, May). *Diagnostic-based psychotherapy: The uniformity myth revisited.* Paper presented at the meeting of the second European Conference on Child and Adolescent Therapy, Oslo, Norway.

Shirk, S., & Russell, R. (1996). *Change processes in child psychotherapy: Revitalizing treatment and research.* New York: Guilford Press.

Shirk, S., Van Horn, M., & Leber, D. (1997). Dysphoria and children's processing of supportive interactions. *Journal of Abnormal Child Psychology, 25,* 239–249.

Silverstone, P. H. (1990). Low self-esteem in eating disordered patients in the absence of depression. *Psychological Reports, 67*(1), 276–278.

*Simmons, C. H., & Parsons, R. J. (1983). Developing internality and perceived competence: The empowerment of adolescent girls. *Adolescence, 18,* 917–912.

*Stark, K., Reynolds, W., & Kaslow, N. (1987). A comparison of relative efficacy of self-control therapy and a behavioral problem-solving therapy for depression in children. *Journal of Abnormal Child Psychology, 15,* 91–113.

Twamley, E. W., & Davis, M. C. (1999). The sociocultural model of eating disturbances in young women: The effects of personal attributes and family environment. *Journal of Social and Clinical Psychology, 18*(4), 467–489.

Unger, J. B., Kipke, M. D., Simon, T. R., Montgomery, S. B., & Johnson, C. J. (1997). Homeless youths and young adults in Los Angeles: Prevalence of mental health problems and the relationship between mental health and substance abuse disorders. *American Journal of Community Psychology, 25*(3), 371–394.

van der Ham, T., van-Strien, D. C., & van Engeland, H. (1998). Personality characteristics predict outcome of eating disorders in adolescents: A 4-year prospective study. *European Child and Adolescent Psychiatry, 7*(2), 79–84.

Vondra, J., Barnett, D., & Cicchetti, D. (1989). Perceived and actual competence among maltreated and comparison children. *Development and Psychopathology, 1,* 237–255.

*Waksman, S. A. (1984). A controlled evaluation of assertion training with adolescents. *Adolescence, 19,* 277–282.

Weissman, A. (1980). Dysfunctional Attitude Scale. In J. Fisher & K. Corcoran (Eds.), *Measures for clinical practice* (pp. 263–266). New York: Free Press.

Weisz, J., Donenberg, G., Han, S., & Kauneckis, D. (1995). Child and adolescent psychotherapy outcomes in experiments and clinics: Why the disparity? *Journal of Abnormal Child Psychology, 23,* 83–10.

Westra, H. A., & Kuiper, N. (1997). Cognitive content specificity in selective attention across four domains of maladjustment. *Behaviour Research and Therapy, 35* (4), 349–365.

*Wilson, N. H., & Pierce, J. P. (1986). Anxiety management training and study skills: Counseling on self-esteem and test anxiety. *The School Counselor, 34,* 18–31.

Zupan, B. A., Hammen, C., & Jaenicke, C. (1987). The effects of current mood and prior depressive history on self-schematic processing in children. *Journal of Experimental Child Psychology, 43*(1), 149–158.

SUGGESTED READINGS

Harter, S. (1999). *The construction of the self: A developmental perspective.* New York: Guilford Press.

Persons, J. (1989). *Cognitive therapy in practice: A case formulation approach.* New York: Norton.

Shirk, S., & Russell, R. (1996). *Change processes in child psychotherapy: Revitalizing treatment and research.* New York: Guilford Press.

9

Treatment of a Sexually Abused Adolescent with Posttraumatic Stress Disorder

ANNE HOPE HEFLIN
ESTHER DEBLINGER

Child sexual abuse is a highly prevalent societal problem that cuts across all ethnic, racial, educational, and socioeconomic groups. Retrospective surveys of adults suggest that approximately 27% of adult females and 16% of adult males suffer sexual victimization by the age of 18 (Elliott & Briere, 1992; Finkelhor, Hotaling, Lewis, & Smith, 1990). More recently, Boney-McCoy and Finkelhor (1995) collected information through telephone interviews regarding prevalence rates among youth between the ages of 10 and 16 in the United States. In that nationally representative sample, 15.3% of the females and 5.9% of the males reported that they had experienced sexual assault. Given the high prevalence of child sexual abuse, it is important that all clinicians who work with children and adolescents have some understanding of the phenomenon of child sexual abuse, its consequences, and treatment programs designed to address its most common sequelae.

Research has demonstrated that sexual abuse survivors may be affected by their abusive experiences in a variety of ways, with some survivors exhibiting minimal, if any, apparent effects, whereas others develop severe social or psychiatric problems. The sequelae of child sexual abuse include externalizing behavior problems such as aggression, delinquent behaviors, sexual acting-out behaviors, running away, and substance abuse. They may also include internalizing problems such as depression, suicide attempts, self-injury, and fears (Anderson, 1981; Beitchmen et al., 1992;

Boney-McCoy & Finkelhor, 1995; Briere & Elliott, 1994; Dembo et al., 1987; Kendall-Tackett, Williams, & Finkelhor, 1993; Sansonnet-Hayden, Haley, Marriage, & Fine, 1987). One of the most common types of difficulties experienced is symptoms of posttraumatic stress disorder (PTSD). Investigations of the prevalence of PTSD among child sexual abuse survivors indicate that from 32% to 48% of clinical samples of sexually abused children meet full criteria for the diagnosis of PTSD (Ackerman, Newton, McPherson, Jones, & Dykman, 1998; Famularo, Kinscherff, & Fenton, 1992; McLeer, Deblinger, Henry, & Orvaschel, 1992), while more than 80% exhibit some PTSD symptoms (McLeer et al., 1992). Thus, it is important that treatment programs developed for children who have been sexually abused include components designed to address any possible PTSD symptomatology.

Recent studies have also demonstrated that sexually abused children are more likely to experience certain patterns of negative cognitions than their nonabused peers. As a group, sexually abused children experience more self-blame for negative events, lower interpersonal trust, beliefs that they are different from their peers and that the world is a dangerous place, and more negative perceptions of sexuality and of their own body images than do nonabused children (Cohen, Deblinger, Maedel, & Stauffer, 1999; Heflin, Mears, & Deblinger, 1996; Heflin, Mears, Deblinger, & Steer, 1997; Mannarino & Cohen, 1996). Furthermore, this pattern of negative cognitions has been related to self-reports of psychological symptomatology (Heflin et al., 1996; Mannarino & Cohen, 1996), thus suggesting the importance of addressing these cognitions in psychotherapy.

The role of nonoffending parents has been recognized as one of the most important variables in mediating the effects of child sexual abuse. Children's postabuse adjustment has been linked with the level of support they receive from nonoffending adults following their disclosure (Conte & Schuerman, 1987; Everson, Hunter, Runyon, Edelson, & Coulter, 1989; Feiring, Taska, & Lewis, 1998; Friedrich, Lueke, Beilke, & Place, 1992; Spaccarelli & Fuchs, 1997). Furthermore, children's postabuse outcomes have been associated with maternal levels of symptomatology, with higher levels of maternal symptomatology linked with higher levels of symptoms among children (Deblinger, Steer, & Lippman, 1999a; Deblinger, Taub, Maedel, Lippmann, & Stauffer, 1997; Runyon, Hunter, & Everson, 1992). Finally, maternal support and emotional distress have been linked not only to children's postabuse symptomatology, but also to children's response to treatment, with higher levels of support and lower levels of maternal distress predicting a more positive response to treatment by children (Cohen & Mannarino, 1996, 1998; Friedrich et al., 1992). In summary, these findings indicate that the amount of support and degree of emotional distress exhibited by nonoffending parents may have an important influence on children's postabuse adjustment and response to treatment. Given the significance of those parental factors, it is important that clinicians look for opportunities to assist nonoffending parents to cope effectively with their own emotional distress and to offer appropriate support for their sexually abused children. Accordingly, the treatment approach described herein includes a major component focused on providing interventions for nonoffending parents.

The treatment of children and adolescents who have experienced sexual abuse is still in its early stages. However, the literature that does exist suggests that an abuse-focused cognitive-behavioral treatment approach may be quite effective in alleviating symptoms of sexually abused children (Berliner & Saunders, 1996; Cohen & Mannarino, 1996, 1997, 1998; Deblinger, Lippman, & Steer, 1996; Deblinger, McLeer, & Henry, 1990; Deblinger, Steer, & Lippman, 1999b; Stauffer & Deblinger, 1996). Deblinger and Heflin (1996) have described this abuse-specific cognitive-behavioral approach in detail in a book titled *Treating Sexually Abused Children and Their Nonoffending Parents*. The approach described in this chapter for an adolescent victim of child sexual abuse draws primarily from this literature.

Also relevant to the treatment of adolescent victims of sexual abuse are the treatment programs focused on providing care to adult rape victims (Foa, Rothbaum, & Ette, 1993; Foa, Rothbaum, Riggs, & Murdock, 1991). Cognitive-behavioral rape treatment programs have largely been based on the strategies of stress-inoculation training and exposure treatment. Stress-inoculation training focuses on the development of coping skills to manage anxiety and fear. Exposure treatment involves reliving the trauma and confronting memories and feelings associated with the traumatic experience.

ADOLESCENT TREATMENT ISSUES

Although the treatment plan outlined in the following case study of an adolescent victim of sexual abuse draws from both treatment programs for child victims of sexual abuse (Deblinger & Heflin, 1996) and programs for adult rape victims (Foa et al., 1993), these treatment programs had to be adapted to be appropriate for adolescents. For example, many of the rape treatment programs for adults include highly focused exposure work that requires great willingness and cooperation on the part of the patient.

Although adult rape victims may be able to tolerate the immediate discomfort of that exposure while focusing on the long-term goal of symptom relief, children and adolescents are less able to commit to such arduous work. Thus, the exposure work we recommend for adolescents is more gradual and less anxiety-provoking at each step. This adaptation is necessary to keep the adolescent involved and committed to therapy. It is also important that the therapist educate the adolescent's parents regarding the rationale for the exposure work and maintain a collaborative relationship with the parents. In the context of such a relationship, the therapist and parents can work together to motivate the adolescent to remain involved in therapy, even at points when the therapy may evoke distressing memories for the adolescent.

Cognitive-behavioral treatment programs developed for younger children also had to be adapted for use with adolescents. The greatest adaptation has to do with the inclusion of a large treatment component focused on sexuality and dating. Although younger children may be provided with basic sex education, that treatment component is expanded significantly for adolescent patients. This increased attention to the issue is felt to be important with adolescents, because issues of sexuality and dating are of such great concern for most adolescents. Furthermore, difficulties with sexual adjustment that have been identified as a potential consequence of child sexual abuse (Briere & Elliott, 1994; Browne & Finkelhor, 1986; Cohen et al., 1999; Heflin et al., 1997; Neumann, Houskamp, Pollock, & Briere, 1996) may first become problematic during adolescence. During this developmental period, most youth are consolidating their attitudes and beliefs regarding sexuality; thus, this seems to be a pivotal time to address these potential problems. It is important that significant efforts be made to understand the adolescent's thoughts and attitudes toward sexuality, to identify how those cognitions influence behaviors, to dispute any maladaptive or dysfunctional thoughts, and to facilitate communication between the adolescent and a nonoffending parent about sexual issues.

THEORETICAL MODEL

The treatment approach utilized in this case study is based on a cognitive-behavioral theoretical model. This model offers a social learning conceptualization of the development, maintenance, and treatment of abuse-related symptoms in sexually abused children and adolescents. The development of PTSD and related symptoms exhibited by sexually abused adolescents can be explained by two-factor learning theory, incorporating both classical and operant conditioning principles (Lyons, 1987). When an adolescent experiences sexual abuse (unconditioned stimulus), he or she often instinctively experiences negative emotions such as fear, shame, or anger (unconditioned response). Classical conditioning occurs when other neutral cues, such as certain clothes, a particular tone of voice, dark, and so on (conditioned stimuli), present at the time of the sexual abuse become conditioned such that they too elicit negative emotions (conditioned responses), even though these cues are inherently innocuous. For example, an adolescent who was sexually abused in the darkness when she was wearing certain clothes may naturally experience fear at the time of the abuse. Unfortunately, she may continue to experience fear whenever she is in the dark or wears that particular outfit, due to the association of these previously neutral cues with the actual abuse. Operant conditioning comes into play when the sexually abused adolescent learns to avoid abuse-related cues in order to reduce the likelihood of experiencing conditioned fear. Each time she avoids the darkness or wearing the particular clothes, she experiences a reduction in fear, and thus her avoidance behaviors are strengthened through negative reinforcement. As avoidance behaviors are repeatedly reinforced, they may generalize, for example, from not wearing the short skirt worn at the time of the abuse to not wearing attractive clothes in general.

Abuse-related memories and thoughts may also become conditioned stimuli that automatically elicit negative emotions as a result of the processes just described. An ever wider range of cues comes to activate these memories, and the stimulus thresholds for activating them are lowered. Thus, it is not surprising that many child sexual abuse victims frequently work hard to avoid thoughts and memories of their own abusive experiences. However, even though adolescents as well as their nonoffending parents often feel that avoidance is an effective coping response because it leads to immediate reductions in anxiety, there is evidence that such behavior is associated with increased long-term symptomatology (Johnson & Kenkel, 1991; Leitenberg, Greenwald, & Cado, 1992; Spaccarelli, 1994). The cognitive-behavioral intervention referred to as "gradual exposure," therefore, is designed to assist sexually abused children and adolescents to gradually confront these anxiety-provoking, inherently innocuous, reminders of their abusive experiences. Through gradual but repeated attempts to confront abuse-related cues, children and adolescents learn that thoughts, memories, and reminders of the abuse are not harmful and need not be avoided.

Sexual abuse also may significantly influence a child's or adolescent's developing cognitive view of the world. As was noted previously, child sexual abuse victims may be prone to developing cognitive distortions, particularly with respect to relationships, sexuality, and personal safety. For example, a child sexual abuse victim may begin to think about interpersonal relationships in negative terms beginning at a very young age (e.g., "You can never trust a man"; "You can't count on anyone but yourself"). Such dysfunctional thoughts about relationships may hinder their development of satisfying relationships during adolescence and adulthood. In fact, there is considerable evidence that survivors of child sexual abuse suffer greater difficulties in interpersonal relationships than individuals without such a history (Briere & Runtz, 1987; Elliott, 1994; Gold, 1986; Russell, 1986). The treatment model described, therefore, incorporates a component on cognitive coping skills that aims to assist adolescents and their parents in effectively identifying and disputing dysfunctional, abuse-related thoughts. Because one's cognitive view of the world is in a constant state of development, it can be influenced by new information and experiences. Thus, this treatment model includes a large educational component designed to provide clients with accurate information regarding sexual abuse, healthy sexuality, and body safety skills.

Finally, the cognitive-behavioral model helps to explain the role of nonoffending parents in the maintenance and treatment of their children's abuse-related difficulties. There is considerable evidence that child and adolescent coping responses are significantly influenced by the models of coping presented by their parents (Seligman, 1991). In addition, the reactions of nonoffending parents to their children's abuse-related behavior problems may significantly influence the improvement or exacerbation of such difficulties. For example, nonoffending parents may inadvertently reinforce abuse-related difficulties by responding with increased or inappropriate attention to problem behaviors. Thus, the proposed treatment aims to (1) teach parents effective behavioral skills for responding to their children's abuse-related disclosures and difficulties and (2) help parents to learn more effective coping skills for managing their own distress, so they can model these skills for their children.

CASE EXAMPLE

Presenting Problem

Michelle is a 14-year-old adolescent who was referred for an evaluation and treatment by child protective services (CPS). She is an only child who has been living with both biological parents in a middle-class suburb. The report from the CPS worker indicated that Michelle had been sexually abused for years by her biological father. Michelle eventually disclosed this abuse to a girlfriend who subsequently told her own mother. This mother called the school guidance counselor, who then made the required report to CPS.

A CPS worker and an investigator from the county prosecutor's office interviewed Michelle at school, where she tearfully and somewhat reluctantly disclosed that her father began fondling her at around age 5 or 6. Over time, the abuse escalated to oral sexual activities and vaginal–penile intercourse, which had been occurring approximately weekly over the past several years. Michelle reported that she attempted to tell her mother, but that her mother did not seem to understand and therefore did little to prevent the ongoing abuse.

Following the interview with Michelle, the CPS worker and the investigator went to Michelle's home and interviewed her mother. Michelle's mother, Harriett, responded to the information about Michelle's disclosure with shock and disbelief. She denied that Michelle had ever told her of the abuse. However, she was clear about her willingness to do whatever was required to keep Michelle at home and to protect her appropriately. Based on Michelle's mother's response, the CPS worker decided to leave Michelle in the home with her mother, contingent on Michelle's father leaving the home and having no contact with Michelle. The child protection agency conducted a joint investigation with the county prosecutor's office which resulted in the substantiation of the sexual abuse allegations and the arrest of Michelle's father on sexual assault charges.

Initial Evaluation

In this case, the psychological evaluation focused on identifying how Michelle and her mother were responding to the crisis precipitated by Michelle's disclosure in order to direct the course of therapy most effectively. The evaluation was completed over the course of three assessment sessions.

Evaluation Sessions with Michelle's Mother

Michelle's mother, Harriett, was interviewed to obtain background information regarding family history; Michelle's medical, developmental, and school history; as well as Harriett's thoughts and feelings regarding the allegations of child sexual abuse. Harriett reported that her husband was the primary wage earner for the family and had been employed for years with the same company in a corporate management position. Harriett had recently accepted a position as an elementary school teacher. Harriett reported that the family had moved a number of times due to her husband's job transfers. They had lived in their current home for approximately 2 years. Harriett described Michelle as a generally compliant and cooperative child who was a good student at school; however, she did acknowledge that Michelle had been exhibiting more anger recently. When asked about her perceptions of the allegations of child sexual abuse, Harriett reported that she was shocked and confused about the entire situation. She said that Michelle did not lie, so she must believe her; however, she said it was hard to imagine her husband as a sexual offender. She became tearful during the interview and said that she did not know what was going to happen to her family. She went on to say that she did not know how she and her daughter would manage, either financially or emotionally, without her husband.

Harriett was asked to complete the following measures of her symptomatology. The Symptom Checklist-90—Revised (SCL-90-R; Derogatis, 1983) was chosen to evaluate her general level of distress. The Trauma Symptom Inventory (TSI; Briere, 1995) was chosen to evaluate her symptoms that were more specific to the allegations of sexual abuse. The Global Severity Index of the SCL-90-R was elevated, indicating that Harriett was experiencing significant distress. The results of the TSI indicated that she was experiencing moderate symptoms of depression and anxiety as well as intrusive and distressing thoughts about the sexual abuse. Although she attempted to avoid thinking about the abuse allegations, those efforts did not alleviate her distress.

Harriett was also asked to respond to the Child Behavior Checklist (CBCL; Achenbach, 1991), which is a measure of children's internalizing and externalizing symptoms as well as their social competence. Harriett's responses to the CBCL indicated that Michelle was experiencing an elevated level of internalizing symptoms, but that her externalizing behaviors were within the normal range. Specific scores on these measures are provided in Table 9.1.

Evaluation Sessions with Michelle

During her initial evaluation session, Michelle was interviewed regarding her school history, friends, and other interests. Subsequently, she was asked what she understood about why her mother brought her to the session. In response to that question, Michelle began to disclose the sexual abuse.

That interview proceeded as follows:

THERAPIST: Why do you think your mom brought you here today?

MICHELLE: Because of what happened with my dad.

THERAPIST: What happened with your dad?

MICHELLE: He used to touch me and do things.

THERAPIST: Can you tell me more about that?

MICHELLE: He touched my private parts.

THERAPIST: Did this happen one time or more than one time?

MICHELLE: Lots of times.

THERAPIST: How old were you when it first happened?

MICHELLE: I'm not sure. I guess I was around 5 or maybe 6. (*At this point, her eyes are downcast and her voice low. Although she seems uncomfortable discussing the abuse, she is able to respond thoughtfully and appropriate to the questions she is asked.*)

THERAPIST: How often would it happen?

MICHELLE: Well, usually it happened when my mom had to go to a meeting at night, usually on Tuesdays. Sometimes on the weekends, too, if she went out shopping, but usually I tried to go with her.

THERAPIST: Where were you when it happened?

MICHELLE: Usually my Dad would call me into his room and tell me to lie down on his bed, and he'd do it there. But sometimes he'd do it out in the family room.

THERAPIST: You said he would touch your private parts. What did he touch them with?

MICHELLE: His hands, mostly.

THERAPIST: And how were your clothes arranged when he would touch you?

MICHELLE: Usually he pulled my pants down or told me to do it.

THERAPIST: How about his clothes?

MICHELLE: Sometimes they were on and sometimes they were off.

THERAPIST: Did he ever touch your private parts with anything besides his hands?

MICHELLE: Yeah.

THERAPIST: What else did he use to touch you?

MICHELLE: Well, he would make me have sex with him. (*At this point in the interview, she begins crying.*)

THERAPIST: Is this hard to talk about?

MICHELLE: (*Nods head to indicate "yes."*)

THERAPIST: I'm really glad that you were able to talk about what has happened because in the long run talking about it will help you feel better. I'm sorry that it's so hard to talk about now, but the more we talk about it the easier it will get. Let's talk a little more and then we can do some other things together.

The therapist did not end the discussion of the abuse while Michelle was in distress out of concern that she would be encouraged to stop discussing the issue whenever she was feeling upset. Thus, the therapist attempted to provide her with support so that she could continue the discussion briefly. Then, they would end the discussion when Michelle was less distressed. Through that experience, Michelle would learn that she could tolerate discussions of the abuse.

THERAPIST: You said that your father would make you have sex with him. Different people mean different things when they say they "have sex." What do you mean by that?

MICHELLE: Well, he would put his private into mine.

THERAPIST: Did that happen one time or more than one time?

MICHELLE: Lots of times. Almost every Tuesday.

THERAPIST: Did he touch you in any other way?

MICHELLE: No, I don't think so.

THERAPIST: Did he ever have you touch him?

MICHELLE: Well, sometimes he would make me rub his private.

Although Michelle was able to discuss the abuse clearly, with significant detail, she was obviously anxious and uncomfortable during the discussion. She became tearful at times and seemed eager to end the discussion. The therapist praised her for her courage in disclosing the abuse and for her willingness to discuss it in spite of the discomfort it precipitated.

Michelle also was asked to complete psychological measures designed to assess her level of depression, anxiety, and posttraumatic stress symptoms related to her sexual abuse experience. She completed the Child Depression Inventory (CDI; Kovacs, 1992), which is a self-report measure of depression. Her responses revealed a mild level of depression. She also completed the State–Trait Anxiety Inventory for Children (STAIC; Spielberger, 1983), which measures both state and trait anxiety. Her scores on those scales were within the normal range. Finally, Michelle completed the Trauma Symptom Checklist for Children (TSCC; Briere, 1996) which includes subscales for anxiety, depression, anger, posttraumatic stress, dissociation, and sexual concerns. Michelle received elevated scores on the subscales for depression, posttraumatic stress, and sexual distress. A review of her responses to individual items revealed that she was bothered by intrusive memories and nightmares related to the abuse, that she tried to avoid thinking of the abuse, and that her perceptions of sexuality were quite negative. Specific scores on these measures are provided in Table 9.1.

Finally, to complete the evaluation process, both Michelle and her mother were interviewed individually regarding any emotional or behavioral symptoms that Michelle might be exhibiting, using the Kiddie Schedule for Affective Disorders and Schizophrenia for School Age Children— Epidemiologic Version (K-SADS-E; Orvaschel, Puig-Antich, Chambers, Tabrizi, & Johnson, 1982). Based on their mutual reports, Michelle met the criteria for the diagnosis of PTSD as well as the diagnosis of dysthymic disorder according to the fourth edition of the *Diagnostic and Statistical Manual of Mental Disorders* (DSM-IV; American Psychiatric Association, 1994). Her symptoms of PTSD included recurrent, distressing memories and dreams of the abuse; attempts to avoid thoughts and reminders of the abuse; feelings of increased distance from other people; problems sleeping and concentrating; and increased anger and irritability. These symptoms had been increasingly evident for the last year. Her symptoms of dysthymic disorder included depressed mood; disturbance of sleep, concentration, and appetite; and feelings of hopelessness. These symptoms had been evident for approximately 2 years.

TABLE 9.1. Pre- and Posttreatment *T*-Scores on Assessment Measures Showing Initial Elevations

	Pretreatment	Posttreatment
Harriett's scores		
SCL-90 Global Severity Index	73	62
Trauma Symptom Inventory (TSI)		
Anxious arousal	66	60
Depression	68	64
Intrusive experiences	70	53
Defensive avoidance	69	48
Michelle's scores		
Child Behavior Checklist (CBCL)		
Internalizing score	71	56
Externalizing score	54	58
Child Depression Inventory (CDI)	65	59
Trauma Symptom Checklist for Children (TSCC)		
Depression	72	63
Posttraumatic stress	84	54
Sexual concerns	74	52

Treatment

Michelle's Treatment

In Michelle's initial therapy session, the evaluation findings were reviewed. Subsequently, the treatment plan was presented to Michelle. The therapist explained that she would be teaching Michelle what is known about sexual abuse because it is generally easier to cope with an experience we know something about and understand. The therapist further stated that she would be teaching Michelle some skills for dealing with her own upsetting feelings about the abuse and her relationship with her father. Michelle was receptive to those recommendations for therapy. However, when the therapist next explained that they would be talking a lot about Michelle's sexual abuse experience in order to help her become more comfortable with her thoughts and memories of the abuse, Michelle expressed some reluctance. The therapist was sympathetic and stated that those discussions would occur gradually, without ever requiring more of Michelle than she could handle. Finally, the therapist explained that they would be discussing sexuality in general, dating relationships, and abuse-response skills. Initially, Michelle and her mother would be seen separately, but eventually they would be seen in joint sessions. The purpose of the joint sessions would be to facilitate communication between Michelle and her mother regarding the sexual abuse, as well as sexuality in general. The therapist stated that her intention was to encourage open communication so that Michelle and her mother eventually could continue the therapeutic process on their own.

Thus, Michelle's treatment plan consisted of a number of different components. These components generally were provided to Michelle in the order in which they are presented in this chapter. However, there is considerable overlap between the therapy components, and during therapy attention sometimes shifted back and forth between the components.

EDUCATION REGARDING CHILD SEXUAL ABUSE

The first component of Michelle's treatment was to provide her with education regarding sexual abuse. The purpose of providing this education was to dispel any distressing misconceptions Michelle might have regarding sexual abuse. Additionally, these educational discussions would allow Michelle to become comfortable discussing sexual abuse in a somewhat general way before focusing specifically on the details of her personal experience.

The sexual abuse education was provided with the use of an information sheet that has been developed specifically for this purpose. The information sheet is written in question-and-answer form. It addresses issues such as what sexual abuse is, who is responsible for the abuse, why sexual abuse occurs, how many and what types of children are abused, how children feel when they have been abused, and why children find it difficult to tell about abuse.

The questions initially were posed to Michelle in order to obtain her responses to them before providing the "correct" response. In that way, it was possible to elicit some of Michelle's inaccurate and distressing perceptions, so that they could be corrected. For example, when asked how many children she believed were sexually abused, Michelle reported that she thought there were probably one or two in each state per year. She was surprised and somewhat relieved to learn that, in fact, as many as one in three girls are sexually abused before they reach adulthood. That information seemed to reduce her sense of isolation and feeling that she was different from everyone else. After eliciting Michelle's own thoughts, the answers provided on the information sheet were discussed with her.

COPING SKILLS TRAINING

The next component of Michelle's treatment was to provide her with some skills for coping with the emotional distress generated by her memories of the abuse. This training in coping skills was provided before engaging Michelle in focused gradual exposure exercises, which were anticipated to be the most taxing aspect of her treatment. Two sessions were devoted to coping skills training early in Michelle's therapy. These skills were used throughout therapy.

The first coping technique offered to Michelle was cognitive coping skills training. This training is based on the work of Beck (1976) and Seligman (1991). To initiate that training, a triangle illustrating the connections between thoughts, emotions, and behaviors was presented to Michelle. Nonabuse-related examples were provided to demonstrate how thoughts may influence our emotions. Michelle was then given a series of hypothetical situations and was asked to practice identifying the thoughts that might elicit the emotions described in those situations. Subsequently, Michelle was taught how to evaluate the accuracy and usefulness of thoughts and how to generate replacement thoughts for those that are not accurate, adaptive, or helpful. Once Michelle had developed basic skills in identifying and challenging the thoughts underlying distressing emotions, her own emotions regarding her sexual abuse experience were elicited. She was encouraged to identify the thoughts underlying these emotions. She and the therapist then analyzed her thoughts for accuracy and adaptiveness. Michelle was able to identify several thoughts that were heightening her level of emotional distress. For example, one of the emotions she initially identified was a feeling of guilt. The following conversation took place as she and the therapist discussed her feeling of guilt, and Michelle learned to identify and dispute the inaccurate thought that was contributing to her guilt.

THERAPIST: When something reminds you about the abuse now, what feelings do you have?

MICHELLE: I guess I mostly just feel bad.

THERAPIST: I'm not sure what you mean by "bad." Can you tell me a little more about which kind of bad feeling you have?

MICHELLE: Well, I just feel guilty about all of it.

THERAPIST: OK, remember how we said that sometimes our thoughts influence how we are feeling? Can you tell me what you are thinking about when you feel guilty?

MICHELLE: I just feel like I must have done something to make my dad decide to do it to me.

THERAPIST: What do you think you might have done?

MICHELLE: I don't know. He used to always yell at me for the clothes I wore, so I guess maybe I wore the wrong kind of stuff.

THERAPIST: What do you think was wrong with your clothes?

MICHELLE: I don't really know. I dress like all the other kids, but he said I was trying to look too grown up, too sexy. He even said sometimes that I made him do it to me because of the way I walked around in really short shorts and miniskirts.

THERAPIST: Well, let's think about that carefully. You said that you dress like other kids?

MICHELLE: Yeah, pretty much.

THERAPIST: And so, do you think that dressing like that has also caused all of them to be sexually abused?

MICHELLE: Well, not all of them, no. Actually, I don't think this has happened to any of my friends.

THERAPIST: So, if dressing like that hasn't caused them to be sexually abused, it doesn't make sense that it caused you to be abused, does it?

MICHELLE: No, I guess not.

THERAPIST: Also, you said that sometimes your father said you *made* him abuse you by the clothes you wore? Think about that statement logically. Can you *control* a person's behavior by the clothes you wear?

MICHELLE: I guess not.

THERAPIST: You don't sound sure. Think about it this way, does anyone make *you* behave a certain way by the clothes they wear?

MICHELLE: No. But, I've heard people say that a girl was asking to be raped when she was wearing really tight or short clothes. I was thinking that I sort of did the same thing.

THERAPIST: I think when people say that, they're suggesting that the clothes you wear send a message to other people about who you are, which makes some sense. But I don't think that a short skirt sends the message that the girl wearing it wants to be sexually abused. It just doesn't make sense to me that every girl who wears a miniskirt wants to have a sexual encounter with every man she sees.

MICHELLE: No, I guess not.

THERAPIST: Michelle, I don't think that the clothes you wore had anything to do with your father sexually abusing you. I think he sexually abused you because he has a problem with touching, not because of anything you did or anything you wore. I think he said that you made him do it to give himself an excuse and make himself feel better about doing something he knew was wrong.

MICHELLE: That makes sense. He always used to be looking for someone to blame for the littlest things.

THERAPIST: Also, I think when you blame yourself for making your father sexually abuse you, you are making yourself feel much worse than you need to feel. Let's try to think of a more accurate thought you could use to replace the thought that you are to blame for the abuse because of the clothes you wore. Can you think of how you could replace that?

MICHELLE: Well, I could say what you did, that my clothes can't *make anyone do something they didn't want to do*, so I couldn't have made my dad abuse me.

THERAPIST: Exactly! Now we need to practice using that replacement thought to get rid of the inaccurate thought that is making you feel badly.

Subsequently, the therapist used role plays to give Michelle opportunities to practice using these cognitive coping skills. The therapist pretended to be a friend of Michelle's who was sexually abused and struggling with the same guilt-producing thought. Michelle was asked to help the friend feel better by disputing her friend's dysfunctional thought. In a similar manner, the therapist worked with Michelle to identify other inaccurate and ineffective thoughts that were causing Michelle distress. The therapist also used cognitive coping homework sheets to structure Michelle's practice of these skills at home. The sheets provide columns for the identification of distressing emotions, the thoughts underlying those emotions, and the replacement thoughts that the patient generates. Michelle completed those sheets and returned them the following session for review. Michelle responded very well to this training.

The therapist also offered Michelle some training in the effective expression of emotions. Michelle acknowledged that she was feeling angry more frequently and with greater intensity than she had previously. Much of that anger was being expressed inappropriately, in outbursts toward her mother. With the therapist's help, she was able to generate some ideas about how she could more effectively express her anger. She began keeping a journal of her feelings and found that writing them down was helpful to her. Additionally, the therapist discussed with Michelle how she could present issues to her mother in a way that allowed Michelle to express her opinion, but did not anger or alienate her mother. The therapist and Michelle did role plays to practice those skills for the appropriate expression of anger.

GRADUAL EXPOSURE

The gradual exposure process followed a hierarchy of increasingly anxiety-provoking stimuli associated with the sexual abuse experience. In work with children and adolescents, this hierarchy is a fluid model, developed as the therapist works with the child. Although adults may be able to identify their level of anxiety associated with various stimuli at the beginning of treatment, children and adolescents are much less able and willing to do that. Thus, the therapist must construct and revise the hierarchy, incorporating his or her own observations of the client's anxiety level, as well as the client's own report of his or her level of distress. In work with Michelle, the therapist began work with the premise that general discussions of sexual abuse would be least anxiety-provoking for Michelle. The next step up the hierarchy would be to include more personalized discussions of Michelle's experience, but not yet focusing on the specific acts of sexual abuse. For example, gradual exposure sessions at this level might focus on general discussions of Michelle's relationship with her father. Subsequently, discussions would move to the specific episodes of abuse, but focused on those which were least distressing. At the top of the hierarchy would be detailed discussions of the most upsetting episodes of the abuse. The final step in the hierarchy would be to share information about the specific episodes of abuse with her mother.

The gradual exposure process with Michelle actually had been initiated during the sessions focused on education regarding sexual abuse and cognitive coping skills because those sessions allowed Michelle to discuss the general topic of sexual abuse, which was not particularly anxiety-provoking. Having completed that work successfully, by the fifth session it was time to move up the hierarchy of anxiety-provoking topics to begin discussing Michelle's own experiences.

As is true for most adolescents, Michelle dreaded the therapy sessions in which she would discuss the specifics of her sexual abuse. She expressed her belief that she felt better when she just didn't think about the abuse. She said that she wanted to forget all about it. The therapist explained that although Michelle might temporarily distract herself from thinking about the abuse, it was unlikely that she would ever truly forget it. Furthermore, the therapist said that, given the fact that Michelle could not truly forget the abuse, the best thing to do would be to find a way to help Michelle be more comfortable with her memories.

The therapist began this work by asking for details of Michelle's disclosure of sexual abuse because that was not likely to be terribly anxiety-provoking. Indeed, Michelle was able to discuss her disclosures to her friend and to investigating professionals without significant distress. However, when she began to discuss her disclosure to her mother, she became much more upset. Michelle was able to label her emotions as sadness as well as anger toward her mother. Through further discussion, it became clear that Michelle was angry with her mother for not being as supportive as she would have liked. Furthermore, she was angry because she believed that she had previously told her mother about what was happening, and her mother had not acted to help her. As that earlier attempt at disclosure was discussed, Michelle realized that she actually had not clarified for her mother what was happening. Indeed, during the earlier disclosure, Michelle, who was angry about being punished by her father, had only told her mother that her father hurt her sometimes. Nonetheless, Michelle expected that her mother would be able to help her or "fix things." Eventually, Michelle was able to understand that her expectations of her mother were unrealistic, although understandable, because many children expect parents to be able to accomplish anything. Michelle was able to recognize that her mother really had no way of knowing that Michelle was referring to sexual abuse. The therapist made mental notes that clearly this was an issue to discuss in the joint sessions.

During the sixth session, the therapist asked Michelle to recall the last episode of sexual abuse she experienced with her father. Michelle became anxious during that discussion and was tearful at times. However, with the support and encouragement of the therapist, Michelle was able to provide details about where, when, and how her father had touched her during the last episode. The therapist also encouraged Michelle to share the thoughts, feelings, and physical sensations she experienced during the abusive interaction. Michelle left that session tired, but composed and proud of her ability to talk about the abuse despite her anxiety.

Future sessions proceeded in a similar manner, with the therapist focusing the discussions on specific episodes of sexual abuse. Because Michelle had experienced so many episodes of abuse, she had a tendency to group episodes together, saying, "It always happened that way." As much as possible, the therapist tried to focus Michelle on specific episodes by linking the episodes with events or occasions such as holidays, birthdays, or the first time her father touched her in a different way. By focusing on specific episodes, the therapist was attempting to have Michelle reexperience the emotions and sensations of that experience. By confronting those often distressing memories, Michelle learned that the memories themselves were not harmful and need not be feared or avoided. During this work, the therapist refrained from asking questions requiring affective or cognitive processing that might distract Michelle from her memories of the episode. Although such questions were important to help Michelle make sense of her experience both emotionally and intellectually, they were saved for different times when they would not interrupt the actual gradual exposure work. During the processing exercises, the therapist encouraged Michelle to use her cognitive coping skills to manage distressing thoughts and feelings generated by the exposure work. Additionally, the therapist pointed out to Michelle how much progress she was making; the conversations seemed to have become easier over the course of several sessions.

Throughout the exposure work, Michelle expressed intense anger toward her father, saying he had never been a real father to her. The therapist responded empathically, expressing her understanding of Michelle's anger. The therapist and Michelle discussed the basis for Michelle's anger and her thoughts regarding any future contact she might have with her father.

Michelle stated adamantly that she did not want to have any contact with him. The therapist wanted to support Michelle, but was also aware that Michelle's feelings might change some over time and thus wanted to give Michelle a sense of the alternative responses that were possible. Thus, the therapist expressed her belief that Michelle should not be forced to have contact with her father and also described various ways in which other survivors of sexual abuse have chosen to respond to their abusers, ranging from having no contact at all, to writing a letter expressing their feelings, to verbally confronting the abuser, to eventually forgiving the abuser. The therapist emphasized that there is no one right way to respond to this situation, except that no one should have to continue to be a victim of abuse.

After four sessions of exposure work, the therapist talked with Michelle about writing a book about her sexual abuse experience, with the possibility of using this book (with identifying information altered) to help younger children cope with a sexual abuse experience. (The therapist had already obtained the permission of Michelle's mother to suggest this possibility to Michelle.) Michelle responded positively to this suggestion and seemed to feel proud of her ability to help younger children. The next several sessions were devoted to writing a book outlining her experience of sexual abuse and how she had coped with this experience successfully. Completing this project gave Michelle a real sense of pride and accomplishment.

EDUCATION ABOUT DATING, SEXUALITY, AND BODY SAFETY SKILLS

Education regarding these topics began during the sessions focused on gradual exposure. In that way, it was possible to shift the discussions away from the anxiety-provoking gradual exposure work from time to time. The primary purposes of this education were to (1) make sure Michelle had appropriate factual information regarding sexuality and abuse-response skills, (2) explore Michelle's beliefs and feelings regarding sexuality and prevent any confusion between the sexual abuse and healthy adult sexuality, and (3) facilitate communication between Michelle and her mother regarding these topics. Much of this work occurred during the joint sessions with Michelle and her mother.

Parent Treatment

During the initial treatment session with Michelle's mother, the evaluation findings and the proposed treatment plan were reviewed. Harriett's individual treatment sessions would essentially follow a process parallel to Michelle's sessions, with the addition of a module focusing on parenting skills. Also during that first treatment session, Harriett was informed that current research suggests that the most important factor influencing the recovery of sexually abused children may be the level of support that they receive from a nonoffending parent (Conte & Schuerman,1987; Everson et al., 1989; Feiring et al., 1998; Friedrich et al., 1992; Spaccarelli & Fuchs, 1997). Thus, her active participation in treatment would be strongly encouraged. At this point, Harriett tearfully broke down, questioning if she could be there for Michelle when she was barely managing to hang on herself.

Harriett was reminded that treatment initially would focus on helping her cope with her own emotional reactions. The therapist emphasized that discovering that your child has been sexually abused is highly traumatic for any parent. Moreover, she would not be asked to participate in sessions with her daughter for quite some time. In fact, joint sessions would not be initiated until she was feeling much less distressed and coping more effectively. However, the importance of her modeling effective coping strategies for Michelle was emphasized because there is evidence linking maternal and child cognitive coping styles (Seligman et al., 1984).

EDUCATION REGARDING CHILD SEXUAL ABUSE

Individual parent sessions began with the provision of some basic information. Michelle's mother had many specific questions about the criminal prosecution, as well as general questions about child sexual abuse. Although some information about the standard procedures of investigation and prosecution was provided, Harriett was directed to the county Victim Witness Coordinator for specific information concerning the current standing of the investigation and the legal steps that could be expected in this case. Harriett also was provided with information about the prevalence, etiology, and impact of child sexual abuse. Much like her daughter, she seemed astounded to learn about the high prevalence rate associated with child sexual abuse. Additional information was provided via a Child Sexual Abuse Fact Sheet specifically designed for parents. The therapist encouraged Harriett to read the information sheet carefully and write down any additional questions she might have for the next session.

COPING SKILLS TRAINING

Many of the early treatment sessions with Harriett focused on her emotional state and coping efforts. She was encouraged to verbalize her feelings and thoughts, particularly those she had been keeping to herself. Although she believed it was unlikely, she acknowledged occasionally thinking that she and her husband would get back together after he served his time. She reported that he had contacted her several times asking for her forgiveness and for her commitment to the marriage. At those times, she experienced a range of feelings toward him, including sympathy, love, frustration, and anger. Michelle's mother seemed relieved to focus on her own needs and seemed comforted by the knowledge that other mothers expressed similar feelings and concerns. However, she was encouraged to postpone making any decisions about reunification until she and her daughter had completed counseling. It was suggested that her husband would need to successfully complete his own course of therapy and be able to accept responsibility for the abuse before any possibility of reunification should be pursued. It was further suggested that with time and counseling she would likely begin to feel stronger and more independent, and then she could make these important decisions from a position of strength rather than weakness. If, at that point, she was still considering reunification, she was encouraged to pursue family therapy to more fully evaluate that possibility.

The cognitive coping model (Seligman, 1991) was presented, utilizing the triangle diagram described earlier. Michelle's mother seemed to quickly grasp the interrelationships between thoughts, feelings, and behaviors. She acknowledged that her thoughts and feelings seemed to fluctuate dramatically, especially when she was at home with too much time to dwell on the situation. She reported that her behavior, particularly toward her daughter, seemed to reflect these erratic thoughts and feelings. She was not always as supportive toward her daughter as she would have liked to be.

As the therapist helped Harriett explore the thoughts that seemed to underlie her most depressed moods, it became clear that some of these moods were driven by dysfunctional thoughts and misconceptions. Harriett, for example, was convinced that she was responsible for her daughter's abuse because of her occasional failure to respond positively to her husband's sexual advances. In addition, she feared that her daughter's inappropriate introduction to sexual activity would lead her to take sexual risks that would ultimately expose her to the HIV virus.

The cognitive coping model was used as follows to help Harriett learn to dispute the thoughts she and the therapist identified as dysfunctional:

THERAPIST: I'd like to focus some time on those thoughts that seem to make you feel really guilty and responsible for your daughter's abuse. Tell me about the last time you were feeling that way.

HARRIETT: Well, I guess it was just yesterday. I was talking to my sister on the phone. She tries to be supportive, but sometimes I think she blames me for this whole thing.

THERAPIST: How did you feel after that phone call?

HARRIETT: Guilty, responsible, absolutely awful.

THERAPIST: What do you recall saying to yourself when you were feeling that way?

HARRIETT: Well, I couldn't stop thinking that if I hadn't turned down my husband's sexual advances maybe he wouldn't have abused Michelle. I keep trying to remember the times when I did say no. It wasn't that often. My husband didn't seem interested in having sex frequently, and when he was interested I was usually delighted. Still, I wonder if he went to Michelle on the occasions that I did say no.

THERAPIST: What else were you thinking?

HARRIETT: I was thinking that maybe if I stayed trimmer he would have been more attracted to me. I just wasn't a good enough wife and I obviously failed as a mother. Why wasn't I there to protect my daughter?

THERAPIST: It's no wonder you are feeling awful; those are pretty harsh things to say to yourself. I bet you wouldn't say those things to a good friend who was in your situation. I want you to try something with me now. I'm going to pretend I'm you and repeat some of the thoughts you just shared. I want you to be my best friend and convince me with the facts you know about child sexual abuse and the knowledge you have about effective cognitive coping that some of my thoughts are hurtful and just plain wrong. Do you think you can do that?

HARRIETT: I'll try.

Michelle's mother responded well to the "best friend" role play. She helped "her best friend" to recognize that her husband gave few, if any, direct indications that he was dissatisfied with their sexual relationship. Moreover, she argued that there were alternatives to sexually abusing a child if he was, in fact, dissatisfied. He could have talked to her about it, suggested counseling, or even had an affair with an adult woman rather than hurting his daughter. Harriett also was able to point out all the things that made her a good wife and a very caring and supportive mother. Harriett was able to use the positive replacement thoughts she generated to dispute her repetitive thoughts of guilt and responsibility for her daughter's abuse.

Unfortunately, Michelle's mother had more difficulty disputing her thoughts concerning her daughter's potential exposure to the HIV virus and other sexually transmitted diseases. She was very concerned that her daughter would become sexually active as a result of the abuse. When pushed, however, she was able to acknowledge that although her daughter was interested in boys, there was no evidence that she was sexually active. In addition, Harriett was informed that young adults who have more knowledge about sex are much less likely to experience sexually transmitted diseases and teenage pregnancy. She was encouraged to dispute her anxiety-provoking thoughts with those facts. Harriett also was comforted by the fact that she and the therapist would provide sex education and information about healthy sexuality to Michelle together during joint sessions. Michelle's mother was asked to monitor and record her thoughts when she felt particularly depressed between sessions. She then used the cognitive coping homework sheets described earlier to dispute the dysfunctional thoughts while replacing them with more accurate and positive thoughts.

PARENTING SKILLS

During the evaluation, Michelle's mother reported that her husband was the disciplinarian in the family. She wondered whether she could effectively discipline Michelle on her own. Harriett expressed particular concern about some of the changes she observed in Michelle's behavior during recent months. She explained that Michelle increasingly exhibited angry outbursts and requested much more independence than ever before. In addition, she expressed concern that Michelle was becoming too interested in boys. She worried that this drive for independence and increased interest in boys might be a precursor to sexual relationships for Michelle.

Harriett's most pressing concerns seemed to be related to Michelle's interest in boys and dating. She was, therefore, asked to provide a great deal of information about the quality and pattern of these interests and behaviors. Harriett reported that she had responded to the seemingly sudden emergence of Michelle's interests with increasing restrictiveness. Not surprisingly, Michelle constantly complained about what she believed was an unreasonably early curfew, as well as her mother's reluctance to allow her to spend time with boys, even in the most closely supervised circumstances.

Michelle, in fact, seemed to interpret the restrictions as punishment for her role in the sexual abuse. Although we planned to address this mother–daughter conflict during joint sessions, Michelle's mother was encouraged to begin the process by exploring what the current adolescent norms seemed to be by consulting other mothers, teachers, and guidance counselors concerning their expectations for curfews and opposite sex interactions. Harriett was encouraged to continue to monitor Michelle's behaviors by requiring that she provide her with basic information concerning whom she was with, where she was, what she was doing, and when she would be home. She was informed that parents who consistently maintain this type of simple information about their children's whereabouts tend to have children with fewer psychosocial problems.

In conjunction with the parenting sessions, Michelle's mother was encouraged to begin reading *Parents and Adolescents Living Together* by Gerald Patterson and Mary Forgatch (1987). Although this book is not specific to the treatment of sexually abused adolescents, it offers a highly effective step-by-step approach for managing conflicts experienced between parents and teenagers. In fact, it is often helpful for parents to recognize that abuse-related behavior problems can be treated with the same methods that are effective in treating other typical problems of adolescence. Although Michelle's angry outbursts may have been a manifestation of the irritability and anger that is frequently a symptom of PTSD, her mood swings also may simply have reflected an exaggeration of the normal struggle that adolescents often experience between their dependency needs and their healthy striving toward autonomy. Regardless of whether Michelle's angry moods were a direct result of the abuse or a response to her mother's increased restrictiveness, it was agreed that her outbursts were inappropriate and dysfunctional. Thus, Harriett was encouraged to begin examining the pattern of angry disputes between herself and her daughter by recording the antecedents and consequences associated with these problematic episodes. The therapist then assisted Harriett in developing an effective plan for eliminating the angry outbursts, which included praising Michelle for appropriate expressions of anger while providing effective consequences for inappropriate angry outbursts. Simultaneously, the therapist taught Michelle more effective means of expressing her anger.

GRADUAL EXPOSURE

For this mother, gradual exposure to specific information concerning her daughter's abuse was provided during the final module prior to the initiation of the joint sessions. Michelle's mother needed considerable time to cope with her own feelings and to regain her confidence as a parent. Because she was reluctant to deal with the specifics of her daughter's abuse, the initial exposure sessions focused on the general circumstances of the abuse, as well as her husband's emotional abusiveness toward herself and Michelle. Ultimately, however, with Michelle's permission, the book Michelle had written about her experiences was gradually shared with her mother. Although Harriett's reactions to this material were highly emotional at first, by the time she began the joint sessions, she had read her daughter's book several times. Eventually, she was able to read this calmly, with pride and respect for her daughter's courage in enduring and writing about the abusive experiences. Michelle's detailed descriptions of how her father used her feelings of love and fear to encourage her cooperation in the sexual abuse seemed to enhance Harriett's empathy for her daughter and clarified her understanding of the dynamics of sexual abuse. Harriett had never discussed the sexual abuse directly with her daughter and was very anxious about doing so in joint sessions.

She was therefore encouraged to participate in role plays in which the therapist played Michelle. Although Harriett's natural instincts during the role plays seemed to be excellent, she was given some guidance to provide more direct support to her daughter in the form of clear and specific praise for her accomplishments in therapy.

Joint Sessions

The joint sessions were viewed as a critical component of Michelle's treatment for a number of reasons. The joint sessions provided an opportunity for Michelle and her mother to communicate openly about the abuse and their feelings regarding Michelle's father. Through that communication, Michelle and her mother were able to clarify any misunderstandings or confusion that existed between them and eliminate any secrets that were hindering their relationship. The sessions also allowed Michelle's mother to assume a more therapeutic role so that the treatment process could continue after the formal therapy sessions were over. The focuses of the joint sessions were as follows: discussions regarding sexuality and dating, abuse-response skills, and gradual exposure.

The joint sessions began during the 12th therapy session. Following individual meetings with both Michelle and her mother, a 20-minute joint session was held. Both Michelle and her mother were quite anxious about meeting jointly. Therefore, it was decided that the initial discussions would be about sex education in general because that would not exacerbate their anxiety. A book regarding sexuality and dating, *Asking about Sex and Growing Up* (Cole, 1988), was presented to them. It was explained that the therapist wanted to encourage them to discuss issues regarding sexuality openly, and that this book would help initially to structure those discussions. During that session, Michelle and her mother took turns reading aloud from that book. They were asked to continue that process for homework. Although some of the information presented regarding anatomy and sexual functioning was a review of information Michelle had received in school, these discussions gave her opportunities to ask questions, express concerns, and openly talk with her mother about these issues.

A similar format was followed for the next several sessions, with a brief joint meeting following Michelle's and Harriett's individual meetings. During these sessions, an attempt was made to explore Michelle's attitudes toward sexuality. Studies suggest that child sexual abuse may be associated with avoidance of sexual activity, as well as with promiscuity (James & Meyerding, 1977; Meiselman, 1978). Cognitive factors may mediate the effects of the abusive experience, and so may determine whether and how the abuse influences later sexual adjustment. Indeed, one study demonstrated that college students who had been sexually abused as children had more negative perceptions of their own sexuality because they were more likely to view themselves as promiscuous than were nonabused women (Fromuth, 1986). Thus, it was thought to be important to explore Michelle's attitudes toward sexuality, with the aim of disputing any inaccurate or dysfunctional beliefs about sexuality.

Through these discussions, it became clear that Michelle was somewhat confused about healthy sexuality. Although she was interested in boys and had some curiosity about the experience of a sexual relationship with a peer, she also was very anxious about such a relationship. She expressed a desire to get married eventually and have children, yet she described sex as being dirty and frightening. In contrast to her mother's concerns, Michelle was not yet sexually active. However, her confusion about sexuality put her at some risk for making poor decisions regarding her own sexuality.

The therapist worked with Harriett to help Michelle make a clear distinction between her own experience of sexual abuse and healthy sexuality between two adults who love and are committed to each other. Although Michelle's mother initially was concerned about describing adult sexuality too positively, for fear of encouraging Michelle to become sexually active, the therapist pointed out during Harriett's individual sessions that Michelle had to overcome a preexisting negative attitude toward sexuality. Harriett felt strongly that she did not want to encourage any premarital sexual activity. The therapist stated that it was appropriate that Harriett communicate her values to Michelle, but that it was also important that Michelle understand that within the right relationship, adult sexuality is a positive thing. Thus, after completing this individual work, Harriett was able to communicate to Michelle during joint sessions that sexuality within a marriage is healthy and positive, while emphasizing that the decision to enter into a sexual relationship is a serious decision that should be made with great thought and care.

The discussions during the joint sessions moved on to the topic of dating and what Michelle and her mother felt were appropriate levels of physical affection in dating relationships. As Michelle began to see that her mother could tolerate those discussions without becoming upset, she became increasingly open. Eventually the conversations turned to the issue of contraceptive methods. Harriett was able to provide Michelle with education regarding contraceptive methods. She acknowledged to Michelle that ultimately it was her decision as to when she became involved in a sexual relationship. Harriett indicated to Michelle that although it was her strong belief that Michelle should wait until marriage to be sexually active, she would like to know if Michelle did decide to enter a sexual relationship, so that she could help her obtain appropriate contraceptives.

The conversations regarding dating naturally led to discussions of abuse-response skills, focusing on aggressive sexual encounters in dating situations, as well as episodes of sexual abuse by adult perpetrators. Michelle was taught about body ownership, her absolute right to say "no" in any situation, the fact that she owed no one anything in terms of sexual touches, and the need to get away and tell someone about inappropriate sexual touches.

Research suggests that modeling and role plays seem to be more effective than didactic instruction in encouraging the use of abuse-response skills (Wurtle & Miller-Perrin, 1992). With this in mind, Michelle and her mother were asked to role play potentially abusive encounters. Like many adolescents in therapy, Michelle initially balked at the idea of participating in "silly" role plays of such unlikely encounters. The therapist responded with the statistics on date rape and participated in a role play with Michelle's mother of a scenario that seemed relevant to Michelle. Ultimately, Michelle joined in on the role plays, first by critiquing her mother's performance and then by outperforming her. Following each role play, Michelle and Harriett were encouraged to share the feelings and thoughts they experienced during each simulated dating interaction. This gave the therapist an opportunity to help Michelle and her mother dispute any dysfunctional or inaccurate thoughts they may have experienced in reaction to the role play (e.g., "Maybe my date touched me like that because he could tell I had been touched before, when my dad abused me").

After four joint sessions devoted to the topics just described, the therapist refocused Michelle and her mother on more formal gradual exposure work. This work began by having Michelle read her book regarding her experience to her mother during a joint session. Michelle's mother responded with praise and admiration for Michelle's courage and hard work.

Then she asked Michelle questions about her experience. This was a pivotal session because it allowed Michelle to see that her mother could tolerate this discussion and, in fact, would be supportive of her. Both Michelle and her mother seemed greatly relieved and proud of themselves at the end of this session.

As sessions progressed, the individual sessions were shortened, allowing more time in the joint sessions. Michelle and her mother continued to discuss specific episodes of the sexual abuse. Another important topic was Michelle's early attempt at disclosure to her mother and her feelings regarding her mother's lack of helpful response at that time. Michelle was able to express her anger toward her mother, and her mother explained her lack of understanding at the time and apologized for not being able to support Michelle.

The final critical issue for discussion concerned their feelings toward Michelle's father and their thoughts regarding future relationships with him. Michelle's mother was honest in expressing her conflicted feelings, but assured Michelle that she would never force Michelle to live with her father again. Michelle stated unequivocally that she did not want to see or talk to her father at that time and was uncertain whether she would ever want any contact with him. They agreed that each of them need some more time to independently resolve their feelings toward him and that they need not share the same feelings. The therapist suggested that they may want to come back to therapy to work on that issue some more after the disposition of the legal charges against Michelle's father became clear. This work reflects the authors' belief that, in incest cases, it often is not possible to completely resolve the feelings of the victim and the nonoffending parent to-ward the perpetrator in an initial course of treatment, particularly before any pending legal actions are completed. Rather, it may be more appropri-ate to allow the family members to gain strength and confidence in their own abilities before they are faced with making a decision regarding whether or not to pursue an ongoing relationship with the offender. If, at a later point, they decide they would like to pursue some type of relationship, and the offender has successfully completed a course of individual therapy and is able to accept responsibility for the abuse, then the family may be encour-aged to return to therapy to obtain some assistance in establishing a healthy relationship that provides safe and appropriate boundaries for everyone.

By the 20th session, the therapist, Harriett, and Michelle were begin-ning to talk about the timing of termination. The therapist, therefore, asked Michelle and her mother to repeat the psychological measures they initially completed, so that their progress could be evaluated. Although Harriett's Global Severity Index score on the SCL-90-R had fallen, it was still mildly elevated, indicating that she continued to experience some distress. Simi-larly, her scores on the TSI indicated that she still had elevated levels of de-pressive and anxious symptoms. However, her scores on the TSI subscales for intrusive experiences and defensive avoidance were no longer in the clinical range, indicating that she was no longer experiencing intrusive and distressing thoughts of the abuse and was not engaging in such frequent avoidant behavior.

When Michelle's responses to her measures were evaluated, her previ-ously elevated scores on the posttraumatic stress and sexual distress sub-scales of the TSCC had dropped below the level of clinical significance. In a pattern similar to that of her mother, Michelle's scores on the depression measures (the depression subscale of the TSCC and the CDI) remained mildly elevated, suggesting that although her posttraumatic stress symp-toms had been successfully reduced, her symptoms of depression were still evident, albeit at a lower level. Interestingly, her mother's responses to the CBCL indicated that she perceived Michelle's internalizing symptoms as having been reduced significantly, as they were no longer in the clinical range. Finally, both Michelle and her mother completed the K-SADS-E. Based on their reports, Michelle no longer met criteria for either PTSD or dysthymia. Although she continued to endorse several depressive symp-toms, they were not sufficient to warrant a diagnosis. Michelle's and Harriett's scores at the end of treatment are presented in Table 9.1.

The therapist summarized the findings and presented them to Michelle and her mother. They discussed the fact that, for both mother and daughter, the symptoms of posttraumatic stress had diminished to the extent that they were no longer problematic. However, the therapist also shared the finding that both mother and daughter continued to exhibit mild symptoms of de-pression, although those symptoms also had been reduced. The therapist dis-cussed the possibility of continued treatment, either as a continuation of the same therapeutic relationship or through participation in a group therapy program at the same facility. Michelle and her mother felt as though they had completed as much work as was possible at that time in individual therapy, but they expressed some interest in the group therapy program.

The therapist explained that the group therapy program was a time-limited 12-session program, offering separate but simultaneous groups for sexually abused youth and their nonoffending parents. She further explained that the groups were very helpful in reducing the sense of isolation that many families experience when struggling with child sexual abuse. She described the groups as offering opportunities for families to support each other and share with each other strategies they have found useful in coping with this experience. Michelle and her mother agreed to participate in the next session of therapy groups.

The therapist supported their decision, as participation in group therapy should help to address issues of isolation and stigma that might be contributing to their ongoing symptoms of depression and anxiety. Participation in the groups also provided a means of gradually reducing their reliance on therapy, without ending the therapeutic process and the provision of support too abruptly. However, the therapist also offered them the possibility of returning to individual treatment if needed in the future, particularly at predictable times of stress, such as the pending trial for Michelle's father.

Thus, based upon the reevaluation, as well as the clients' sense of progress, it was decided to taper down the individual therapy process by spreading out the final sessions. Session 21 was scheduled for 2 weeks later, and the final session for 1 month after that. Those last two sessions consisted largely of joint meetings with Harriett and Michelle in which their work in therapy was reviewed, their progress was emphasized, accomplishments were praised, and suggestions were made for continuing the therapeutic work at home. For example, they were encouraged to continue discussing sexuality, dating, and issues related to the sexual abuse. In addition, they were urged to utilize the cognitive coping exercises to continue to combat depressive thoughts and feelings. Finally, they were encouraged to contact the therapist if at any point they felt it might be useful to come back for further sessions.

SUMMARY

The treatment model presented in this chapter can be tailored to address the wide range of difficulties presented by adolescent survivors of sexual abuse. However, to effectively apply the intervention described, the clinician should be skilled in the application of cognitive-behavioral interventions and knowledgeable in the area of child sexual abuse. The interventions described are flexible and should be chosen based on the individual needs of the child and family. For example, in some cases, behavior-management training may not be necessary. However, in other cases, the parent may benefit from the parenting skills training. It should be noted, however, that we believe that direct discussion of the trauma and related thoughts and feelings should be regarding as central to the effective treatment of posttraumatic stress symptoms resulting from child sexual abuse. Interestingly, however, this is the aspect of treatment that tends to be met with the greatest resistance. Most adolescents and parents enter therapy with the expectations that psychotherapy will help them feel better. It is therefore quite disconcerting to some clients that the proposed gradual exposure exercises may cause some degree of discomfort. For some clients, this is simply unacceptable, and they may choose a less directive approach for treatment for themselves and their families. However, therapists can usually overcome such natural resistance by establishing a healthy and collaborative therapeutic relationship and explaining the treatment rationale in clear, sensitive, and developmentally appropriate terms to both parents and children.

A strength of this model is the heavy emphasis on involving the nonoffending parent as a therapeutic agent. However, it is important to consider referral to another individual therapist if the parent seems to be grappling with personal or marital issues that require greater focus and attention than the child's therapist can provide. It is our contention that involving a nonoffending parent in the treatment of his or her child can extend the benefits of therapy beyond the therapy hour, as well as beyond the point of termination. In fact, there was no question in the case study described that Michelle's mother contributed dramatically to her daughter's recovery and positive adjustment.

Finally, it should be noted that, although this case study describes a short-term treatment approach, child sexual abuse cases can be very complex and may require follow-up counseling periodically. It is therefore important to offer parents and children anticipatory guidance to assist them in identifying when additional counseling might be needed. Parents and children may need additional assistance in coping with their anxiety associated with the case going to court or when family reunification issues are being considered. Although the initial course of therapy is intended to provide clients with the necessary skills for coping with future stressors on their own, families are often comforted to know that therapeutic resources are available if needed.

REFERENCES

Achenbach, T. M. (1991). *Manual for the Child Behavior Checklist 4–18 and 1991 Profile*. Burlington: Department of Psychiatry, University of Vermont .

Ackerman, P., Newton, J., McPherson, W. B., Jones, J., & Dykman, R. (1998). Prevalence of posttraumatic stress disorder and other psychiatric diagnoses in three groups of abused children (sexual, physical, and both). *Child Abuse and Neglect, 22*(8), 759–774.

American Psychiatric Association. (1994). *Diagnostic and statistical manual of mental disorders* (4th ed.). Washington, DC: Author.

Anderson, L. S. (1981). Notes on the linkage between the sexually abused child and the suicidal adolescent. *Journal of Adolescence, 4,* 157–162.

Beck, A. (1976). *Cognitive therapy and the emotional disorders.* New York: International Universities Press.

Beitchman, J. H., Zucker, K. J., Hood, J. E., DaCosta, G. A., Akman, D., & Cassavia, E. (1992). A review of the long-term effects of child sexual abuse. *Child Abuse and Neglect, 16,* 101–118.

Berliner, L., & Saunders, B. (1996). Treating fear and anxiety in sexually abused children: Results of a controlled, two year follow-up study. *Child Maltreatment, 1*(4), 294–309.

Boney-McCoy, S., & Finkelhor, D. (1995). Psychosocial sequelae of violent victimization in a national youth sample. *Journal of Consulting and Clinical Psychology, 63*(5), 726–736.

Briere, J. N. (1995). *Trauma Symptom Inventory professional manual.* Odessa, FL: Psychological Assessment Resources.

Briere, J. N. (1996). *Trauma Symptom Checklist for Children professional manual.* Odessa, FL: Psychological Assessment Resources.

Briere, J. N., & Elliott, D. M. (1994). Immediate and long-term impacts of child sexual abuse. *The Future of Children, 4*(2), 54–69.

Briere, J., & Runtz, M. (1988). Symptomatology associated with childhood sexual victimization in a nonclinical adult sample. *Child Abuse and Neglect, 12,* 51–59.

Browne, A., & Finkelhor, D. (1986). Impact of child sexual abuse: A review of the research. *Psychological Bulletin, 99,* 66–77.

Cohen, J. A., & Mannarino, A. P. (1996). A treatment outcome study for sexually abused preschool children: Initial findings. *Journal of the American Academy of Child and Adolescent Psychiatry, 35*(1), 42–50.

Cohen, J. A., & Mannarino, A. P. (1997). A treatment study for sexually abused preschool children: Outcome during a one-year follow-up. *Journal of the American Academy of Child and Adolescent Psychiatry, 36*(9), 1228–1235.

Cohen, J. A., & Mannarino, A. P. (1998). Interventions for sexually abused children: Initial treatment outcome findings. *Child Maltreatment, 3*(1), 17–26.

Cohen, J. B., Deblinger, E., Maedel, A. B., & Stauffer, L. B. (1999). Examining sex-related thoughts and feelings of sexually abused and nonabused children. *Journal of Interpersonal Violence, 14*(7), 701–712.

Cole, J. (1988). *Asking about sex and growing up.* New York: Beech Tree Books.

Conte, J. R., & Schuerman, J. (1987). Factors associated with an increased impact of child sexual abuse. *Child Abuse and Neglect, 2,* 201–211.

Deblinger, E., & Heflin, A. H. (1996). *Treating sexually abused children and their nonoffending parents: A cognitive behavioral approach.* Thousand Oaks, CA: Sage.

Deblinger, E., Lippmann, J., & Steer, R. (1996). Sexually abused children suffering posttraumatic stress symptoms: Initial treatment outcome findings. *Child Maltreatment, 1*(4), 310–321.

Deblinger, E., McLeer, S. V., & Henry, D. (1990). Cognitive behavioral treatment for sexually abused children suffering posttraumatic stress: Preliminary findings. *Journal of the American Academy of Child and Adolescent Psychiatry, 29,* 747–752.

Deblinger, E., Steer, R., & Lippmann, J. (1999a). Maternal factors associated with sexually abused children's psychosocial adjustment. *Child Maltreatment, 4*(1), 13–20.

Deblinger, E., Steer, R., & Lippman, J. (1999b). Two-year follow-up study of cognitive behavioral therapy for sexually abused children suffering post-traumatic stress symptoms. *Child Abuse and Neglect, 23*(12), 1371–1378.

Deblinger, E., Taub, B., Maedel, A., Lippmann, J., & Stauffer, L. (1997). Psychosocial factors predicting parent reported symptomatology in sexually abused children. *Journal of Child Sexual Abuse, 6,* 35–49.

Dembo, R., Dertke, M., LaVoie, L., Borders, S., Washburn, M., & Schmeidler, J. (1987). Physical abuse, sexual victimization and illicit drug use: A structural analysis among high risk adolescents. *Journal of Adolescence, 10,* 13–33.

Derogatis, L. R. (1983). *The SCL-90–R: Administration, scoring, and procedures manual II.* Baltimore: Clinical Psychometric Research.

Elliott, D. M. (1994). Impaired object relations in professional women molested as children. *Psychotherapy, 31,* 79–86.

Elliott, D. M., & Briere, J. (1992). Sexual abuse trauma among professional women: Validating the Trauma Symptom Checklist—40 (TSC-40). *Child Abuse and Neglect, 16*(3), 391–398.

Everson, M. D., Hunter, W. M., Runyon, D. K., Edelson, G. A., & Coulter, M. L. (1989). Maternal support following disclosure of incest. *American Journal of Orthopsychiatry, 59*(2), 197–207.

Famularo, R., Kinscherff, R., & Fenton, T. (1992). Psychiatric diagnoses of maltreated children: Preliminary findings. *Journal of the American Academy of Child and Adolescent Psychiatry, 31,* 863–867.

Feiring, C., Taska, L., & Lewis, M. (1998). Social support and children's and adolescents' adaptation to sexual abuse. *Journal of Interpersonal Violence, 13,* 240–260.

Finkelhor, D., Hotaling, G., and Lewis, I., & Smith, C. (1990). Sexual abuse in a national survey of men and women: Prevalence, characteristics, and risk factors. *Child Abuse and Neglect, 14,* 19–28.

Foa, E., Rothbaum, B. O., & Ette, G. S. (1993). Treatment of rape victims. *Journal of Interpersonal Violence, 8,* 156–276.

Foa, E., Rothbaum, B. O., Riggs, D. S., & Murdock, T. B. (1991). Treatment of PTSD in rape victims: A comparison between cognitive-behavioral procedures and counseling. *Journal of Consulting and Clinical Psychology, 59,* 715–723.

Friedrich, W. N., Luecke, W. J., Beilke, R. L., & Place, V. (1992). Psychotherapy outcome of sexually abused boys: An agency study. *Journal of Interpersonal Violence, 7*(3), 396–409.

Fromuth, M. E. (1986). The relationship of childhood sexual abuse with later psychological and sexual adjustment in a sample of college women. *Child Abuse and Neglect, 10,* 5–15.

Gold, E. R. (1986). Long-term effects of sexual victimization in childhood: An attributional approach. *Journal of Consulting and Clinical Psychology, 54,* 471–475.

Heflin, A. H., Mears, C., & Deblinger, E. (1996, November). *Coping style, attribu-*

tional style, and symptomatology among sexually abused adolescents. Poster presented at the annual meeting of the Association for the Advancement of Behavior Therapy, New York.

Heflin, A. H., Mears, C., Deblinger, E., & Steer, R. (1997, June). *A comparison of body images and views of sexuality between sexually abused and nonabused girls.* Poster presented at the annual meeting of the American Professional Society on the Abuse of Children, Miami, FL.

James, J., & Meyerding, J. (1977). Early sexual experience as a factor in prostitution. *Archives of Sexual Behavior 7*, 31–42.

Johnson, B. K., & Kenkel, M. B. (1991). Stress, coping, and adjustment in female adolescent incest victims. *Child Abuse and Neglect, 15*, 293–305.

Kendall-Tackett, K. A., Williams, L. M., & Finkelhor, D. (1993). Impact of sexual abuse on children: A review and synthesis of recent empirical studies. *Psychological Bulletin, 113*(1), 164–180.

Kovacs, M. (1992). *Children's Depression Inventory manual.* Toronto: Multi-Health Systems.

Leitenberg, H., Greenwald, E., & Cado, S. (1992). A retrospective study of long-term methods of coping with having been sexually abused during childhood. *Child Abuse and Neglect, 16*, 399–407.

Lyons, J. A. (1987). Post-traumatic stress disorder in children and adolescents: A review of the literature. *Developmental and Behavioral Pediatrics, 8*(6), 349–356.

Mannarino, A., & Cohen, J. (1996). Abuse-related attributions and perceptions, general attributions, and locus of control in sexually abused girls. *Journal of Interpersonal Violence, 11*(2), 162–180.

McLeer, S. V., Deblinger, E., Henry, D., & Orvaschel, H. (1992). Sexually abused children at high risk for post-traumatic stress disorder. *Journal of the American Academy of Adolescent and Child Psychiatry, 31*(5), 875–879.

Meiselman, K. C. (1978). *Incest: A psychological study of causes and effects with treatment recommendations.* San Francisco: Jossey-Bass.

Neumann, D. A., Houskamp, B. M., Pollock, B. M., & Briere, J. (1996). The long-term sequelae of childhood sexual abuse in women: A meta-analytic review. *Child Maltreatment, 1*(1), 6–16.

Orvaschel, H., Puig-Antich, J., Chambers, W. J., Tabrizi, M. A., & Johnson, R. (1982). Retrospective assessments of child psychopathology with the Kiddie SADS-E. *Journal of the American Academy of Child and Adolescent Psychiatry, 21*, 392–397.

Patterson, G., & Forgatch, M. (1987). *Parents and adolescents living together: Part 1. The basics.* Eugene, OR: Castalia.

Runyon, D. K., Hunter, W. M., & Everson, M. D. (1992). *Maternal support for child victims of sexual abuse: Determinants and implications* (Final report for the National Center for Child Abuse and Neglect). Washington, DC: U. S. Department of Health and Human Services.

Russell, D. E. H. (1986). *The secret trauma: Incest in the lives of girls and women.* New York: Basic Books.

Sansonnet-Hayden, H., Haley, G., Marriage, K., & Fine, S. (1987). Sexual abuse and psychopathology in hospitalized adolescents. *American Academy of Child and Adolescent Psychiatry, 26*, 753–757.

Seligman, M. (1991). *Learned optimism.* New York: Knopf.

Seligman, M., Peterson, C., Kaslow, N. J., Tanenbaum, R. L., Alloy, L. B., & Abramson, L. (1984). Attributional style and depressive symptoms among children. *Journal of Abnormal Psychology, 93,* 235–238.

Spaccarelli, S. (1994). Stress, appraisal, and coping in child sexual abuse: A theoretical and empirical review. *Psychological Bulletin, 116*(2), 340–362.

Spaccarelli, S., & Fuchs, C. (1997). Variability in symptom expression among sexually abused girls: Developing multivariate models. *Journal of Clinical Child Psychology, 26*(1), 24–35.

Speilberger, C. D. (1983). *Manual for the State–Trait Inventory for Children.* Palo Alto, CA: Consulting Psychologists Press.

Stauffer, L. B., & Deblinger, E. (1996). Cognitive behavioral groups for nonoffending mothers and their young sexually abused children: A preliminary treatment outcome study. *Child Maltreatment, 1*(1), 65–76.

Wurtle, S. K., & Miller-Perrin, C. L. (1992). *Preventing child sexual abuse: Sharing the responsibility.* Lincoln: University of Nebraska Press.

SUGGESTED READINGS

Berliner, L., & Elliott, D. M. (1996). Sexual abuse of children. In J. Briere, L. Berliner, J. Bulkley, C. Jenny, & T. Reid (Eds.), *The APSAC handbook on child maltreatment* (pp. 51–71). Thousand Oaks, CA: Sage.

Chaffin, M., Bonner, B. L., Worley, K. B., & Lawson, L. (1996). Treating abused adolescents. In J. Briere, L. Berliner, J. Bulkley, C. Jenny, & T. Reid (Eds.), *The APSAC handbook on child maltreatment* (pp. 119–139). Thousand Oaks, CA: Sage.

Cohen, J. A., & Mannarino, A. P. (1998). Interventions for sexually abused children: Initial treatment outcome findings. *Child Maltreatment, 3*(1), 17–26.

Deblinger, E., & Heflin, A. H. (1996). *Treating sexually abused children and their nonoffending parents: A cognitive behavioral approach.* Thousand Oaks, CA: Sage.

Deblinger, E., Lippmann, J., & Steer, R. (1996). Sexually abused children suffering posttraumatic stress symptoms: Initial treatment outcome findings. *Child Maltreatment, 1*(4), 310–321.

10

Treatment of Adolescent Eating Disorders

WAYNE A. BOWERS
KAY EVANS
DANIEL LeGRANGE
ARNOLD E. ANDERSEN

Cognitive-behavioral therapy (CBT) is a recommended intervention for treating eating disorders, including anorexia nervosa (AN) and bulimia nervosa (BN) (American Psychiatric Association, 2000; Wilson & Fairburn, 2002). Research on CBT has consistently shown it to be an effective treatment for bulimia nervosa (Agras, Schneider, Arnow, Raeburn, & Telch, 1989; Agras et al., 2000; Wilson & Fairburn, 1993; Wilson, Rossiter, Kleifield, & Lindholm, 1986) and anorexia nervosa (Pike, 2000; Wilson & Fairburn, 1993). Fairburn and Cooper (1989) have developed a CBT model that can be considered a standard of care for outpatient treatment of bulimia nervosa. Treatment results have been positive whether delivered in small groups or through individual sessions, and long-term follow up studies indicate that therapeutic gains are maintained over time (Fairburn et al., 1995). Although detailed treatment manuals have yet to be published for treating anorexia nervosa, several authors have developed CBT programs for this disorder (Garner, Vitousek, & Pike, 1997; Wilson, Fairburn, & Agras, 1997). It is worth acknowledging that research on CBT for AN has lagged behind that for BN. It has been suggested that the delay in developing interventions for AN may be related to the complex and often unyielding nature of this disorder (Vitousek, 1991). In the same way, studies and case reports describing the use of CBT with children and adolescents with eating disorders are relatively uncommon. Work in this area lags behind that with adults.

247

This chapter will focus on the ways in which cognitive-behavioral models can inform the treatment of children and adolescents with eating disorders. It will present a general theoretical model for understanding eating disorders as well as a cognitive-behavioral model that has recently been developed for treating anorexia nervosa. We will briefly review group and family therapy interventions that have proven useful for treating AN and will discuss how they can be applied to adolescents and children. Particular attention will be paid to interventions designed to address distortions in body image which commonly accompany eating disorders. When appropriate, specific interventions will be described and supportive empirical data will be cited.

COGNITIVE-BEHAVIORAL THERAPY OF EATING DISORDERS

One of the defining clinical features of an eating disorder is the attempt to achieve significant weight loss through restrictive eating. This is often accompanied by compulsive exercise, and is sometimes complicated by binge eating, self-induced vomiting, or laxative abuse. Weight loss is driven by a profound fear of gaining weight and an overvalued desire to be thin. The weight loss may become life-threatening as the avoidance of eating and the binge–purge behavior becomes progressively more frequent and severe. Distortion of body size and shape, cessation of menstrual cycles with extreme weight loss, and social withdrawal are common features of these disorders. Other psychiatric and medical problems complicate the treatment of eating disorders. Children and adolescents with eating disorders frequently manifest comorbid psychiatric disorders such as depression, obsessive–compulsive disorder, anxiety, and personality vulnerabilities. Suicidal ideation and self-destructive gestures are not uncommon and can complicate treatment. Additionally, there can be medical complications related to starvation, weight loss, and extreme or long-term binge–purge behavior (Garner & Garfinkel, 1997).

Children and adolescents with AN and BN often view their difficulties as egosyntonic. That is, they view their behavior as reasonable and do not acknowledge that they have a problem. The use of food, whether restrictive dieting or overeating, is often viewed as a means of establishing control over their environment (i.e., home, parents, friends, life circumstance, society) and weight. They frequently view attempts to change how they eat or what they weigh as reflecting others' jealousy or desires to control them. The treatment of children and adolescents with eating disorders is made more difficult by the fact that their participation in therapy is often involuntary. As a result, they are often noncompliant with the treatment process. This lack of a collaborative therapeutic rapport can lead to longer durations of treatment and, in the case of AN, may necessitate inpatient management.

Wilson et al. (1997) developed a cognitive-behavioral model for BN. They proposed that patients with eating disorders believe their shape and weight are of such fundamental importance that both must be kept under strict control. Binge eating, from a cognitive-behavioral perspective, represents a secondary response to extreme dietary restraint. Beliefs and values regarding thinness and weight are postulated to play a primary role in the maintenance of the condition. CBT for BN, as such, is directed at altering dysfunctional beliefs and values concerning food, body shape, and weight that maintain the disorder (Cooper & Fairburn, 1984; Wilson et al., 1997).

Cognitive-behavioral models of AN view the disorder as multiply determined (Garfinkel & Garner, 1982; Garner, 1985). Eating disorder symptoms stem from the interaction of sociocultural, individual, and familial factors (Garner et al., 1997). The cognitive-behavioral model conceptualizes eating disorders from a developmental perspective, and emphasizes the role of cognition as a moderator of distressed emotions and resultant abnormal behavior (Garfinkel & Garner, 1982; Garner, 1985; Garner & Bemis, 1982; Garner et al., 1997; Vitousek & Orimoto, 1993; Wilson et al., 1997). The model acknowledges that genetic, neurochemical, and endocrine factors may play a role in the etiology and maintenance of eating disorders (Grice et al., 2002; Klump, McGue, & Iacono, 2000; Wade, Bulik, Neale, & Kemdler, 2000). The ways in which cognitive, socioenvironmental, and biological factors interact in contributing to vulnerability for eating disorders, however, are not well understood. The cognitive-behavioral model, then, views AN as a final common pathway of multiple events and experiences (Garfinkel & Garner, 1982). It conceptualizes AN as stemming from an interacting series of events or experiences contributing to the cognitively vulnerable adolescent's belief that weight loss will alleviate distress and dysphoria (Bowers & Andersen, 1994; Garfinkel & Garner, 1982; Garner & Bemis, 1982, 1985). It is believed, then, that a range of factors may contribute to the vulnerable individual's developing the belief that "it is absolutely essential that I be thin." This belief serves as a proximal risk factor for the development of AN. This belief is rigidly held and is typically associated with maladaptive tacit beliefs, attitudes, and assumptions about the meaning of body weight, shape, and personal competency. Dieting, weight loss, and attaining thinness become factors that these individuals manipulate in an attempt to exercise control over their internal and external environments (Garner & Bemis, 1982, 1985). Additionally, thinness is often reinforced by the compliments of others and by an enjoyable sense of success and personal efficacy. The individual then attempts to further decrease food intake and is reinforced for additional weight loss. Although continued weight loss may be perceived as evidence that one has control over an important outcome in one's life, it can also lead to social ostracism. This criticism may be threatening to the individual's sense of control and self-worth. Protracted weight loss, as such, can lead the individual to withdraw from friends, family, and peers.

DEVELOPMENTAL CONSIDERATIONS

Studies of the effectiveness of cognitive-behavior therapy for treating eating disorders have tended to use adult samples. As noted, the treatment of children and adolescents with eating disorders has not received extensive empirical attention. Studies completed to date suggest that family-based interventions can be effective for treating youth with eating disorders (Crisp et al., 1991; Dare, Eisler, Russell, & Szmukler, 1990; Eisler et al., 2000; Hall, 1987). However, there is no a priori reason to believe that cognitive and behavioral factors that serve as the focus of treatment in clinical work with adults should not play a role in CBT with youth.

CBT with adults emphasizes the central role of cognitive contents and processes in the development of eating disorders, and focuses on assisting patients to change maladaptive or distorted perceptions and beliefs that accompany these conditions. Cognitive and behavioral techniques are employed to teach patients to become more aware of their perceptions of specific events and to aid them in monitoring and reevaluating recurrent, maladaptive patterns of thinking. The ultimate goal is to develop alternative ways of looking at day-to-day events and to provide the individual with more effective strategies for coping with distressing events as they arise (Reinecke, 1992).

In addition to developing alternative ways of seeing the world and coping with life events, CBT attempts to change developmental templates or schemas (Freeman, 1993). Schemas may be defined as relatively enduring, tacit mental representations that serve to guide the selection, perception, encoding, storage, and retrieval of information. They influence how phenomena are perceived, conceptualized, and recalled (Freeman & Reinecke, 1995). Schemas, which are established during infancy and childhood, influence an individual's perceptions, attributions, beliefs, and information-processing style. Schemas that are strongly held are resistant to rational disputation and may become central to the way the patient defines him- or herself and others. Self-schemas, or self-representational systems, have been found to strongly influence the processing of personally meaningful information, as well as information related to personal performance, self-esteem, and self-worth. They may, as such, play a role in the development and maintenance of eating disorders. As a consequence, changing maladaptive schemas plays an important role in CBT of eating disorders, as it does in the treatment of depression and Axis II disorders among adults.

ADAPTATIONS OF COGNITIVE THEORY AND TECHNIQUE

The social, emotional, and cognitive skills of children and adolescents are not as well developed as those of adults. With this in mind, it is often necessary to modify standard cognitive therapy techniques when working with youth (Braswell & Kendall, 1988; Finch, Nelson, & Ott, 1993; Kendall & Braswell, 1985; Matson, 1989; Meyers & Craighead, 1984; Reinecke, 1992; Zarb, 1992). Adaptations include attempting to develop alternative ways of thinking (i.e., encouraging the use of adaptive self-statements), rather than emphasizing rational disputation of cognitive distortions. In addition, an emphasis is placed on understanding the role that parents and peers play in the development of the child. Children develop in a social context. Parents, peers, and media influence the development of adaptive problem-solving skills, affect regulation capacities, and beliefs among children. CBT acknowledges that the child's social environment may play a role in the development of maladaptive beliefs about the self, weight, and appearance. Thus, clinical practice with children and adolescents requires that we attend to the social, emotional, and cognitive developmental level of the patient. Adolescents, for example, often demonstrate cognitive egocentrism in that they may not have consolidated the ability to engage in formal operational thought (Shirk, 1988). This may be reflected in tendencies to view their difficulties as uniquely important, and to feel that others are as acutely aware of their shortcomings and difficulties as they are (Elkind, 1966). Adolescent egocentrism, in conjunction with an inability to use hypothetico-deductive reasoning to evaluate the validity and adaptiveness of their thoughts and actions, can limit the effectiveness of standard cognitive therapy techniques with youth.

Adolescence is a time when abstract reasoning skills, the capacity for self-observation and self-understanding, an awareness of motives, an ability to evaluate hypothetical alternatives, a sensitivity to inconsistencies and discrepancies between beliefs, and an ability to use abstract principles as guides for behavior emerge in their mature form. Schrodt and Wright (1987) suggest that cognitive therapy can be used to nurture the development of adaptive skills such as these. Studies indicate that negative expectancies, maladaptive beliefs, cognitive distortions, problem-solving deficits, and negativistic attributional style may play a role in the development and maintenance of behavioral and emotional problems among youth (Kendall & MacDonald, 1993). Schrodt and Wright (1987) propose that attempts to develop rational and flexible modes of thinking may be associated with an improvement in self-concept and self-esteem, as well as a reduction in behavioral and emotional symptoms. A goal of treatment, then, is to substitute immature and maladaptive reasoning with more mature, flexible, and adaptive cognitive processes.

The active, goal-oriented, here-and-now focus of CBT is well suited for work with adolescents. The collaborative problem-solving approach of cognitive therapy helps to counter difficulties that adolescents can have in engaging in a working relationship with adult therapists. The egalitarian, empirical approach of CBT encourages healthy skepticism. If the therapist can convey to the patient that his or her perception of a situation is but one possible alternative, and if the teenager can be encouraged to reciprocate by looking at his or her own thoughts with the same critical eye, then collaborative empiricism can be attained.

CBT stresses the importance of focusing on specific target symptoms and developing specific treatment goals. Families of adolescents with eating disorders are often chaotic—family instability, high levels of expressed emotion, and feelings of ambivalence are not uncommon. With this in mind, CBT explicitly attempts to reduce conflict among family members. Beliefs, expectations, attributions, and assumptions held by family members that may contribute to the child's distress are explored and resolved. Direct attempts are made to develop communications skills and effective parenting practices and to encourage negotiation and empathic support within the family. Treatment is most effective when the family, the adolescent, and the treatment team work together in a collaborative manner. We address not only the dysfunctional attitudes, cognitive distortions, and maladaptive behavior patterns demonstrated by the child, but also those demonstrated by other family members.

As in work with adults, the process of CBT with adolescents involves bringing automatic thoughts, schemas, assumptions and perceptual processes into awareness. As noted, adolescents vary in their capacity for self-reflection and in their metacognitive capacity to "think about thinking." With this in mind, asking teenagers to create a diary—to put their thoughts into writing—can help them gain a more objective view of situations as well as insight into maladaptive or distorted perceptions.

CBT of eating disorders with adolescents is similar, in many ways, to work with adults. Interventions focus on rectifying specific beliefs, attributions, and cognitive distortions that contribute to the eating disorder. Cognitive and behavioral techniques are employed to teach adolescents to anticipate potentially distressing situations, and to be more aware of their thoughts, feelings, and behaviors. As with adults, adolescents learn to identify and label their emotions, as well as recurrent patterns of thinking. Socratic questioning is used to assist the adolescent in evaluating the validity of automatic thoughts. For those adolescents who do not yet have the ability to reflect productively on their thoughts, emotions, and motivations, an emphasis is placed on developing logical alternatives for their maladaptive thoughts (Reinecke, 1992).

Behavioral interventions are often used in treating adolescents with eating disorders. For patients with severe AN, the initial interventions are primarily behavioral in nature. The degree of emphasis placed on the use of behavioral techniques varies with the severity of the disorder. When working with adolescents with AN, it is important to assess the degree of accompanying cognitive impairment. Attempts are made to evaluate their capacity for self-reflection, their social problem-solving skills, the rigidity of their beliefs and schemas, and their ability to engage in hypothetico-deductive reasoning. With more cognitively impaired individuals, initial sessions may emphasize the use of behavioral interventions. Behavioral techniques such as activity scheduling, mastery and pleasure activities, mood monitoring, and graded behavioral task assignments can increase their awareness of how their behavior contributes to and maintains their distress. Behavioral assignments are selected such that they are appropriate for the patient's level of understanding and motivation. Some adolescents, for example, may experience difficulty understanding complex ideas or procedures. Accordingly, behavioral tasks should be developed and practiced during the therapy session before the adolescent attempts them alone. Similarly, it is important that the patient understands the rationale for each assignment. Behavioral interventions such as activity scheduling and mood monitoring can be particularly helpful when used during food-related activities. Mastery and pleasure ratings also may be used to challenge the patient's beliefs about being fat or out of control. Graded task assignments can be used to complete difficult tasks. For example, a patient with AN might be encouraged to plan steps needed to finish a meal. This might begin with making a list of steps, then encouraging them to simply *imagine* each successive step in the sequence leading to the desired outcome. They subsequently would be encouraged to eat a small amount of a "prohibited food" in the presence of the therapist, and then to discuss the accompanying thoughts and emotions.

The cognitive techniques used in working with adolescents with eating disorders are also similar to those used in treating adults. Thought records, guided imagery, identification and labeling of cognitive distortions, and rational disputation are much the same. As noted, however, less emphasis is placed on identification and resolution of tacit assumptions and schemas. Adolescents often have not developed and consolidated an articulated set of beliefs about themselves, their world, and their future. A psychosocial approach for understanding adolescents' schemas has been developed by Freeman (1993). Based upon Erikson's developmental framework, Freeman discusses cognitions related to each stage of development. His formulation is similar, in many ways, to other developmentally informed models of cognitive therapy, in that he emphasizes the social context in which individuals function. He notes that individuals develop within the social context of home, school, church, and peers. The effect of each on a given individual is determined by the person's ability to assimilate and integrate the socialization demands of each of these domains. From this perspective, it becomes possible to change existing schemas and to assist the adolescent in developing more adaptive tacit beliefs by identifying and addressing salient demands in each domain.

Adaptations to the "standard" cognitive therapy model (Beck, Rush, Shaw, & Emery, 1979; J. Beck, 1995) are necessary when working with individuals with eating disorders. Garner and Bemis (1985) recommend that several specific features of eating disorders be addressed. These include (1) the relative intractability of the disorder (including reluctance to enter into treatment), (2) interaction between physical and psychological elements, (3) prominence of deficits in self-concept, (4) idiosyncratic beliefs related to food and weight, and (5) the patient's beliefs regarding the desirability of retaining certain symptoms (e.g., low body weight, control over others). Several standard CBT interventions can be used to address these features. These include (1) monitoring thoughts and feelings and increasing the individual's awareness of automatic thoughts, (2) becoming aware of the relationships between thoughts, feelings, and dysfunctional behaviors, (3) identifying negative automatic thoughts and challenging these cognitions, (4) increasing the ability to accept more appropriate interpretations, and (5) identifying and modifying underlying schemas that maintain the disorder.

As noted, CBT for youth with eating disorders places a greater emphasis on working with parents and other important persons in a child's life. This stance is consistent with evidence supporting the effectiveness of family therapy for treating youth with eating disorders. With this in mind, active attempts are made to understand how parents may inadvertently contribute to their child's difficulties. This may take the form of identifying maladaptive beliefs the parents may be conveying to their child, and of addressing maladaptive parenting practices. Coercive and controlling attempts to have the child eat, even when done with the best of intentions, are worthy of clinical attention. Behavioral interventions, including contingency management for weight gain, can play an important role in the treatment of children with AN.

GROUP INTERVENTIONS

Group psychotherapy can be quite useful for treating eating disorders (Andersen, Bowers, & Evans, 1997; Bowers, 2000; Bowers, Evans, & Andersen, 1997; Garner & Garfinkel, 1997). Three types of groups have been found effective for treating eating disorders. These can be integrated with individually based cognitive-behavioral approaches in developing a more comprehensive and effective treatment program.

Psychoeducational Group

Studies indicate that outpatient psychoeducational group therapy can be effective in changing some behaviors associated with BN, including frequency of vomiting and bingeing (Laessle et al., 1991; Olmsted et al., 1991; Ordman & Kirschenbaum, 1986). Psychoeducational interventions are also commonly used in day treatment and inpatient treatment programs. Psychoeducational groups typically have two goals: (1) to provide information on basic principles of cognitive therapy and on the relationship of beliefs and attitudes to eating disorders, and (2) to provide information on the effects of the disorder itself. In accomplishing the first goal, the psychoeducational group explores various aspects of cognitive therapy (e.g., cognitive distortions, automatic thoughts) in a didactic fashion and their relationship to the eating disorder. Attempts are made to teach patients the basic concepts of cognitive therapy and provide information about the effects of the disorder. After each group, homework assignments using these concepts are given to patients to complete before the next session. The objectives of this group are that the patient will:

- Be able to define cognitive therapy.
- Understand basic cognitive therapy principles (e.g., cognitive triad, assumptions, automatic thoughts, cognitive distortions, schemas, core beliefs).
- Demonstrate the ability to rate his or her mood.
- Be able to identify automatic thoughts that he or she experiences.
- Be able to use reframing techniques for changing negative automatic thoughts.
- Be able to identify at least two cognitive distortions that he or she experiences.
- Demonstrate the ability to use the Daily Record of Dysfunctional Thoughts.
- Apply problem-solving skills to his or her life experiences.
- Be able to appropriately use at least one behavioral technique (e.g., activity scheduling, mastery and pleasure, graded task assignments, cognitive rehearsal, assertiveness, and role playing).
- Be able to appropriately use at least one cognitive therapy intervention (e.g., identifying automatic thoughts, challenging automatic thoughts, reattribution techniques, advantages–disadvantages, and homework).

Ancillary areas covered may include self-concept and self-esteem, values clarification, feelings identification, and rational problem solving. Materials on the nature and consequences of eating disorders may also be presented. This might include information on the effects of starvation, how the disorder functions psychologically, and the social and media views of an individual's appearance (Garner, 1997; Garner, Rockert, Olmsted, Johnson, & Coscina, 1985). Group leaders use a range of instructional techniques, including didactic approaches, role plays, discussions, practice sessions, homework, and creative expression exercises (e.g., artwork) in presenting the material. Reading materials, such as *Mind over Mood* (Greenberger & Padesky, 1995), a workbook describing specific cognitive and behavioral techniques, might also be assigned. Groups typically meet once a week, with sessions lasting from 60 to 90 minutes. Outcomes are measured by satisfactory completion of homework assignments, active participation in group discussions, activities that reflect an understanding of the material being taught, and level of participation in treatment outside of the group.

Cognitive Group Therapy

Group CBT for eating disorders introduces techniques derived from standard cognitive therapy in a process-oriented framework (Bowers, 2000). Group therapy is increasingly recognized as an effective and economical tool for treating eating disorders (Hall, 1985). A blend of process-oriented approaches (Yalom, 1995) and cognitive-behavioral principles (Bowers, 2000; Lee & Rush, 1986; White & Freeman, 2000) can be quite effective. Blending these two models gives the group leader latitude to deal with personal and interpersonal issues as they arise. Integrating the palliative factors of group therapy with problem-oriented cognitive therapy principles allows the clinician to focus on cognitive and developmental factors involved that may be maintaining the eating disorder. The group can influence the patients' perceptions and permit patients to assist each other's recovery through self-disclosure and confrontation of symptomatic behavior, distorted ideas, and negative attitudes.

When working with an eating disorder group, some of the goals are explicit whereas others are implicit and more personal. Explicit goals include change in disordered eating (i.e., bingeing, purging, restriction of dietary intake, overexercise), whereas others are more subtle (e.g., expression of emotion, assertiveness, overcoming fear of interpersonal relationships). The group explicitly attempts to facilitate change. Each member of the group is aware of other members' goals, and it is expected that they will discuss, challenge, and support other members regarding their goals. Individuals' goals are often addressed through the group process. Group members may, for example, wish to focus on being open with others and becoming more aware of their own cognitive distortions, automatic thoughts, schemas, and core beliefs. These issues may be discussed as they become evident in the group process. The group process brings to light many of these "subtle goals" while at the same time helping members to become aware of common cognitive aspects of their disorder. This is accomplished through self-disclosure and confrontation of symptomatic behavior, distorted ideas, and negative attitudes.

Although eating disorder therapy groups may be diagnostically homogeneous, this is not mandatory. It is possible to include patients with both AN and BN in groups so long as common themes and concerns are identified and addressed. Shared cognitive themes include cognitive distortions, automatic thoughts, schemas, and core beliefs related to weight, appearance, perfectionism, self-concept, and need for control.

Whereas psychoeducational groups provide didactic information about cognitive therapy, the cognitive therapy group focuses on facilitating cognitive, emotional, and behavioral change by using those concepts. As in other forms of group therapy, an emphasis is placed on the interactions between group members. This leads to an understanding of how behavior within the group may reflect how each member functions in the outside world. This allows group members to identify maladaptive beliefs and cognitive processes as they become apparent during the session. The group creates a supportive atmosphere in which members increase their awareness of maladaptive beliefs and cognitive processes in the here and now. The group also provides an opportunity for members to practice identifying cognitive distortions, automatic thoughts, schemas, and core beliefs for themselves and other patients as they occur within the group.

According to Yalom (1995), therapy groups can be effective for several reasons. They instill hope, provide feelings of "universality," offer opportunities for altruism and interpersonal learning, impart information, develop social skills, and provide for a corrective recapitulation of the primary family unit. Patients who struggle with AN frequently are not aware, for example, that there are many others who experience similar difficulties. Participating in group therapy with others suffering from similar symptoms allows individuals to overcome feelings of shame and their desire for secrecy. They can begin to express their feelings of frustration or helplessness about their relationship with food. It is possible to instill a sense of hope by showing that it is possible to change these seemingly unresolvable issues surrounding food and weight (Lee & Rush, 1986; Yalom, 1995). The power to help others, frequently unnoticed by those who see themselves as struggling, can allow group members to move away from being self-focused and facilitate their experiencing a sense of altruistic self-worth. Thus, the group provides its members the opportunity both to observe and contribute to solving others' problems, and to understand themselves (Yalom, 1995).

A cognitive therapy group challenges maladaptive views of the world that patients have established. Much of the group work is directed toward helping patients understand how their cognitions affect their mood and consequent behaviors. Another healing factor is the ability of group members to identify in others the ramifications of their own eating disorder. As patients help each other identify and change negative cognitions, they come to resolve their own problems by seeing themselves reflected in others. The cognitive therapy group explicitly focuses on identifying and changing maladaptive beliefs and attitudes that members have established. By participating in the group, patients begin to understand how the AN has worked for them and can begin to explore alternative methods of satisfying their emotional needs. As group members help each other in confronting their negative cognitions, they come to recognize their own maladaptive beliefs. They can come to resolution by seeing their issues reflected by others in the group.

Body Perception Group

Body image is the picture of our body that we form in our mind. It is the way the body appears to ourselves. Evidence indicates that patients with eating disorders maintain distorted perceptions of their weight and shape (Vitousek & Orimoto, 1993). Our experience has been that patients who do not resolve these distorted body perceptions may not engage in the recovery process. Rather, they tend to maintain their eating disorder as a means of avoiding weight gain. Resolving body image issues alone will not "cure" an eating disorder. If these misperceptions are not dealt with effectively, however, they can stand in the way of recovery. Body perception treatment must attend to a number of distortions. These include how the patients see themselves, how they believe others perceive them, and how their bodies actually function versus myths and mispeceptions that they hold as truths. Each of these issues must be addressed in order for the patients to maintain gains they have achieved in the treatment of their eating disorder.

The body perception group focuses on helping patients understand their body distortions and how these distortions sustain their eating disorder. This process can be one of the most difficult aspects of treatment. In a body perception group, patients are supportive yet confrontational with one another. They help each other recognize these distortions and bring their perceptions into the realm of reality. It can be difficulty to completely resolve an individual's distorted body image. Through participation in a body perception group, patients learn to diminish the impact of their distorted perceptions on their behavior and to put these perceptions into a proper, more adaptive, perspective.

Cognitive therapy can be effective in helping patients challenge their maladaptive beliefs and establish reasonable alternatives. It is not unusual, however, to find that patients with eating disorders have not thought through how they developed these perceptions and beliefs, and whether they recognize them as distortions. When patients are challenged to provide a rationale for their maladaptive beliefs and distorted perceptions, they are frequently surprised to find that they cannot offer any validation.

The purpose of the group is to help patients change distorted perceptions of their bodies. Patients have difficulty accepting their bodies before the onset of the illness, during the illness, and during the recovery process. We recognize that patients often find it difficult to accept their bodies during the recovery process. For many of them the changes that their bodies are undergoing are quite significant. During treatment for AN, some patients will almost double their weight. This is a significant change for them, both visually and physically. We acknowledge the significance that these changes hold for them. To do otherwise would be less than honest. We work diligently with the patients to understand that honesty is the key to recovery. They must experience us being honest with them in order to feel comfortable doing the same with us.

The body perception group is not activity oriented. We do not draw pictures around the patients' bodies, nor do we have them play with butter (as a way to help them deal with anxieties about fat). As this is a cognitive-behavioral group, our approach is based on collaborative empiricism. Patients are given homework assignments that bring forth their personal concerns. These problems are then brought to the body perception group, where the therapist and other group members deal with them in a cognitive-behavioral context. This type of group can cut across a continuum of care that includes inpatient, partial, intensive outpatient, and individual outpatient care. In the body perception group the patients are encouraged to express their feelings about their bodies and the thoughts that lead to these feelings. The patients are then assisted to follow a path to better understanding of these thoughts and the evidence or lack of evidence for them.

The group sessions focus on helping patients to identify the distorted thoughts and perceptions they have regarding their bodies and how to deal with their bodies in a healthy, adaptive manner. Patients typically come to treatment with many distortions that they have gathered from society or their families. They are taught to keep a daily record of their dysfunctional thoughts and perceptions, and to reframe these thoughts. Although patients readily learn the technique of rational disputation, they often try to "think" distorted thoughts through without writing them out in a thought record. This approach, however, is not optimal. We encourage patients to integrate the actual writing process into their lives. The process of putting one's thoughts on paper, and of looking at one's thoughts and perceptions as objects to be evaluated, can be quite helpful. Simply reflecting on the process is typically ineffective. Thinking about one's automatic thoughts and distorted perceptions does not, on its own, assist the patient in replacing them. Schemas are addressed in a similar manner as part of the body perception group.

Patients in cognitive therapy are taught that food and weight are not the true problems. Rather, discomfort with emotional concerns is the problem. Difficulties managing negative emotions and stressful life events become associated with distorted body perceptions and maladaptive beliefs about weight and shape, as patients feel that they can control these areas of their life. Focusing upon weight and shape allows them to avoid the pain of dealing with other, more critical, emotional concerns. We work with them to understand their true concerns, rather than accepting body image distortion as the primary problem. We regularly suggest to patients that when body perception becomes a concern for them, they ask themselves, "What is the real problem?" This approach is consistent with the standard cognitive therapy technique of encouraging patients to recognize social and environmental triggers for the activation of automatic thoughts.

Patients with eating disorders often have a poor understanding of diet and metabolism. With this in mind, we explore with patients their beliefs about how their bodies function as a means of identifying additional distorted thoughts and beliefs. Patients are often surprised to learn, for example, that if rhesus monkeys are allowed to overeat on one day, they will eat less the next to balance their caloric intake. Similarly, if monkeys are prohibited from eating on one day, they will overeat the next. Caloric intake, in short, is maintained homeostatically. Patients are then encouraged to allow their bodies to "normalize their intake." They are encouraged to adopt the view that thoughts and emotions should not be used to manage weight. We also discuss the way in which body fat is regulated and explain the weight restoration process. There are many distorted beliefs associated with body perception concerns. Only with frank discussion do these issues come to light.

The group setting allows patients to provide support for one another. Quite often, patients are able to recognize that their distorted beliefs and perceptions do not apply to others. They can, as a result, see others in a realistic light. It is often helpful for patients to verbalize their thoughts and feelings so that they can see how others react. It is also helpful for them to know that others in the group have thoughts and feelings similar to their own. Group members are encouraged to help each other reframe their maladaptive thoughts and perceptions. In the process, they help themselves. Put another way, they begin to listen to themselves as they validate others.

Group therapists need to be patient and to tolerate repetitiveness. It can be difficult for patients to accept new concepts and ways of thinking. Stressful events can precipite the reactivation of negative schemas and the recurrence of maladaptive beliefs. These must be reframed again and again, until it becomes natural for the patients to do this for themselves without assistance.

Body perception groups also serve to increase patients' awareness of the ways in which thoughts and feelings influence one another. Patients come to learn that, when they experience negative thoughts about their bodies, there typically is an underlying emotional concern which has precipitated it. Patients learn that they use eating and diet as a way of feeling in control physically when they feel out of control emotionally. A common example of this phenomena is the patients' statement that they "feel fat." They are conceptually fusing perceptions of shape and weight with affective states. When this occurs, the therapist can note that "fat" is not an emotion, and can encourage them to reexamine the emotions they *are* experiencing and how these feelings may be related to thoughts about weight, shape, and diet. Patients are then encouraged to explore how these thoughts and feelings may be related to problems that are occurring in their life. The body perception group, then, assists patients in applying cognitive-behavioral skills they have learned to a specific symptom of the eating disorder—distorted body image.

FAMILY TREATMENT STRATEGIES

Cognitive-behavioral approaches for treating AN among adolescents have received little study, and relatively little has been written about the use of cognitively based family therapy for treating this disorder. Attempts have been made, however, to adapt approaches developed for treating adults with AN for work with youth (Bowers, Evans, & Andersen, 1997; Dattilio, 1994; Teichman, 1992). Family therapy has received the strongest empirical support as an approach for treating AN (Dare, 1983; Dare & Eisler, 1997; Eisler et al., 2000). Family-based interventions can be integrated into a comprehensive cognitive-behavioral approach for treating adolescents with AN.

Clinical Trials of Family Therapy for Eating Disorders

The first controlled treatment studies involving the families of adolescent AN patients were conducted in the mid-1980s at the Maudsley Hospital in London. The Maudsley group regarded family involvement as an essential part of treatment for adolescents with AN. They viewed parental involvement in the treatment as fundamental for building a therapeutic alliance between the treatment team, the family, and the patient (Dare, 1983). The Maudsley approach to treating adolescents with AN has been shaped by a series of controlled trials comparing family therapy with individual supportive psychotherapy. These findings suggest that family therapy can be effective for adolescents with a short history of AN (Russell, Szmukler, Dare, & Eisler, 1987). The beneficial effects of family therapy were maintained at 5-year follow-up (Eisler et al., 1997). A comparison of two forms of family therapy (conjoint and separated family treatment) indicate that adolescents with AN do well in outpatient family therapy, even without prior hospitalization, when parents participate in treatment (Eisler et al., 2000; LeGrange, Eisler, Dare, & Russell, 1992). Taken together, these findings suggest that parental involvement can be beneficial in treating adolescents with AN.

Compared to the treatment of adolescents with AN, much less is known about the treatment of adolescents with bulimia nervosa (BN). Although AN and BN are distinct syndromes, overlap in symptomatology is common. Therefore, treatments that have proved to be effective for adolescent AN might also be beneficial in working with adolescents with BN. From a developmental perspective, one can argue that adolescent patients with BN and AN share similar challenges (e.g., the negotiation of individuation, separation from their families, sexuality, the development of an adult identity, etc.). Moreover, patterns of cognitive distortions, maladaptive beliefs, and information-processing deficits appear to be similar between these groups. Therefore, it is reasonable to suggest that adolescent patients with BN still living with their families of origin may benefit from family therapy.

There are theoretical and clinical arguments for involving family members in the treatment of adolescents with BN. Parents' feelings of shame, guilt, and blame can exacerbate the symptomatic behavior of their child. Family interventions can be used to address these concerns. Moreover, family therapy offers an opportunity to share information about the condition with the parents and the adolescent, and to discuss difficulties surrounding meals and the impact of the eating disorder on family relationships. Adolescents with BN typically deny that their behavior is problematic. They do not appreciate the seriousness of their illness. This necessitates that the parents ensure that the adolescent receives treatment. Robin and colleagues (1995) characterized the anorexic teen as "out of control" and "unable to take care of herself." If we characterize bulimic youth in similar terms, it places a responsibility on the parents to work to restore healthy eating in their offspring.

A manual for psychotherapeutic interventions with families for adolescent AN has recently been developed (Lock, LeGrange, Agras, & Dare, 2001). This manual incorporates elements of the Maudsley treatment program that have been found effective for a subgroup of AN patients (Eisler et al., 1997, 2000). The protocol underscores the central role of parents as a resource in the treatment of adolescent patients with AN. Unlike more traditional family therapy models in which the patient is seen as having developed a problem in response to external factors (e.g., genetic, physiological, familial, or sociocultural), and treatment is aimed at the individual to counteract the effects of these external causative factors, the Maudsley approach focuses on the eating disorder per se. This treatment emphasizes the parents' ability to help the adolescent overcome the "intrusion" of the AN in the adolescent's normal development.

Viewing parents in this way is important theoretically, and distinguishes this approach from other family and individual therapies for AN. The main focus of treatment is the empowerment of the parents in order to succeed in refeeding their starving child. It is only after the eating disorder has been successfully addressed that the parents will hand control over eating back to the adolescent. It is at this point that the family will begin to discuss other issues.

The Maudsley Approach

The theoretical foundation of the Maudsley approach is the view that the adolescent is embedded in the family, and that the parents are critical determinants of the ultimate success of treatment. The eating disorder is seen as interfering with normative adolescent development. Therefore, the parents should take an active role in their child's treatment (i.e., removing the AN), while at the same time showing respect for the adolescent. Respect for the adolescent is demonstrated in several ways. It is, for example, reflected in parents' attempting to distinguish the illness from the patient. Their otherwise healthy child, from this perspective, is seen as being "dominated" by the AN. The parents attempt, then, to play an active role in the treatment and to encourage adaptive behavior. This component of the Maudsley approach is similar, in many ways, to that employed in CBT of obsessive–compulsive disorder among children (March & Mulle, 1998). The Maudsley approach emphasizes the importance of attending to the tasks of normal adolescent development. Parents assist their adolescent with these developmental tasks once the eating disorder has been alleviated. This means, however, that meaningful work on other family conflicts or disagreements may be deferred until the eating disorder has been addressed.

The Maudsley approach differs from other treatment programs in several key ways. First, as noted, the adolescent is not viewed as being in control of the behavior. Rather, the eating disorder is seen as controlling the adolescent. Second, the treatment aims to correct this position by increasing parental control over the adolescent's eating. Third, the Maudsley approach strongly advocates that the therapist should primarily focus his or her attention on the task of weight restoration. The Maudsley approach, in contrast to more traditional family systems approaches (e.g., Minuchin et al., 1975), tends to "stay with the eating disorder" for a longer period of time and addresses it more directly. The therapist is not distracted from the central therapeutic task—keeping the parents focused on refeeding their adolescent so as to break the grip of the eating disorder.

In summary, family therapy can be effective in treating adolescents with AN of short duration. In the majority of cases, recovery is possible without admission to hospital. Successful restoration of an adolescent's health depends on the parents' ability to refeed the child. The parents' responsibility is similar to that of the nursing staff of a specialist inpatient unit. Controlled studies indicate that weight, as well as psychosocial functioning, can be restored for most adolescent patients in a relatively short period of time (Eisler et al., 2000; LeGrange et al., 1992; Russell et al., 1987). Most important, however, is the fact that the benefits of the treatment described here have been demonstrated for this subgroup of patients for up to 5 years (Eisler et al., 1997).

The Maudsley approach to family therapy for adolescent AN proceeds through three clearly defined phases.

Phase I. Regulating the Patient's Food Intake: Sessions 1–12

The overall technique and main strategy is to engage the family in a sympathetic, grave, portentous, but warm manner about the seriousness of their daughter's condition. The aim is to raise parental anxiety and concern about the eating disorder so that they can take appropriate action to return the adolescent's weight to normal. At the same time the therapist will make every effort to reduce parental guilt about having caused the eating disorder. In addition, it is important to engage the patient sympathetically for what the parents will be putting her through in the refeeding process (LeGrange, 1999).

SETTING UP TREATMENT

The therapist's initial task—before the first session can commence—is to set up the family meeting. By setting up the initial family meeting, the therapist begins the process of defining and enhancing parental authority with regard to the management of the crisis. This is time-limited treatment, and success depends to a large extent on the therapist's ability to make a powerful connection with the family. Given the formidable task at hand, the initial telephone contacts are crucial for the successful outcome of this process. It is therefore essential that it is the therapist who schedules the first face-to-face meeting by contacting the family him- or herself once a referral has been received. From the onset of treatment, which commences with the initial telephone contacts, the therapist adopts a grave, concerned tone in order to convey the seriousness of the illness to the family. It may be useful for the therapist, even at this early point, to acknowledge that the parents are demoralized and therefore skeptical of their capacity to be supportive. Encouraging the parents to make sure that the entire family is present for family therapy is a first step they can take to change these feelings.

By calling to schedule the initial family meeting, the therapist attempts to achieve two goals—first, to establish that there is a crisis in the family (i.e., the eating disorder) and begin the process of defining and enhancing parental authority around management of the crisis, and, second, to define the context of treatment, that is, a treatment team (e.g., psychologist/psychiatrist, dietician) and medical monitoring (clinic nurse/pediatrician). Consequently, the therapist begins by putting forward a convincing request that all those living in the same household should attend. Despite alternative suggestions by family members, the therapist should insist that a whole-family consultation is the only way to address the grave family dilemma. Therefore, this meeting will include the parents and all their children. Even adult children who may be in full-time employment but are living at home are required to attend. In addition, any extended family member such as a grandparent, uncle, or aunt who may be living in the same household should be included in this meeting. If the grandparents are not living with the patient and her family, but the patient spends a significant amount of time with them (e.g., the patient spends several hours per day with her grandparents after school and before her parents return from work), then the therapist may want to include these relatives in treatment as well.

THE PRELIMINARY EVALUATION

Before beginning treatment it is necessary to evaluate the client's complaints. The assessment should cover four areas: the nature of the eating disorder, associated comorbid psychopathology, current family functioning, and the family's response to the adolescent with AN. In addition, the adolescent should be medically evaluated to investigate and, if necessary, treat common medical conditions associated with AN (Lock et al., 2001).

In an evaluation interview with an adolescent with AN, it is important to convey support and warmth, while avoiding undo familiarity. Interviews can begin in a general way, with an open-ended question about the patient's family, schoolwork, interests, and activities. Gradually, the interview should be focused more on eating behaviors and problems. The therapist should explore initial triggers for the eating problem, which may include such events as comments on weight (either on being overweight or a compliment on looking thinner), onset of menses, dating, family conflicts, increased pressures to achieve at school, or increased competition with peers. In addition, the therapist should carefully inquire into the manner of weight loss. These include caloric, fat, and protein restriction as well as amount of food eaten. The therapist should then inquire about other methods of weight loss including exercise, laxative use, purging, and diuretic use. The therapist should ask about binge eating and carefully distinguish between the occurrence of a "true binge" (eating significantly more that the average person in finite period) and a "subjective" binge. A subjective binge to a person with AN might consist of two crackers and a half a cup of juice. It is also important that the therapist inquire about loss of menses. Because AN often is complicated by depression and anxiety disorders, the interviewer should screen for these disorders as well.

In the interview with parents it is advisable for both parents to be present, especially when both are involved in the care the child. Not only does this begin to reinforce the parental alliance, it also provides important information that otherwise might be unavailable. At times, one parent may be more involved with the patient and may see things differently from the more distant parent. On the other hand, if one of the parents has been overly distant, this interview can serve as a way to reinforce greater involvement with the problem at hand. Important areas of inquiry would be to ask the parents how they see the development of AN as occurring: When did they first recognize there was a problem? What efforts have they made to help? Are they concerned with other problems such as depression, anxiety, or other changes in behavior? It is important to ask about their thoughts and feelings regarding their child's eating patterns. Often, the therapist finds that the parents portray a much more disturbed pattern of eating than the patient herself describes. The parents should also provide a general picture of their child's emotional and physical development. This can be important insofar as temperamental variables, family problems, and family concerns regarding weight and shape may contribute to their child's difficulties.

THE FIRST FACE-TO-FACE MEETING

The main goals of the therapist's first face-to-face meeting with the family are to establish the seriousness of the adolescent's illness and to begin the process of engaging the family in treatment. To do so, the therapist has five aims: (1) Engage the patient and family through a sincere, warm, and foreboding tone; (2) take a history of the illness and use this information to demonstrate the seriousness of the illness; (3) orchestrate an "intense scene" regarding the patient's illness (i.e., that circumstances are serious, appropriate action ought to be taken immediately, and that the best chance of success is to have the parents take charge); (4) separate or externalize the illness from the patient, sympathize with the patient in a way that acknowledges the possibility of an "underlying problem," and support the adolescent's autonomy in areas outside the refeeding arena; and (5) summarize the central therapeutic goal. The reasons for summarizing the therapeutic goal are to leave the family with a sense of responsibility to take on the task of refeeding their daughter, to alert them not to engage in discussions about diet foods, and to emphasize that they should nourish the client given her profound state of malnutrition.

THE REMAINDER OF PHASE I

For the remainder of Phase I, treatment is almost entirely focused on the eating disorder, and may include a family meal. The family meal provides the therapist with an opportunity for direct observation of family interaction patterns around eating. With younger patients, the therapist makes careful and persistent requests for united parental action directed toward eating. In addition, the therapist directs the discussion in such a way as to create a strong parental alliance around their efforts at reinforcing healthy eating in their child on the one hand, and to align the patient with the sibling subsystem on the other. This phase is characterized by attempts to absolve the parents of responsibility for causing the illness, and by complimenting them on the positive aspects of their parenting of their children.

Thus, Phase I of treatment attempts to reestablish appropriate parental roles in the family system, particularly as it is related to the patient's eating behaviors. Therapy at this point is focused exclusively on the eating disorder and its symptoms. Families are encouraged to work out for themselves the best way to refeed their anorexic child. Attempts are made to maintain the parents' focus on the eating disorder, to maintain continued support for the parents in their efforts to refeed their daughter, and to mobilize the siblings to support their sister through this process.

Phase II. Negotiations for a New Pattern of Relationships: Sessions 13–17

The beginning of Phase II of treatment is signaled when the patient accepts parental demands to increase food intake and begins to experience steady weight gain. The therapist advises the parents to accept that the main task now is a continued return of their child to physical health. A goal at this point is to maintain a regular schedule of meals with a minimum of tension. Family therapy sessions focus on the effects of other family problems on the parents' task of supporting steady weight gain in the patient. The task for the therapist becomes one of assisting the parents and the adolescent to bring about a careful and mutually agreed-upon transfer of responsibility in this domain back to the adolescent. Once eating ceases to be the focus of discussions, the family is able to begin talking about adolescent issues that came to the fore during the time of weight restoration. In addition, other issues and concerns that the family has can now be brought forward for review. This, however, occurs only in relation to the effect these issues have on the parents in their task of assuring regular eating in the absence of anorexic symptoms.

Phase III. Adolescent Issues and Termination: Sessions 18–20

Phase III is initiated when the patient maintains a stable weight, regular menses have resumed, and any binge–purge symptoms have abated. The central theme here is the establishment of a healthy adolescent or young adult relationship with the parents in which the illness does not constitute the basis of interaction. This entails working toward increased personal autonomy for the adolescent, more appropriate family boundaries, and the need for the parents to reorganize their life together after their children's prospective departure.

All sessions are 60 minutes in duration, except for the family meal, where the clinician should usually allow 90 minutes. Phase I of treatment typically lasts between 3 and 5 months, with sessions scheduled at weekly intervals. The spacing of sessions should be based on the patient's clinical progress. During Phase II, the therapist may schedule sessions every 2nd–3rd week, whereas monthly sessions are scheduled toward the conclusion of treatment during Phase III.

CASE EXAMPLE

Presenting Concerns

Sally was a 13-year-old seventh grader who was admitted to our psychiatric inpatient eating disorders unit. She had been previously treated through emergency room visits for malnutrition and dehydration and had been tube fed in the past. Upon admission she was very cachetic and emaciated in appearance, and appeared to have difficulty concentrating and making decisions. Sally was ruminating about food, and had a strong desire to be thin. She demonstrated motor hyperactivity and restlessness, which continued throughout treatment. She obsessed about what she was going to eat, what she had just eaten, and whether she was going to vomit, use laxatives, or exercise to get rid of the food. Sally also expressed difficulty accepting that her behaviors were disrupting her life.

Sally lived with her parents and three siblings. A straight-A student, Sally was extremely active in sports, particularly basketball, and was considered an outstanding athlete. She was originally diagnosed with AN in October 1999, with a reported onset related to the onset of her menstrual cycle. At this time she began making comments about not wanting to grow up. She also was afraid of having adult responsibilities. Following the onset of her menses she drastically reduced her eating and drinking and began to lose significant amounts of weight. She was in constant motion, posturing, and at times and she would not sit unless directed to do so. She wore braces and would use her tongue to pack her braces with food so that she could later brush the food away during her dental hygiene time. Her behavior during meals included shredding her food, wiping food on her napkin or placemat, spitting food particles on hands or clothes, and holding her food in her mouth for long periods of time. She would drop food on the floor, on her clothing, around her tray and plate, and on her chair. Initially she had to be directed to eat, chew, swallow, and not pick at her food. She made negative comments about the food, such as "this food is nasty," and exhibited negative self-talk, such as " I cannot do this." Sally needed to be observed continuously in order to prevent her from overexercising and carrying out other eating disorder behaviors. She reported having constant urges to exercise, and in general she was experiencing racing thoughts.

Initial Assessment

Our multidisciplinary treatment team evaluated Sally. The team included psychiatrists, psychologists, psychiatric nurses, social workers, educators, and occupational and activities therapists. She was given a thorough physical, a psychiatric examination, and a battery of psychological tests. This was to assess cognitive and motivational factors that might be contributing to her eating disorder, as well as her level of intellectual functioning and personality characteristics. Nursing and social services assessed family functioning and her ability to relate to others on the inpatient unit. Occupational and activities therapy assessed her understanding of exercise and leisure activities and coping skills and food related activities.

Upon admission Sally was 5'3" tall and weighted 69.7 pounds—this was 59% of her ideal body weight. She was started on a weight restoration program and was discharged within a target weight range of 115–119 pounds. Psychological testing revealed an adolescent who was in the high average range of intellectual functioning, with no cognitive impairment. She was experiencing moderate, self-reported symptoms of depression. Sally's testing was consistent with individuals who have many somatic concerns, who overreact to stressful situations, and who are seen as self-centered, egocentric, and immature. She demonstrated strong needs for attention and was psychologically naïve, with little insight into her illness. Additionally, her testing demonstrated that she had feelings of dissatisfaction, hopelessness, low self-confidence, and a sense of inadequacy. The results of tests specifically related to her eating disorder (Eating Attitudes Test and Eating Disorders Inventory–2) were consistent with individuals who have been diagnosed with an eating disorder. This suggested an intense concern about being fat, eating, and being out of control. She also had a strong desire to be perfect and believed that her personal achievements needed to be superior. She was concerned that others would be critical of her if she did not accomplish every task and that only the highest standards of personal performance were acceptable. She did not adequately understand her own internal awareness of her body and misperceived physical sensations, and also was confused and apprehensive in responding to emotional states. There was an indication of a desire to retreat to the security of childhood to avoid the psychological and biological experiences related to being an adult. Sally had a strong tendency to seek virtue through pursuit of spiritual ideals like self-discipline and control of bodily urges. She was also impulsive in her behaviors and engaged in behaviors via her eating disorder that were destructive to herself and to her relationship with others, particularly her family and friends.

Diagnosis and Formulation

Diagnostically, Sally met the criteria for anorexia nervosa of the *Diagnostic and Statistical Manual of Mental Disorders*, fourth edition (DSM-IV; American Psychiatric Association, 1994). These problems were superimposed on family issues, extremely high personal expectations, a perfectionist personality style, and a struggle with fear of maturation. Family issues relevant to Sally's recovery included a need to strengthen the marital relationship, problems with an intense focus on dieting, health problems with obesity, and lack of quality family time. The family had difficulty with the expressions of emotional content, and both Sally and her parents had difficulty allowing one another to express their feelings without the other taking responsibility for those feelings, particularly if the feeling was negative.

Sally acknowledged that she would put tremendous pressure on herself to meet exceedingly high expectations. Consequently, she felt bad about herself when she could not live up to those expectations. This shift in mood and negative self-evaluation led to greater control over food. She frequently described herself as "never good enough," although she excelled athletically and academically. She realized that she used sports to cope with stress. When she became too weak to participate in sports, she instead focused on weight, shape, size, and food.

Sally also pursued self-improvement activities to be perceived as a "better person" rather than as a way of building her own self-confidence. Perfectionism was equated with confidence, and she would accept nothing less. She was clear regarding her academic role but very uncertain how she fit into her social and family roles. Sally was extremely guarded with others and seemed to perceive emotional distance as necessary for safety. She described her family members as quite detached and emotionally distant from one another, and Sally did not feel supported or as though she even fit in with her family.

Given the information about Sally, the treatment team began to conceptualize her problems as follows:

Behavioral coping strategies

Restriction of diet
Increased amounts of exercise
Intense focus on academic perfection

Cognitive distortions

Dichotomous thinking
Catastrophizing
Mind reading

Automatic thoughts

"I'll never be good enough for my parents, I am a failure."
"I must be a better person."
"I'm obese."

Assumptions

"If I don't control my weight, then I'm a failure."
"If I express my emotions, then others will be angry with me."
"If I don't get good grades, then I won't be loved."
"If I put myself first, then I'm a selfish person."

Schemas

"Showing emotions will mean negative outcomes."
"I can show only positive emotions."
"Criticism from others means I'm no good."

All of Sally's concerns were exacerbated by her weight loss. She used her diet and restricted emotions as a way to control her future, her world, and herself. When her weight was low she felt in control and saw herself as achieving her high expectations. Attempts to assist her in gaining and maintaining an adequate weight were seen as threats to her personal world and future. She felt that others were attempting to remove the one thing that she felt confident about, being able to be thinner than others around her (Figure 10.1).

Course of Treatment

Weight restoration was accomplished by starting Sally on 1,200 calories per day for 4 days and then increasing by 500 calories approximately every 4 days until 3,500 calories were taken each day. Following the patient's attaining target range, a maintenance level of calories was determined. The patient was medically stable upon admission, although she appeared emaciated and was moderately dehydrated. Her electrolytes were checked and monitored to ensure there were no abnormalities.

Situation	Emotions	Automatic thoughts	Rational response
Reducing her exercise	Sad, anxious	I'm a bad person if I don't stay in shape.	Being in shape is not who I am.
Eating a snack	Anxious	If I gain weight, I'll be out of control.	My weight is not who I am.

FIGURE 10.1. Sally's Record of Dysfunctional Thoughts.

Initially the patient was tearful and noncompliant, and took 2–3 hours to finish a meal. Within a reasonable amount of time, the patient was able to eat within protocol guidelines and to do so without dissolving into tears. As her malnutrition began to resolve, she was able to actively participate in the cognitive work and began to make progress in understanding her illness and behaviors. She continued to maintain a high motor activity level throughout her treatment.

Sally's inpatient treatment was on a unit designed to use cognitive therapy as the primary psychotherapeutic intervention. The unit has many principles of a cognitive therapy inpatient setting (Bowers, 1993; Wright, Thase, Beck, & Ludgate, 1993). The unit nursing staff is familiar with the therapeutic interventions of cognitive therapy using group and individual therapy. Other members of the treatment team (psychiatrists, family therapist, occupational therapist, recreational therapist) also use primarily a cognitive model when working with these patients.

The main psychotherapeutic interventions on the unit are a psychoeductional group, group cognitive therapy, and family therapy. Each is designed to blend with the other three psychotherapies. The psychoeducational group explores various aspects of cognitive therapy (i.e., cognitive distortions, automatic thoughts) in a didactic fashion. Group cognitive therapy combines Beck's theory and interventions in a process-oriented framework (Bowers, 2001; Bowers & Andersen, 1994). Family therapy maintains a cognitive framework designed to work with family communications and schemas (Dattilio, 1994; Teichman, 1992). Patients are involved in some form of cognitive therapy for at least 3 hours per day.

Sally developed good knowledge of the therapeutic skills required to work on changing her thoughts, feelings, and behaviors. However, she was not able to apply these concepts to her life. Sally's inability to practice the skills she had learned was directly related to her reluctance to try anything new. This reluctance was fueled by her fear of being imperfect, which would bring on feelings of worthlessness. The difficulty in using her skills was also related to her automatic thoughts, basic assumptions, and schemas regarding herself and her role within her family. Creating or enhancing knowledge of how to change is one potential reason CBT can be effective in the treatment of AN. Additionally, cognitive therapy provides a structure for change in those individuals who do not have as good grasp on what it takes to apply these therapeutic skills to their lives. Sally expressed concern and fear over the amount of work she would need to do to recover from her eating disorder.

Sally began most of her days in a psychoeducational cognitive therapy group. It was in this group that the cognitive and behavior skills that would accompany group were described and discussed. This group specifically works on identification of automatic thoughts, cognitive distortions, basic assumptions, and schemas. It details various ways to monitor and identify these concepts as well as providing a forum for each group member to learn and assist others in how to change their thoughts, feelings, and behaviors.

Sally had difficulty in becoming adept at cognitive skills. She often needed assistance by others in the group on the use of various interventions. However, the assistance that was offered was actually a way to have her emotions come to the surface. It became apparent that Sally put others in the group first. Putting others first created a great deal of emotional distance, so she would not violate her basic assumptions.

Group sessions suggested ways for Sally to monitor her thoughts, feelings, and behaviors in situations that created mood shifts. This was particularly helpful to decrease her perfectionist stance. She was helped to increase her awareness of her own shortcomings by identifying reccurring patterns in thoughts regarding her performance and the standards that she set for herself. By challenging her thoughts she was able to express herself more emotionally and develop close relationships with other patients on the unit. She also decreased her strong need to be thin as a way to control her world.

The cognitive therapy group became a place for Sally to use her new skills in order to explore changing some of her current developmental patterns and modifying the underlying schemas that maintained her disorder. By interacting with other group members who encouraged her expression of feelings, Sally was able to challenge the idea that a close relationship meant giving up on her own person. She began to understand her fear of becoming emotionally close and to challenge her thoughts that an intimate relationship was always painful. Additionally, Sally was able to acknowledge that expressing her emotions did not always lead to negative outcomes. She also experienced how being angry, sad, or frightened was a way to open and strengthen close bonds with others. The group gave Sally a forum to be an adolescent without the responsibility of taking care of others. She could be herself and display both strong and weak aspects of her character.

Throughout her hospitalization, Sally was constantly involved with cognitive therapy so that this information was repeated in a variety of settings. Cognitive principles were included in family therapy, and group therapy as well was translated into hands-on experience in occupational therapy, recreational therapy, and her daily interactions with other patients and staff on the unit. The milieu strengthened Sally and helped her generalize her learning, thereby improving her chances of using it with her parents and friends outside of the hospital setting.

Sally's initial outcome was extremely positive, and she was able to demonstrate many changes in her behaviors during her first hospitalization. At discharge she felt that she had learned how to use the skills for change and equally important how to communicate them to others. She was able to identify how her own thoughts and perceptions contributed to her eating disorder and interfered in her life. She made significant changes in how she interacted with food and her world. However, it would take four more in-patient stays and a referral to another program, in which the family could learn how to provide the structure that she needed in her home, before she was able to attempt to live at home successfully.

Follow-Up and Relapse Prevention

This case is typical of the adolescent population that presents for treatment of eating disorders. The care of the adolescent is complicated in that it involves many developmental issues that are not present in the adult population. As with this patient, it is essential that the parental team be involved in the treatment, because they will have to be able to provide care and supervision of the adolescent when she returns home. It is imperative that the patient's cognitive processing be explored and the issues identified that will need to be reframed if the patient is to successfully recover. The intensity of this patient's disease points out the necessity of the team's being able to remain objective despite the difficulty presented by managing the behaviors with the patient. It is also important to remember the parameters of normal adolescence so that treatment allows for the normal behaviors one expects at that age. It is a time of striving for independence and a time for adolescents to explore their own power. Peer relationships are important and must be acknowledged and maintained, for this is the world that we want the adolescent to return to and engage fully in.

In this case, the patient and her family will continue to have extensive treatment work to do. The family was ill-prepared to cope with their daughter's illness, and even though the family was willing to work with the treatment team—as was their daughter—the work was arduous and overwhelming for all of them. This situation requires skill and commitment on the part of the treatment team, as the family and patient rely on the team to help them keep recovery in perspective. So many of the adolescents and their families come to treatment expecting a "quick cure," and it is difficult for them to accept the reality of the recovery process. This particular case required that the patient be placed out of the home for part of the treatment, not because the family was inappropriate, but because they were unable to cope with the amount of time and effort it takes to supervise an adolescent with this level of illness. It became apparent in time that the family was going to have to be trained to provide supervision in the home, as no amount of verbal direction was going to prepare them for the actual techniques needed in the home to keep this patient well. Consequently, the patient and her family were referred to the eating disorders outpatient program at the University of Chicago to gain further family therapy.

We have seen many cases similar to the one described here, and eventually, with consistent treatment, the patients are able to recover and return to healthy, productive lives. The treatment team has to keep this end point in perspective and continually offer this hope to the patient and family. Adolescence is a time of struggle, and the occurrence of an eating disorder at this time makes it even more difficult for the patient and family.

Every patient that is discharged from our continuum of care must have follow-up treatment established prior to leaving our program. It is essential for recovery to continue the work that has been started. It is imperative for the patients and their families to understand that the experience they have just participated in is only the beginning of treatment, not the end point. Adolescents need their parents to be strong enough to assist them in continuing their recovery process. Parents need to be supported by the treatment team in their efforts to keep their children in treatment even though the adolescent—through the very nature of adolescence—may struggle against this directive. It is also important for the parents to know that the therapy sessions are for the adolescent and not for the parent, as many parents in the struggle will feel a need to invade the therapy process in order to get their own needs met. It is important for these parents to establish individual or couple therapy. Adolescents are a challenging population to work with, but they offer a rewarding experience as well. Aftercare is extremely important to the continued success of the patient in the battle against AN. Support and structure are needed within the therapeutic relationship to be able to maintain progress. Also, it is important that continued work be done to assist the patient to recognize the cognitive distortions, basic assumptions, and schemas that have contributed to the eating disorder.

CONCLUSIONS

The principles and interventions of cognitive therapy can be applied effectively in treating eating disorders among adolescents. The structure of cognitive therapy allows for individualized care and developing strategies that fit the patient's needs. Although developed to address cognitive, behavioral, social, and developmental factors associated with eating disorders, these approaches are entirely consistent with the assumptions and principles of "standard" forms of CBT (Beck et al., 1979; J. Beck, 1995). These approaches endeavor to alter maladaptive schemas, to encourage healthy eating patterns, to improve family interactions, and to support normative development among youth.

Treating adolescents with eating disorders can be challenging. The level of cognitive understanding and social maturity of the patient can hinder progress. It is important to be cognizant of the patient's level of cognitive development, capacity for abstract reasoning, cognitive flexibility, and motivation when selecting an intervention. As we have seen, close cooperation with parents increases the likelihood of therapeutic improvement. It is critically important to have the parents accept and be actively involved in the treatment process. Cognitive family therapy can be very helpful in this regard, as can enlisting the parent to act as adjunct cognitive therapists with their child.

Future research must examine the effectiveness of CBT for treating adolescents with eating disorders, as well as how individual, group, and family therapy interventions can be integrated in treating these disorders. Our clinical experience suggests that adolescents and their families often respond positively to cognitive-behavioral concepts and are able to use techniques based on these models in overcoming eating disorders. Although small in number, the results of outcome studies are promising. Individual, group, and family approaches to cognitive therapy, then, are promising approaches for understanding and treating eating disorders among youth.

REFERENCES

Agras, W. S., Schneider, J. A., Arnow, B., Raeburn, S. D., & Telch, C. F. (1989). Cognitive-behavioral treatment with and without exposure plus response prevention in the treatment of bulimia nervosa: A reply to Leitenberg and Rosen. *Journal of Consulting and Clinical Psychology, 57*, 778–779.

Agras, W. S., Walsh, J., Fairburn, G. G., Wilson, G. T., & Kraemer, H. C. (2000). A multicenter comparison of cognitive-behavioral therapy and interpersonal psychotherapy for bulimia nervosa. *Archives of General Psychiatry, 57*(5), 459–466.

American Psychiatric Association. (1994). *Diagnostic and statistical manual of mental disorders* (4th ed.). Washington, DC: Author.

American Psychiatric Association. (2000). Practice guidelines for the treatment of patients with eating disorders (revision). *American Journal of Psychiatry, 157*(1, Suppl.), 1–39.

Andersen, A. E., Bowers, W. A., & Evans, K. K. (1997). Inpatient treatment of anorexia nervosa. In D. M Garner & P. E. Garfinkel (Eds.), *Handbook of treatment for eating disorders* (2nd ed., pp. 327–353). New York: Guilford Press.

Beck, A. T., Rush, A. G., Shaw, B. F., & Emery, G. (1979). *Cognitive therapy of depression*. New York: Guilford Press.

Beck, J. (1995). *Cognitive therapy: Basics and beyond*. New York: Guilford Press.

Bowers, W. A. (1993). Cognitive therapy for eating disorders. In J. H. Wright, M. E. Thase, A. T. Beck, & J. W. Ludgate (Eds.), *Cognitive therapy with inpatients: Developing a cognitive milieu* (pp. 337–356). New York: Guilford Press.

Bowers, W. A. (2000). Eating disorders. In J. White & A. Freeman (Eds.), *Cognitive-behavioral group therapy for specific problems and populations* (pp. 127–148). Washington, DC: American Psychological Association.

Bowers, W. A. (2001). Eating disorders. In J. R. White & A S. Freeman (Eds.), *Cognitive-behavioral group therapy for specific problems and population* (pp. 127–148). Washington, DC: American Psychological Association.

Bowers, W. A., & Andersen, A. F. (1994). Inpatient treatment of anorexia nervosa: Review and recommendations. *Harvard Review of Psychiatry, 4*, 193–203.

Bowers, W. A., Evans, K. K., & Andersen, A. E. (1997). Inpatient treatment of eating disorders: A cognitive milieu. *Cognitive and Behavioral Practice 4*, 291–323.

Braswell, L., & Kendall, P. (1988). Cognitive-behavioral methods with children. In K. Dobson (Ed.), *Handbook of cognitive-behavioral therapies* (pp. 167–213). New York: Guilford Press.

Cooper, P. J., & Fairburn, C. G. (1984). Cognitive behavior therapy for anorexia nervosa: Some preliminary findings. *Journal of Psychosomatic Research, 28*, 493–499.

Crisp, A. H., Norton, K., Gowers, S., Halek, C., Bowyer, C., Yeldhan, D., Levett, G., & Bhat, A. (1991). A controlled study of the effect of therapies aimed at adolescents and family psychopathology in anorexia nervosa. *British Journal of Psychiatry, 159*, 325–333.

Dare, C. (1983). Family therapy for families containing an anorectic youngster. In *Understanding anorexia nervosa and bulimia: Report of the fourth Ross Conference on Medical Research*. Columbus, OH: Ross Laboratories.

Dare, C., & Eisler, I. (1997). Family therapy for anorexia nervosa. In D. M. Garner & P. E. Garfinkel (Eds.), *Handbook for treatment of eating disorders* (2nd ed., pp. 307–324). New York: Guilford Press.

Dare, C., Eisler, I., Russell, M. R., & Szmukler, G. I. (1990). The clinical and theoretical impact of a controlled trial of family therapy in anorexia nervosa. *Journal of Marital and Family Therapy, 16*, 39–57.

Dattilio, F. M. (1994). Families in crises. In F. M. Dattilio & A. Freeman (Eds.), *Cognitive-behavioral strategies in crises intervention* (pp. 278–301). New York: Guilford Press.

Eisler, I., Dare, C., Hodes, M., Russell, G., Dodge, G., & LeGrange, D. (1997). A five-year follow-up of a controlled trial of family therapy in severe eating disorders. *Archives of General Psychiatry, 54*, 1025–1030.

Eisler, I., Dare, C., Russell, G. F. M., Hodes, M., Dodge, E., & LeGrange, D. (2000). Family therapy for adolescent anorexia nervosa: The results of a controlled comparison of two family interventions. *Journal of Child Psychology and Psychiatry, 41*(6), 727–736.

Eisler, I., Dare, C., Russell, G. F. M., Szmukler, G. I., LeGrange, D., & Dodge, E. (1997). Family and individual therapy in anorexia nervosa. A 5-year follow-up. *Archives of General Psychiatry, 54*, 1025–1030.

Elkind, D. (1966). Egocentrism in adolescence. *Child Development, 38*, 1025–1034.

Fairburn, C. G., & Cooper, P. J. (1989). Eating disorders. In K. Hawton, P. M. Salkovskis, J. Kirk, & D. M. Clark (Eds.), *Cognitive behavioral therapy for psychiatric disorders* (pp. 160–192). New York: Oxford University Press.

Fairburn, C. G., Norman, P. A., Welch, S. L., O'Conner, M. E., Doll, H. A., & Peveler, R. C. (1995). A prospective study of outcome in bulimia nervosa and the long-term effects of three psychological treatments. *Archives of General Psychiatry, 52*, 304–312.

Finch, A., Nelson, W., & Ott, E. (Eds.). (1993). *Cognitive-behavioral procedures with children and adolescents: A practical guide*. Boston: Allyn & Bacon.

Freeman, A. (1993). A psychosocial approach to conceptualizing schematic development for cognitive therapy. In K. T. Kuehlwein & H. Rosen (Eds.), *Cognitive therapies in action* (pp. 54–87). New York: Jossey-Bass.

Freeman, A., & Reinecke, M. (1995). Cognitive therapy. In A. Gurman & S. Messer

(Eds.), *Essential psychotherapies: Theory and practice* (pp. 182–225). New York: Guilford Press.

Garfinkel, P. E., & Garner, D. M. (1982). *Anorexia nervosa: A multidimensional perspective*. New York: Brunner/Mazel.

Garner, D. M. (1985). Individual psychotherapy for anorexia nervosa. *Journal of Psychiatry Research, 19,* 423–433.

Garner, D. M. (1997). Psychoeducational principles in treatment. In D. M. Garner & P. E. Garfinkel (Eds.), *Handbook of treatment of eating disorders* (2nd ed., pp. 145–177). New York: Guilford Press.

Garner, D. M., & Bemis, K. M. (1982). A cognitive behavioral approach to anorexia nervosa. *Cognitive Therapy and Research, 6,* 1–27.

Garner, D. M., & Bemis, K. M. (1985). Cognitive therapy for anorexia nervosa. In D. M. Garner & P. E. Garfinkel (Eds.), *Handbook of psychotherapy for anorexia nervosa and bulimia* (pp. 107–146). New York: Guilford Press.

Garner, D. M., & Garfinkel, P. E. (Eds.). (1997). *Handbook of treatment for eating disorders* (2nd ed.). New York: Guilford Press.

Garner, D. M., Rockert, W., Olmsted, M. P., Johnson, C. J., & Coscina, D. V. (1985). Psychoeducational principles in the treatment of bulimia and anorexia nervosa. In D. M. Garner & P. E. Garfinkel (Eds.), *Handbook of psychotherapy for anorexia nervosa and bulimia* (pp. 513–572). New York: Guilford Press.

Garner, D. M., Vitousek, K. M., & Pike, K. M. (1997). Cognitive-behavioral therapy for anorexia nervosa. In D. M. Garner & P. E. Garfinkel (Eds.), *Handbook of treatment for eating disorders* (2nd ed., pp. 94–144). New York: Guilford Press.

Greenberger, D., & Padesky, C. A. (1995). *Mind over mood: A cognitive therapy treatment manual for clients*. New York: Guilford Press.

Grice, D. E., Halmi, K. A., Fichter, M. M., Strober, M., Woodside, D. B., Treasure, J. T., Kaplan, A. S., Magistretti, P. J., Goldman, D., Bulik, C. M., Kaye, W. H., & Berrettini, W. H. (2002). Evidence for susceptibility gene for anorexia nervosa on chromosome 1. *American Journal of Human Genetics, 70,* 787–792.

Hall, A. (1985). Group psychotherapy for anorexia nervosa. In D. M. Garner & P. E. Garfinkel (Eds.), *Handbook of psychotherapy for anorexia nervosa and bulimia* (pp. 213–239). New York: Guilford Press.

Hall, A. (1987). The place of family therapy in the treatment of anorexia nervosa. *Australian and New Zealand Journal of Psychiatry, 21,* 568–574.

Kendall, P., & Braswell, L. (1985). *Cognitive-behavioral therapy for impulsive children*. New York: Guilford Press.

Kendall, P., & MacDonald, J. (1993). Cognition in the psychopathology of youth and implications for treatment. In K. Dobson & P. Kendall (Eds.), *Psychopathology and cognition*. San Diego: Academic Press.

Klump, K. L., McGue, M., & Iacono, W. G. (2000). Age differences in genetic and environmental influences on eating attitudes and behavior in preadolescent and adolescent female twins. *Journal of Abnormal Psychology, 109*(2), 239–251.

Laessle, R. G., Beumont, P. J. V., Butow, P., Lennerts, W., O'Connor, M., Pirke, K. M., Touyz, S. W., & Waadi, S. (1991). A comparison of nutritional management and stress management in the treatment of bulimia nervosa. *British Journal of Psychiatry, 159,* 250–261.

Lee, N. F., & Rush, A. J. (1986). Cognitive-behavioral group therapy for bulimia. *International Journal of Eating Disorders, 2,* 599–615.

LeGrange, D. (1999). Family therapy for adolescent anorexia nervosa. *Journal of Clinical Psychology, 55*, 727–740.

LeGrange, D., Eisler, I., Dare, C., & Russell, G. F. M. (1992). Evaluation of family therapy in anorexia nervosa: A pilot study. *International Journal of Eating Disorders, 12*, 347–357.

Lock, J. D., LeGrange, D., Agras, W. S., & Dare, C. (2001). *Treatment manual for anorexia nervosa.* New York: Guilford Press.

March, J., & Mulle, K. (1998). *OCD in children and adolescents: A cognitive-behavioral treatment manual.* New York: Guilford Press.

Matson, J. (1989). *Treating depression in children and adolescents.* New York: Pergamon Press.

Meyers, A., & Craighead, W. (Eds.). (1984). *Cognitive-behavior therapy with children.* New York: Plenum Press.

Minuchin, S., Baker, B. L., Rosman, B. L., Liebman, R., Milman, L., & Todd, T. C. (1975). A conceptual model of psychosomatic illness in childhood. *Archives of General Psychiatry, 32*, 1031–1038.

Olmsted, M. P., Davis, R., Garner, D. M., Rockert, W., Irvine, M. J., & Eagle, M. (1991). Efficacy of a brief group psychoeducational intervention for bulimia nervosa. *Behavior Research and Therapy, 29*, 71–83.

Ordman, A. M., & Kirschenbaum, D. S. (1986). Bulimia: Assessment of eating, psychological adjustment, and familial characteristics. *International Journal of Eating Disorders, 2*, 865–878.

Pike, K. M. (2000, May). *How do we keep patients well? Issues of relapse prevention.* Paper presented at the 9th International Conference on Eating Disorders, New York.

Reinecke, M. A. (1992). Childhood depression. In A. Freeman & F. M. Dattilio (Eds.), *Comprehensive casebook of cognitive therapy* (pp. 147–158). New York: Plenum Press.

Robin, A. L., Siegel, P. T., & Moye, A. (1995). Family versus individual therapy for anorexia: impact on family conflict. *International Journal of Eating Disorders, 17*, 313–322.

Russell, G. F. M., Szmukler, G.I., Dare, C., & Eisler, I. (1987). An evaluation of family therapy in anorexia nervosa and bulimia nervosa. *Archives of General Psychiatry, 44*, 1047–1056.

Schrodt, G. R., & Wright, J. H. (1987). Inpatient treatment of adolescents. In A. Freeman & V. Greenwood (Eds.), *Cognitive therapy: Applications in psychiatric and medical settings* (pp. 69–82). New York: Human Sciences Press.

Shirk, S. (Ed.). (1988). *Cognitive development and child psychotherapy.* New York: Plenum Press.

Teichman, Y. (1992). Family therapy with acting out adolescents. In A. Freeman & F. M. Dattilio (Eds.), *Comprehensive casebook of cognitive therapy* (pp. 147–158). New York: Plenum Press.

Vitousek, K. (1991, November). *Current status of cognitive-behavioral treatment of anorexia nervosa.* Paper presented at the 25th annual convention of the Association for Advancement of Behavior Therapy, New York.

Vitousek, K., & Orimoto, L. (1993). Cognitive-behavioral models of anorexia nervose, bulimia nervosa, and obesity. In K. Dobson & P. Kendall (Eds.), *Psychopathology and cognition* (pp. 191–243). San Diego: Academic Press.

Wade, T. D., Bulik, C. M., Neale, M., & Kemdler, K. S. (2000). Anorexia nervosa and major depression: Shared genetic and environmental risk factors. *American Journal of Psychiatry, 157,* 469–471.

White, J. R., & Freeman, A. S. (2000). *Cognitive-behavioral group therapy for specific problems and populations.* Washington, DC: American Psychological Association.

Wilson, G. T., & Fairburn, C. G. (1993). Cognitive treatments for eating disorders. *Journal of Consulting and Clinical Psychology, 61,* 261–269.

Wilson, G.,T., & Fairburn, C. (2002). Treatments for eating disorders. In P. Nathan & J. Gorman (Eds.), *A guide to treatments that work* (2nd ed.). New York: Oxford University Press.

Wilson, G. T., Fairburn, C. G., & Agras, W. S. (1997). Cognitive behavioral therapy for bulimia nervosa. In D. M. Garner & P. E. Garfinkel (Eds.), *Handbook of treatment for eating disorders* (2nd ed., pp. 67–93). New York: Guilford Press.

Wilson, G. T., Rossiter, E. M., Kleifield, E. I., & Lindholm, L. (1986). Cognitive-behavioral treatment of bulimia nervosa: A controlled evaluation. *Behaviour Research and Therapy, 24,* 277–288.

Wright, J. H., Thase, M. E., Beck, A. T., & Ludgate, J. H. (1993). *Cognitive therapy with inpatients: Developing a cognitive milieu.* New York: Guilford Press.

Yalom, I. (1995). *The theory and practice of group psychotherapy* (4th ed.). New York: Basic Books.

Zarb, J. (1992). *Cognitive-behavioral assessment and therapy with adolescents.* New York: Brunner/Mazel.

SUGGESTED READINGS

Fairburn, C. G. (Ed.). (1995). *Overcoming binge eating.* New York: Guilford Press.

Garner, D. M., & Garfinkel, P. E. (Eds.). (1997). *Handbook of treatment for eating disorders* (2nd ed.). New York: Guilford Press.

Lock, J. D., LeGrange, D., Agras, W. S., & Dare, C. (2001). *Treatment manual for anorexia nervosa.* New York: Guilford Press.

11

Treatment of Academic Skills Problems

KATHY L. BRADLEY-KLUG
EDWARD S. SHAPIRO

Traditionally, student achievement has been viewed as a product of a student's ability and the quality of teaching, schools, and home environment. Within the last two decades, however, researchers and educators have begun viewing a student's self-regulated learning strategies as essential to his or her academic success. Self-regulated learning strategies refer to a student's ability to control his or her behavior, allowing the student to employ specific strategies and evaluate his or her performance on specific learning tasks (Miranda, Villaescusa, & Vidal-Abarca, 1997).

According to self-regulation theorists, possessing the strategies to self-regulate ultimately affects a student's academic achievement. Even high-ability students often do not achieve optimally because of their failure to control their own cognitive, affective, and motor activities (Zimmerman, 1986). These regulation strategies are based on a proactive perspective, with the goal of reducing the number of students who may fail. In other words, the focus shifts to teaching students *how* to learn rather than *what* to learn.

Self-regulation theorists view students as active participants in their learning, possessing the ability to plan, organize, self-instruct, self-monitor, and self-evaluate their academic behavior. Once viewed as a fixed characteristic, self-regulation has come to be seen as a set of context-specific processes that are selectively used to control one's behavior (Zimmerman, 1986). The self-regulatory process chosen by a student depends on several variables, including motivation, training, and time. Some of the most researched methods of self-regulation include goal setting, self-instruction, and self-monitoring (De La Paz, 1999).

Cognitive-behavioral therapy can be effective in improving the self-regulatory behavior of students. Through these procedures students are taught various methods to aid them as they encounter new curricula and learning environments. There are two types of cognitive-behavioral therapy procedures applied to academic skills problems: one that emphasizes antecedent control and one that emphasizes control of consequences.

In antecedent control, the point of the intervention occurs prior to the occurrence of the academic behavior. Here, an emphasis is placed on the cognitive events that precede the behavioral difficulty. Self-instructional training (Meichenbaum & Goodman, 1971; Miller & Brewster, 1992) and strategy training (Graham & Harris, 1999) are examples of cognitive-behavioral therapy techniques for academic skills problems that focus on antecedent control.

In control of consequences, interventions are made after the behavior has occurred. Emphasis is on the analysis and response to the academic skill problem. Use of self-monitoring and self-management interventions (Shapiro & Cole, 1994) represent examples of cognitive-behavioral therapy procedures that are based on control of consequences.

The purpose of this chapter is to provide an overview of several methods of self-regulation, including self-instruction, self-monitoring, and self-management. An example of a specific strategy training model for academic skills is then presented. Finally, two case studies are presented to illustrate the application of these concepts to children in a general education classroom.

OVERVIEW OF COGNITIVE-BEHAVIORAL THERAPY FOR ACADEMIC PROBLEMS

Self-Instruction

Lev Vygotsky, a developmental psychologist, investigated the interaction between thought and behavior. Specifically, he studied the role of private speech as a mechanism for bringing behavior under control of an individual. He proposed that this inner, private speech develops progressively in children, beginning with their behavior being under the control of the external environment. The next stage in the development involves talking out loud and bringing behavior under verbal control. In the final stage children verbally regulate their behavior through internal or silent speech (Vygotsky, 1962).

Influenced by such investigations on the controlling effects of speech and thought on behavior, Meichenbaum and Goodman (1971) conducted an early study of self-instruction to enhance student performance during independent learning tasks. Their intent was simple—to teach impulsive children to think before they act. Through training in this strategy, children were taught to self-verbalize statements both overtly and covertly in situations including error–correction, guidance, problem solving, and reinforcement (Wood, Rosenberg, & Carran, 1993). The basic tenet behind the self-instructional model is to teach students to become more cognizant of the demands of a specific task, which will then lead to an understanding and ability to monitor their use of strategies. The end goal is to enable the students to be in control of their learning (Graham & Wong, 1993). Although many of the early studies in self-instructional training focused on non-academic tasks, a review by Miller and Brewster (1992) reported positive applications of self-instructional training to reading and mathematics skills.

Training in self-instruction consists of several steps and can vary from being very task specific to focusing on more general problem-solving strategies. Initially, the strategy is described and modeled by the trainer. Then the student practices the strategy both overtly and covertly using verbal self-instructions. In the last stage of the training the child receives feedback from the trainer and is required to self-evaluate. Tied to the correct performance of the strategy may be external contingencies such as incentives (Fox & Kendall, 1983).

Studies have found self-instructional training to be effective for students with learning disabilities (LD) as well as those who fail to effectively self-regulate their behavior when encountering certain academic tasks. Specifically, this strategy has been effective across a number of academic areas, including reading comprehension, handwriting, and mathematics.

The effectiveness of self-instructional training versus didactic instruction was investigated by Graham and Wong (1993). In their study, 45 average readers and 45 poor readers across grades 5 and 6 were randomly assigned to one of three groups: didactic teaching of a strategy, self-instruction, or control (no training). Students in the first two groups learned a mnemonic strategy called 3H (Here, Hidden, and in my Head). These students were taught to think of these three terms when asked to answer text-explicit and text-implicit comprehension questions. Those students in the self-instruction group learned three additional questions to ask themselves as they used the 3H strategy. Results of this study indicated that students in both the didactic teaching group and the self-instruction group improved in their reading comprehension performance. Further analysis showed that the self-instructional training was more effective than didactic teaching in enhancing and maintaining comprehension performance.

Miranda and colleagues (1997) investigated the effects of a self-instruction strategy on the reading comprehension of 40 fifth- and sixth-grade students with learning disabilities. The children were taught five prompts to cue them when they were reading: (1) Stop, (2) Think and Decide, (3) Check, (4) Confirm, and (5) Evaluate. The instructor first modeled the strategy for the children, and then each child practiced until he or she was successful. Students were also taught specific reading comprehension strategies such as previewing and activation of previous knowledge. Results demonstrated that the children taught the self-monitoring strategy showed greater gains from pretest to posttest, as compared to students with learning disabilities in a no-treatment control group, on measures assessing main idea, recall, and cloze (filling in the blank with an appropriate word).

Self-Monitoring

Self-monitoring can be defined as "the act of systematically observing and recording aspects of one's own behavior and internal and external environmental events thought to be functionally related to that behavior" (Cone, 1999, p. 411). The most commonly used forms of self-monitoring include self-monitoring of attention (SMA) and self-monitoring of performance (SMP; Reid, 1996). SMA requires the student to assess whether or not he or she is paying attention, while SMP involves the student's assessment of some aspect of academic performance. Both forms of self-monitoring have been used to impact the academic productivity of students with academic skill problems.

Reid (1993) provided the following specific steps for the implementation of a self-monitoring procedure in a classroom: (1) select the behavior, (2) collect baseline data, (3) obtain willing cooperation from the student, (4) instruct the student in the procedure, (5) have the student independently perform the self-monitoring procedure, and (6) evaluate the effectiveness of the intervention. Readers are referred to Rankin and Reid (1995) for an example of how these steps may be used in practice.

Shapiro and Cole (1999) categorized self-monitoring of academic skills problems into two areas: (1) procedures that involve the recording of discrete behaviors related to academic outcomes and (2) procedures that focus on the metacognitive processes underlying academic tasks. Several studies supporting the efficacy of self-monitoring of discrete academic behaviors have been reported. An investigation conducted by Lalli and Shapiro (1990), for example, found that self-monitoring was an effective strategy for teaching sight-word acquisition to elementary-age students with learning disabilities. In a similar manner, Carr and Punzo (1993) taught three male students with behavior disorders/emotional disturbances to self-monitor in three academic areas: reading, mathematics, and spelling. Students made gains in academic accuracy, productivity, and on-task behavior across all subject areas. Self-monitoring of performance also was found to have a positive effect on the spelling achievement and on-task behavior of young adolescents (Reid & Harris, 1993).

Studies focusing on the use of self-monitoring as part of a larger instructional strategy technique can be found in the work of Graham and colleagues in their Self-Regulated Strategy Development (SRSD) model (Graham & Harris, 1999; Harris & Graham, 1994; Sexton, Harris, & Graham, 1998). This model and the research investigating the efficacy of techniques based on it will be described later in this chapter.

One of the areas of discussion in the self-monitoring literature revolves around the most appropriate developmental age to begin teaching this self-regulating skill. Schwartz (1997) proposes teaching early elementary-age students basic self-monitoring skills as a primary part of early literacy instruction. When children first learn to read, for example, they are taught to listen and see if what they read made sense. This is the beginning of teaching basic self-monitoring skills. If the child then goes back and rereads and self-corrects his or her error or asks for assistance from the teacher, the student has demonstrated the successful implementation of the strategy. An example of the integration of this type of strategy instruction in reading can be found in the *Reading Recovery* program (Clay, 1993).

Reid (1996) provided an extensive review of the literature on the effectiveness of self-monitoring strategies with students with learning disabilities. Although there are a number of studies demonstrating the positive impact of self-monitoring on academic *productivity* (e.g., Lloyd, Bateman, Landrum, & Hallahan, 1989; Maag, Reid, & DiGangi, 1993; Reid & Harris, 1993), the impact of self-monitoring on academic *accuracy* has not been consistently demonstrated in the literature. Specifically, many studies to date have failed to assess and report data on both rates of productivity and accuracy. Additionally, self-monitoring alone will not affect a student's accuracy if the student presents with a skills deficit rather than a performance problem. As Reid (1996) points out, self-monitoring does not teach a task specific skill, it teaches students to be cognizant of their performance. Therefore, in order to improve the accuracy of students who demonstrate a skill deficit in reading comprehension, a specific comprehension strategy would need to be taught to address the skill deficit in combination with a self-monitoring strategy to enhance overall performance.

Self-Management

Self-management may be best viewed as a collection of strategies that might include self-assessment, self-recording, self-evaluation, self-monitoring, and self-instruction (McDougall, 1998; Prater, 1994). The use of self-management strategies in special education with students who have academic skills problems is relatively common. In contrast, there are relatively few published studies investigating the use of these interventions in the general education setting. McDougall (1998) completed a comprehensive review of the literature focusing on the use of self-management interventions with students with disabilities in the general education setting. Although over 240 studies have been conducted investigating the efficacy of self-management with students with disabilities, only 14 of those studies were based on individuals in the general education population. Overall, the 14 studies reviewed demonstrated positive outcomes in the areas of social and academic performance for the students involved. Clearly, self-management strategies should be more carefully studied for their impact on children with special needs who are included in the general education setting.

Most self-management interventions focus on developing a specific academic skill area and are employed directly in classroom settings. Callahan, Rademacher, and Hildreth (1998) demonstrated a modification of a self-management strategy to improve academic performance. In their study, 26 sixth- and seventh-grade at-risk students and their families participated in a homework program that involved training both students and parents in the components of a self-management intervention. The dependent variables in the study were the percentage of completed math assignments handed in and the percentage correct of those problems completed. A multiple-baseline across groups design was used to assess the effectiveness of the intervention. After collection of baseline data, training sessions were held for both parents and students. The students were taught the following steps: (1) self-monitor homework start and end times and the location and time of homework completion, (2) self-record the number of problems correct and incorrect, (3) self-reinforce based upon the accuracy of the self-monitoring step, and (4) self-instruct and set goals for the completion of the next assignment. The parents' role was to collect data from Step 1, check the accuracy of the assignments upon completion, and compare the student and parent ratings. Students could earn "matching points" for accuracy in their ratings that could be exchanged for items on a pre-established reinforcement menu. Students also earned points at school for completing their math homework assignments and for returning their rating and matching forms to the teacher. Results indicated that both homework completion rates and accuracy improved for the students. Additionally, both the parents and students indicated satisfaction with the strategy, and reported that the strategies generalized to homework assignments other than those targeted in the study (Callahan et al., 1998).

Carrington, Lehrer, and Wittenstrom (1997) found similar success with a self-management strategy titled *Winning at Homework*. Designed to incorporate the principles of distributed practice, the Premack principle, immediate reinforcement, and paradoxical intention, this intervention can be tailored to the developmental level of the child. The basic tenet of this strategy is that brief periods of uninterrupted homework are immediately followed by a reinforcing activity, that is, play. An electronic timer is used with the child to signal the end of each work/play period. These authors found that with the implementation of this self-management strategy, parent report of severity of homework-related problems was reduced for their sample of children. A question that requires further investigation is whether or not the use of this strategy has an impact on school performance.

McDougall and Brady (1998) conducted a study of the effectiveness of behavioral self-management (BSM) interventions on the math fluency (digits correct per minute) and on-task behavior of five fourth-grade students with and without disabilities in general education classrooms. Students were nominated for participation in the study due to their poor performance in math and limited academic engaged time during independent math assignments. Using a multiple-baseline across subjects design, students were taught two multiple-component self-management strategies within an alternating treatments schedule. Both self-management strategies included the same components of self-monitoring, self-graphing, self-determination of reinforcement, and self-administration of reinforcement. The difference between the two types of self-management strategies was that one focused on monitoring attention and the other focused on monitoring productivity.

Fluency and accuracy data were collected on daily math assignments. Fading of the self-management package was conducted by first lengthening the self-monitoring intervals, then removing the self-recording forms, and then eliminating either the self-graphing or self-reinforcement components. Maintenance data were collected for approximately 2 weeks. Results indicated that all students increased their math fluency and engaged time with the implementation of this self-management package, and that four out of the five students continued to demonstrate improvements as components of the package were gradually removed (McDougall & Brady, 1998).

A Specific Model of Self-Regulated Strategy Instruction

Although the previously discussed cognitive-behavioral strategies have shown success in students with academic skill problems, it is noted that those strategies are most successful if the student learned a skill and is having difficulty performing that skill consistently. The Self-Regulated Strategy Development (SRSD) model is an example of a model designed for the purposes of teaching students a task-specific strategy for a particular academic problem in conjunction with more general self-regulatory strategies such as goal setting, self-monitoring, and self-instruction (Graham & Harris, 1999). The six specific components of SRSD, illustrated in the studies that follow, provide opportunities for students to "develop the background knowledge to use the strategy, establish the benefits of learning the strategy, observe how the strategy is used, memorize the steps of the strategy, practice using the strategy with teacher support, and apply the strategy independently" (p. 259).

Sexton, Harris, and Graham (1998) investigated the effectiveness of the SRSD model with six students with learning disabilities from a fifth- and sixth-grade team. All students were selected specifically because their teacher indicated that they had problems in the area of writing. A multiple-baseline across subjects design was used to assess the effectiveness of the intervention. Specifically, each student was taught a writing strategy based on the mnemonic TREE (Topic sentence, note Reasons, Examine reasons, and note Ending). Embedded within the instruction of this strategy were the basic components of the SRSD model as follows: (1) develop and activate background knowledge, (2) discuss it: instructional goals and significance, (3) model it, (4) memorize it, (5) support it, and (6) perform independently. Results of this study demonstrated that the intervention package had a positive impact upon the students' writing performance. In addition, data collected on attributions of writing success indicated that students were more likely to attribute their success to personal effort after intervention. Students also reported a greater awareness of the importance of strategy use upon completion of the study.

Graham and Harris (1999) reported similar findings in a study with a 12-year-old boy with a learning disability. This student was reported to have severe writing difficulties and lacked strategies for planning, organizing, and revising his writing. The six components of the SRSD model were used to teach the student a specific writing strategy for opinion essays know as DARE (Determine your premise; Assemble reasons to support your premise; Reject arguments for the other side; and End with a conclusion). An additional writing strategy for stories also was taught to the student using the same procedures. The student demonstrated improvements in his overall writing ability after learning the strategies and also changed his previously negative attitude about writing to one that was more positive and confident in his own capabilities. De La Paz (1999) reported similar results in a study of middle school students with and without learning disabilities who improved the quality of their writing after learning a specific strategy through the SRSD model.

Limitations of Cognitive-Behavioral Therapy

There are many methodological shortcomings with research completed on cognitive-behavioral therapy for academic skills problems. Research in this area has been criticized for its lack of clarity in the explanation of the methodology used in the various studies. Some studies, for example, have used multi-component treatment packages, rather than just self-instructional training or self-monitoring. Unless the specific components of these packages are identified and thoroughly explained, replication of results may be limited (Meador & Ollendick, 1984).

Lack of long-term follow-up data has also been identified as a major limitation in this literature. This is a concern, as cognitive-behavioral therapy was suggested as a way of overcoming the limited maintenance of gains observed with strict behavioral interventions. Moreover, even though a particular intervention may be highly successful in one setting or with one specific skill, that intervention may need to be modified in order to meet the curricular demands and needs of individual students (Gerber, 1986).

Finally, the amount of structure required to teach a student to utilize cognitive-behavioral strategies may vary. Gerber (1986) speculates that the amount of structure needed is inversely proportional to the cognitive maturity of the prospective learner. A number of prerequisite skills may be necessary for students to grasp the skills and apply them independently in the natural environment (Graham & Wong, 1993).

One of the strongest and most important criticisms of cognitive-behavioral therapy is the lack of data to support its generalization to tasks outside of the specific task used in the training. Most studies find that self-instruction works on the task used during initial instruction but does not generalize without programming the instruction to other stimuli.

Despite its limitations, a sufficiently strong data base exists to support the use of cognitive-behavioral therapy for the remediation of academic skills problems. The procedures appear to be applicable across academic domains, including both content and basic skill areas. As such, cognitive-behavioral therapy can be an effective and potentially important technique for use by school personnel with a broad group of students who possess all types of learning needs.

CASE EXAMPLES

Steven[1]

Background

Steven was a 9-year-old boy enrolled in the fourth grade. His classroom teacher, Mrs. Powell, referred him to the school's pre-referral intervention team due to concerns with academic progress. Specifically, his teacher reported that Steven was working below grade level in math.

Teacher Interview

According to Mrs. Powell, Steven was performing below his peers in mathematics assignments using the *Silver Burdette and Ginn* fourth-grade curriculum. An examination of Steven's permanent products in math showed no pattern of errors. Rather, many of his errors appeared to be due to care-

---

[1]Many thanks to Danielle Perkins, graduate student in school psychology at the University of South Florida, for the use of this case.

less mistakes. Mrs. Powell noted that Steven was "bright" and could do the assignments, but had a difficult time focusing. Steven was not a behavior concern, although sometimes he could be manipulative. Mrs. Powell's goal was for Steven to progress through the math curriculum at a more consistent pace.

Student Interview

Steven was interviewed using The Instructional Environment System–II (TIES-II; Ysseldyke & Christenson, 1994) semistructured student interview. Steven stated that he understood the expectations set by Mrs. Powell and the assignments given. He stated that math, science, and social studies presented the most difficulties for him, although he still believed he was good at math. Steven stated that he enjoyed doing addition and subtraction problems, but did not like doing timed multiplication tables.

Direct Observations

A 20-minute systematic observation using the Behavioral Observation of Students in Schools (BOSS; Shapiro, 1996) was conducted to determine the percentage of 15-second intervals Steven was actively (e.g., completing math problems) and passively (e.g., watching the teacher demonstrate problems on the board) engaged in the assigned task. Off-task behaviors included times when Steven was not engaged in the assigned academic task.

During this observation Steven was on-task (i.e., actively or passively engaged) 75% of the total intervals observed, which was less than his peers at 94.5% of the intervals observed. Steven's off-task motor and verbal behaviors were minimal, 1.4% and 2.8% of intervals, respectively. Steven was off-task passive during 25% of the intervals observed. He frequently looked around the room aimlessly. This behavior was most apparent during independent seatwork, and when Steven had completed an assignment and was awaiting further instructions.

Direct Assessment

A curriculum-based assessment (CBA) was conducted to determine Steven's instructional level in mathematics. Timed probes were given in the areas of addition, subtraction, and multiplication. Steven was administered one to four randomly selected single skill math probes in each area. Furthermore, Steven was found to be functioning at the second-grade instructional level in addition. In an examination of errors, no consistent pattern was found. In subtraction, Steven attained an instructional level on the first-grade probes. His performance on the first-grade probes, however, was inconsistent with his demonstration of skills on permanent products in the classroom which showed that he could correctly compute problems at the second-grade level. Once again, no specific pattern of errors was evident, and many of Steven's errors appeared to be due to carelessness. It was noted that Steven depended upon using his fingers to perform even the most basic calculations.

Summary of Assessment Data

Based upon the data collected in the interviews, observations, and direct assessment, it appeared that Steven was performing well below grade level in basic math skills. Specifically, it appeared that Steven had not reached a level of automaticity in basic addition and subtraction facts. Data also indicated that Steven had not developed effective self-monitoring strategies for completing math problems, which contributed to his careless errors. Based upon these data, it was determined that Steven would benefit from interventions in math focusing on basic skill development and automaticity of these skills. Additionally, Steven would benefit from instruction in a self-correction strategy.

Intervention Recommendations

In consultation with the teacher, it was determined that Steven needed to practice basic addition and subtraction facts repeatedly to increase fluency. It was recommended that Steven and a peer drill each other on basic addition, subtraction, and multiplication facts using flashcards three times per week. Another strategy that was recommended for Steven involved teaching him effective self-monitoring strategies for mathematics. Specifically, Steven needed a strategy for going back and self-checking his answers on math assignments. A cue card was developed by the examiner to be placed on Steven's desk as a reminder of the steps for completing a math problem (see Figure 11.1). These steps were collaboratively developed by the examiner and Mrs. Powell. Steven was taught to use this strategy when completing all math assignments.

The teacher instructed Steven in the use of the cue card using a self-instructional procedure as outlined originally by Meichenbaum and Goodman (1971) (see Figure 11.2). Mrs. Powell told Steven that whenever he was about to begin a math assignment he was to look at the cue card attached to his desk. She then explained each step of the procedure and used the first few problems on a math assignment to model the procedure, verbalizing each step as she proceeded. Mrs. Powell then asked Steven to follow along and perform the task while she continued to say the steps aloud.

1. Read the directions.

2. Look at the problem and identify the sign (addition, subtraction, multiplication, division).

3. Think about how to complete the problem. (Do I need to borrow? Carry?)

4. Work out the problem.

5. Check the problem to make sure it's correct.

6. If problem is correct, place a slash through problem number. If problem is incorrect, go back to Step 2.

FIGURE 11.1. Steven's math cue card.

Steven next was asked to verbalize the steps as he worked through a problem. When he had successfully completed this task, she instructed Steven to verbalize and complete a series of math problems. When Steven demonstrated that he could follow the steps, Mrs. Powell then instructed him to complete another series of problems while whispering the steps to himself. Finally, Steven was asked to say the steps silently to himself as he continued to practice with his teacher.

Progress Monitoring of Intervention Outcomes

Data continued to be collected on Steven's accuracy of assignment completion throughout the intervention. Results of the procedure are shown in Figure 11.3. During baseline, Steven demonstrated a range of 4% to 37% correct on classroom assignments. After the self-monitoring intervention was implemented, Steven's percentage correct on classroom math assignments ranged from 40% to 100%. Due to the end of the school year, addi-

Teacher	Student
1. Self-talks and performs task.	Observes.
2. Self-talks.	Performs task.
3. Observes student and cues if needed.	Self-talks and performs task.
4. Observes student.	Subvocalizes self-talk and performs task.
5. Observes student.	Performs task silently.

FIGURE 11.2. Self-instruction steps for the teacher and Steven.

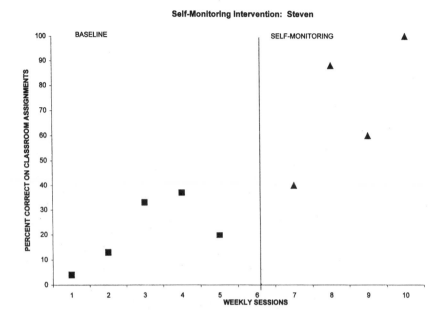

FIGURE 11.3. Results of self-instruction intervention for Steven.

tional data points could not be collected to further evaluate Steven's performance.

Based upon these data, it appeared that the self-monitoring strategy was effective for Steven. Specifically, by the end of the data collection period Steven had met his teacher's expectations (85% or higher) on his classroom assignments in math. When asked about usefulness of this self-monitoring strategy, both the teacher and Steven indicated that they liked the intervention and would continue to use it.

In conclusion, the implementation of a self-monitoring procedure focusing on discrete academic skill outcomes (percentage correct on math classroom assignment) was successful for this student. This is an example of a case where the student had the skill to perform the academic task, but did not perform accurately because he made numerous careless errors. The self-monitoring intervention provided Steven with a structured method of approaching math problems and prevented him for making careless mistakes by incorporating a step that required him to go back and check his work. Because Steven's academic performance improved, both he and the teacher chose to continue using the intervention beyond the data collection period.

Christy[2]

Background

Christy, an 8-year-old girl, was referred to the pre-referral intervention team by her second-grade teacher, Mr. Smith. The presenting concerns included off-task behavior and inconsistent progress in spelling and writing.

Teacher Interview

When discussing his concerns about Christy's performance in spelling, Mr. Smith indicated that Christy could learn a spelling word and orally tell him its meaning. However, on the spelling test on Fridays, Christy was unable to spell the same word correctly. Furthermore, Mr. Smith reported that Christy's mother had been working on spelling at home with Christy.

In the area of writing, Mr. Smith reported that Christy had no difficulty with expressing thoughts or creativity. He indicated that the length and depth (e.g., plot, setting) of her stories were inconsistent. Although Christy did not use capitalization or punctuation in her writing, she could immediately identify a missing period or noncapitalized letter when prompted. Mr. Smith noted that Christy was distractible in class and that she experienced difficulty concentrating. These difficulties may have contributed to her fluctuating levels of academic performance.

Classroom Observation

The Behavioral Observation of Students in Schools (Shapiro, 1996) was utilized to collect data on Christy's behavior. It consisted of a 20-minute observation that quantified Christy's academic engaged time and off-task behaviors. During the large group vocabulary instruction by the teacher, Christy was actively engaged 31% and passively engaged 46% of the intervals observed. Peer comparison indicated a total of 56% engagement. Christy was off-task motor 10% of the intervals and passively off-task 14% of the intervals observed. A peer comparison of the intervals included 12% off-task motor and 33% off-task passive.

---

[2]Many thanks to J. Elizabeth Chesno Grier, doctoral student in school psychology at the University of South Florida, for the use of this case.

Student Interview

Christy was interviewed one afternoon before the commencement of the direct assessment. She perceived herself as "pretty good" in reading and math. She acknowledged, however, experiencing difficulty with spelling and writing. Christy indicated that she enjoyed working in groups with her peers.

Direct Assessment

Survey level assessment (SLA) was administered for spelling and written expression to ascertain Christy's instructional level in these academic areas. Her performance was then monitored for 5 weeks to determine her consistency of performance.

SPELLING

Christy was given three lists of spelling words taken from grade 2 material. Christy was given 7 seconds to spell each of 10 words. The total number of correct letter sequences per minute was then calculated. Christy's median for total letter sequences correct was 19, which may be classified at the frustrational level. The mean total percentage of words correct across the three lists was calculated as 33%.

During the progress monitoring period, Christy's performance in spelling increased from a median score of 19 letter sequences correct per minute to a range of 29 to 36 letter sequences correct per minute (falling between grade 1–2 expectancy levels).

WRITTEN EXPRESSION

Christy was given three story starters in which she had 1 minute to think about what she planned to write and 3 minutes to write. Her writing samples were then examined for total number of words written. Christy's median total words written was 31 and her median words spelled correctly was 17. These results indicated that Christy was currently working within second-grade-level expectations. At the request of her teacher, Christy's progress in written expression was monitored for 5 weeks.

Although Christy's performance in written expression during SLA was at the second-grade level, her performance was consistently at the first-grade level during progress monitoring. In addition, the number of words she spelled correctly in her writing decreased. Weaknesses in Christy's writing included patterns in lack of capitalization, lack of punctuation, poorly constructed sentences, poor spacing between words, and inaccurate spelling. Strengths consisted of sensible sentences, appropriate margins, and mostly legible words.

Summary of Assessment Data

Based upon the data collected during SLA and progress monitoring in spelling and written expression, it appeared that Christy was functioning below the second-grade level in both academic areas. In spelling, although a number of errors were demonstrated, no specific error patterns emerged. Similarly in written expression, Christy demonstrated difficulty in being able to write words to express her thoughts, as well as problems with spelling, mechanics, and overall organization.

Intervention Recommendations

In consultation with Mr. Smith, several intervention strategies were developed for Christy. In the area of spelling, it was determined that Christy would benefit from a self-correction technique to improve her accuracy. Using a sheet of paper with six columns (see Figure 11.4), Christy was instructed to fold the sheet over so that she could not see the first column (model word). Next, the teacher read a list of spelling words aloud and Christy was asked to write each word in the second column on the sheet. Once the list of words had been presented to Christy, she was directed to compare her spelling with the correct spelling of each word in the model word column. If her spelling was correct, she was to write "yes" in the correct column. If her spelling was incorrect, she was to write "no" in the correct column and write the correct spelling of the word three times in the remaining columns on the sheet. This Cover–Copy–Compare self-management technique (McLaughlin & Skinner, 1996) was selected to help teach Christy to spell by comparing words to a model, identifying spelling mistakes, correcting mistakes, and practicing correct spelling. The strategy was introduced by the consultant to Christy and practiced with her until she had grasped the concept. Christy and the consultant met once per week to practice the strategy with the classroom spelling list for that week. The process also was outlined in a letter sent home to Christy's parents to provide additional practice at home.

In the area of written expression, it was decided that Christy would benefit from a simple story grammar to help her organize and plan her story (Grossen & Carnine, 1991). For instance, she would answer the following four questions before she began to write so she would have a plan for her story: (1) Who is the story about? (2) What problem does he or she have? (3) How does he or she try to fix the problem? (4) What happens in the end? This strategy was rehearsed with the consultant demonstrating examples of responses to each question. Then the consultant provided exam-

Blank Chart

Model Word	Word	Correct?	Correction	Correction	Correction

Example

Model Word	Word	Correct?	Correction	Correction	Correction
book	book	Yes			
table	tabl	No	table	table	table
chair	chare	No	chair	chair	chair
movie	movie	Yes			
building	bilding	No	building	building	building

FIGURE 11.4. Christy's self-correction sheet for spelling. This chart can be used with a spelling self-management strategy. The student will fold the model word over so that he or she cannot see the words. Then the teacher, parent, peer, or a tape recording will read the words for the student to spell. Then the student can correct his or her spellings using the model.

ples of how to integrate the responses to each question into a story. Christy then practiced with the consultant until she demonstrated an understanding of the questions and could produce three different stories. Finally, a cue card with the four questions was prepared for her to keep in her desk and to use as a reference for her writing assignments.

It was determined that Christy also would benefit from learning the COPS strategy: Capitalization, Organization, Punctuation, and Spelling (Lovitt, 1995). The consultant worked with Christy to help her learn this strategy. First, the four terms of the COPS strategy were explained to Christy. Next, she was provided with a writing sample, and the consultant demonstrated how it could be edited by reviewing the sample for capitalization, organization, punctuation, and spelling. Christy then was provided with her own writing sample and was asked to verbalize the steps as she proceeded to edit the sample. The last component of the training involved Christy's using the steps to critique her own writing while saying each step quietly to herself. Mr. Smith agreed to remind Christy to follow this strat-

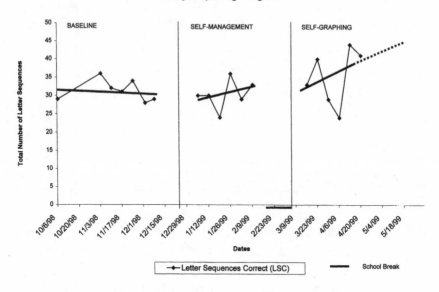

FIGURE 11.5. Results of self-regulation strategy in spelling for Christy.

egy and to have a note card taped to her desk with those components listed on it as a reminder to her when she was given a writing assignment. With the use of this note card, Christy was instructed to self-correct all written assignments before submitting them to her teacher. Weekly written expression probes were administered to Christy to assess the efficacy of these writing strategies.

Follow-Up

SPELLING

After 4 weeks of the intervention, Christy did not consistently meet her short-term goal of writing 30–39 letter sequences correct per minute with an accuracy rate of 80% or above (see Figure 11.5). In fact, her accuracy rate was consistently below 60%. Therefore, an additional strategy of self-graphing was implemented in addition to the spelling intervention. Christy was taught how to graph her total letter sequences correct after the consultant scored her paper. By the end of an additional 4 weeks, Christy had met her long-term goal of the letter sequences correct by writing 40 or more letter sequences correct per minute (see Figure 11.5). Although her accuracy rate had increased, it was not 85% or above as projected in the long-term

goal. However, Mr. Smith indicated that he was pleased with Christy's accuracy on his spelling tests in class, which now ranged from 60% to 100%.

WRITTEN EXPRESSION

After 5 weeks, Christy had not met her short-term goal of writing 36 words
per 3 minutes, which was the criterion for grade 2. In fact, Christy's performance had deteriorated. It was concluded by both teacher and consultant
that Christy spent more time thinking about the story components and
writing mechanics as opposed to writing the story. As a result, the overall
words written in 3 minutes decreased. In order for Christy to achieve her
long-term goal of writing 37 or more words per 3 minutes, which was the
criterion for grade 3, her written expression interventions were modified.
First, a self-graphing strategy was implemented. Since Christy had been
taught how to graph her performance in spelling, she quickly learned how
to graph the number of words written after her passage was scored by the
consultant. The consultant also discussed with Christy the importance of
writing as much about the story as she could. Christy continued to review
the story map components and writing mechanics with the consultant as
well as have them visually present during writing. By the end of an additional 5 weeks, Christy met her long-term goal (see Figure 11.6). In

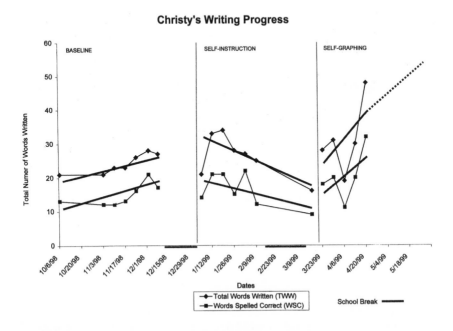

FIGURE 11.6. Results of self-regulation strategy in written expression for Christy.

addition, the number of correctly spelled words used in the story increased in Christy's writing.

In conclusion, this case demonstrated the successful use of several different self-regulation strategies for this student. The importance of collecting frequent progress monitoring data is evident in this case, as the initial intervention did not result in the expected changes. However, upon analysis of the data and discussion with the student and teacher, simply adding the component of self-graphing resulted in improvements in the appropriate direction of successful performance.

DISCUSSION

These cases illustrate several strategies one could select in the area of cognitive-behavioral interventions for academic skills problems. Although these two cases resulted in successful outcomes, it is important to recognize that not all students may respond as positively to these strategies. Students may vary in the degree to which they are willing to accept the "talk out loud to yourself" part of a self-instruction procedure. Indeed, some students are highly resistant to using this type of procedure, and it is unwise to persist in trying to apply the self-instruction technique. In addition, some students may follow the step-by-step procedures of a cognitive-behavioral intervention procedure during training, but fail to use the steps appropriately in the classroom. If the strategy is not implemented correctly, it is possible for the student to become frustrated and to view the experience negatively. Therefore, it is important for the teacher to be included in the training to provide opportunities for the student to practice his or her newly learned skills, and provide reinforcement when those skills are applied correctly.

In general, the use of cognitive-behavioral therapy for improving academic skills has significant potential for effecting positive outcomes in students. As a procedure that teaches skills directly applicable to academic learning, these techniques clearly offer an important and potentially valuable resource for school personnel in preventing academic failure. It is important for practitioners to be aware, however, of the limitations of research in this area. Although cognitive-behavioral therapy appears promising, continued efforts to examine the ways in which it can be used to remediate academic skills deficits are needed.

REFERENCES

Callahan, K., Rademacher, J. A., & Hildreth, B. L. (1998). The effect of parent participation in strategies to improve the homework performance of students who are at risk. *Remedial and Special Education, 19,* 131–141.

Carr, S. C., & Punzo, R. P. (1993). The effects of self-monitoring of academic accuracy and productivity on the performance of students with behavioral disorders. *Behavioral Disorders, 18,* 241–250.

Carrington, P., Lehrer, P. M., & Wittenstrom, K. (1997). A children's self-management system for reducing homework-related problems: Parent efficacy ratings. *Child and Family Therapy, 19,* 1–22.

Clay, M. M. (1993). *Reading Recovery: A guidebook for teachers in training.* Portsmouth, NH: Heinemann.

Cone, J. D. (1999). Introduction to the special section on self-monitoring: A major assessment method in clinical psychology. *Psychological Assessment, 11,* 411–414.

De La Paz, S. (1999). Self-regulated strategy instruction in regular education settings: Improving outcomes for students with and without learning disabilities. *Learning Disabilities Research and Practice, 14,* 92–106.

Fox, D. E., & Kendall, P. C. (1983). Thinking through academic problems: Application of cognitive-behavior therapy to learning. In T. R. Kratochwill (Ed.), *Advances in school psychology* (Vol. 3., pp. 269–301). Hillsdale, NJ: Erlbaum.

Gerber, M. M. (1986). Cognitive-behavioral training in the curriculum: Time, slow learners, and basic skills. *Focus on Exceptional Children, 18,* 1–12.

Graham, S., & Harris, K. R. (1999). Assessment and intervention in overcoming writing difficulties: An illustration from the self-regulated strategy development model. *Language, Speech, and Hearing Services in Schools, 30,* 255–264.

Graham, L., & Wong, B. Y. (1993). Comparing two modes of teaching a question-answering strategy for enhancing reading comprehension: Didactic and self-instructional training. *Journal of Learning Disabilities, 26,* 270–279.

Grossen, B., & Carnine, D. (1991). Strategies for maximizing the reading success in the regular classroom. In G. Stoner, M. R. Shinn, & H. M. Walker (Eds.), *Intervention for achievement and behavior problems* (pp. 333–355). Bethesda, MD: National Association of School Psychologists.

Harris, K. R., & Graham, S. (1994). Constructivism: Principles, paradigms, and integration. *Journal of Special Education, 28,* 233–247.

Lalli, E. P., & Shapiro, E. S. (1990). The effects of self-monitoring and contingent reward on sight word acquisition. *Education and Treatment of Children, 13,* 129–141.

Lloyd, J. W., Bateman, D. F., Landrum, T. J., & Hallahan, D. P. (1989). Self-recording of attention versus productivity. *Journal of Applied Behavior Analysis, 22,* 315–324.

Lovitt, T. C. (1995). *Tactics for teaching* (2nd ed.). Columbus, OH: Merrill.

Maag, J. W., Reid, R., & DiGangi, S. A. (1993). Differential effects of self-monitoring attention, accuracy, and productivity. *Journal of Applied Behavior Analysis, 26,* 329–344.

McDougall, D. (1998). Research on self-management techniques used by students with disabilities in general education settings. *Remedial and Special Education, 19,* 310–320.

McDougall, D., & Brady, M. P. (1998). Initiating and fading self-management interventions to increase math fluency in general education classes. *Exceptional Children, 64,* 151–166.

McLaughlin, T. F., & Skinner, C. H. (1996). Improving academic performance through self-management: Cover, copy, and compare. *Intervention in School and Clinic, 32,* 113–118.

Meador, A. E., & Ollendick, T. H. (1984). Cognitive behavior therapy with children: An evaluation of its efficacy and clinical utility. *Child and Family Behavior Therapy, 6,* 25–44.

Meichenbaum, D., & Goodman, J. (1971). Training impulsive children to talk to themselves: A means of developing control. *Journal of Abnormal Psychology, 77,* 115–126.

Miller, G. E., & Brewster, M. E. (1992). Developing self-sufficient learners in reading and mathematics through self-instructional training. In M. Pressley, K. R. Harris, & J. T. Guthrie (Eds.), *Promoting academic competence and literacy in school* (pp. 169–222). New York: Academic Press.

Miranda, A., Villaescusa, M. I., & Vidal-Abarca, E. (1997). Is attribution retraining necessary? Use of self-regulation procedures for enhancing the reading comprehension strategies of children with learning disabilities. *Journal of Learning Disabilities, 30,* 503–512.

Prater, M. A. (1994). Improving academic and behavior skills through self-management procedures. *Preventing School Failure, 38,* 5–9.

Rankin, J. L., & Reid, R. (1995). The SM rap—or, here's the rap on self-monitoring. *Intervention in School and Clinic, 30,* 181–188.

Reid, R. (1993). Implementing self-monitoring interventions in the classroom: Lessons learned from research. *Monograph in Behavioral Disorders: Severe Behavior Disorders of Children and Youth, 16,* 43–54.

Reid, R. (1996). Research in self-monitoring with students with learning disabilities: The present, the prospects, the pitfalls. *Journal of Learning Disabilities, 29,* 317–331.

Reid, R., & Harris, K. R. (1993). Self-monitoring of attention versus self-monitoring of performance: Effects on attention and academic performance. *Exceptional Children, 60,* 29–40.

Schwartz, R. M. (1997). Self-monitoring in beginning reading. *The Reading Teacher, 51,* 40–48.

Sexton, M., Harris, K. R., & Graham, S. (1998). Self-regulated strategy development and the writing process: Effects on essay writing and attributions. *Exceptional Children, 64*(3), 295–311.

Shapiro, E. S. (1996). *Academic skills problems: Direct assessment and interventions* (2nd ed.). New York: Guilford Press.

Shapiro, E. S., & Cole, C. L. (1994). *Behavior change in the classroom: Self-management interventions.* New York: Guilford Press.

Shapiro, E. S., & Cole, C. L. (1999). Self-monitoring in assessing children's problems. *Psychological Assessment, 11,* 448–457.

Vygotsky, L. (1962). *Thought and language.* New York: Wiley.

Wood, D. A., Rosenberg, M. S., & Carran, D. T. (1993). The effects of tape-recorded self-instruction cues on the mathematics performance of students with learning disabilities. *Journal of Learning Disabilities, 26,* 250–258.

Ysseldyke, J., & Christenson, S. (1994). *The instructional environment system–II.* Longmont, CO: Sopris West.

Zimmerman, B. J. (1986). Becoming a self-regulated learner: Which are the key subprocesses? *Contemporary Educational Psychology, 11,* 307–313.

SUGGESTED READINGS

Maag, J. W., Rutherford, A. B., & DiGangi, S. A. (1992). Effects of self monitoring and contingent reinforcement on on-task behavior and academic productivity of learning-disabled students: A social validation study. *Psychology in the Schools, 29,* 157–172.

Reid, R. (1996). Research in self-monitoring with students with learning disabilities: The present, the prospects, the pitfalls. Journal of *Learning Disabilities, 29,* 317–331.

Shapiro, E. S., & Cole, C. L. (1994). *Behavior change in the classroom: Self-management interventions.* New York: Guilford Press.

Shapiro, E. S., Duman, S. L., Post, E. E., and Levinson, T. S. (2002). Self-monitoring procedures for children and adolescents. In M. R. Shinn, H. M. Walker, & G. Stoner (Eds.), *Interventions for academic and behavior problems: II. Preventive and remedial approaches* (pp. 433–454). Bethesda, MD: National Association of School Psychologists.

12

Treatment of Family Problems

NORMAN B. EPSTEIN
STEPHEN E. SCHLESINGER

The hallmark of family therapy is its attention to *interpersonal* factors that make it difficult or impossible to resolve people's difficulties by treating the people involved solely on an individual basis. Very commonly, families identify problems by describing the undesirable behavior of one member, rather than viewing their difficulties as the result of problems in interactions among members. However, the initial explanation that they may offer for consulting a therapist does not necessarily turn out to be, on closer examination, the actual basis of their distress. This chapter describes a variety of intra- and interpersonal factors that are important in a cognitive-behavioral approach to the assessment and treatment of family problems. Although it can be tempting to focus on cognitions and behaviors of one family member that appear to contribute to a family problem, the chapter emphasizes that it often is the combination of cognitions and behaviors of two or more members that results in relationship problems.

Cognitive-behavioral approaches to family therapy are rooted in cognitive mediation models of individual functioning (e.g., Beck, 1976; Ellis, 1962), which stress that an individual's emotional and behavioral reactions to life events are shaped by the particular interpretations that the person makes of the events, rather than solely by objective characteristics of the events themselves. Therapists who have applied cognitive mediation principles to couples (e.g., Baucom & Epstein, 1990; Beck, 1988; Dattilio & Padesky, 1990; Ellis, Sichel, Yeager, DiMattia, & DiGiuseppe, 1989; Epstein, 1982; Epstein & Baucom, 1998, 2002; Jacobson, 1984; Rathus & Sanderson, 1999; Schlesinger & Epstein, 1986) and to families (e.g., Dattilio, 1994, 1998; Epstein & Schlesinger, 1991; Epstein, Schlesinger, & Dryden, 1988; Huber & Baruth, 1989; Schwebel & Fine, 1994) have focused on how the behaviors of family members constantly serve as "life events" that are interpreted and evaluated by other family members.

In a cognitive-behavioral view of family relationships, cognitions, behaviors, and emotions are seen as exerting *mutual* influences upon one another. For example, a cognition (e.g., inferring that one's child is *willfully* disobeying one's orders) can produce emotions (e.g., anger) and behaviors (e.g., spanking). In contrast, an emotion (e.g., anger) can influence cognitions (e.g., selectively noticing unpleasant actions by one's child and overlooking positive ones) and behaviors (e.g., yelling, rather than speaking in a firm but calm manner). Finally, a behavior (e.g., withdrawing from one's family members) can affect one's emotions (e.g., decreased feelings of intimacy, due to few shared pleasant activities with the other family members) or cognitions (e.g., drawing the conclusion, "I must not care about them any longer, or else I would not be acting this way").

Consistent with a systems approach to family therapy (e.g., Watzlawick, Beavin, & Jackson, 1967), cognitive-behavioral approaches include a premise that members of a family simultaneously influence and are influenced by each other. Consequently, a behavior on the part of one member leads to behaviors, cognitions, and emotions in other members, and in return the other members' responses elicit cognitions, behaviors, and emotions in the former individual. Once such a *cycle* among family members is in motion, a dysfunctional cognition, behavior, or emotion at any point can lead to a negative spiral. For example, if one member misinterprets another's behavior as due to malicious intentions and therefore responds by disparaging the other, the other member may in turn think, "I try my best, and all I get in return is criticism" and may therefore leave the house in anger. Then, the first individual might interpret the other's withdrawal in a negative manner, such as "Well, he [she] obviously can't stand being caught trying to take advantage of me." Each member experiences and reacts to his or her cognitions about the other person as if they represent the absolute truth, and conflict can escalate quickly, as in this example.

When more than two individuals are involved in an interaction, the events that members observe, as well as the resulting cognitions about those events, become more complex than is the case with dyadic interactions (Epstein & Schlesinger, 1991). Each family member may observe at least four kinds of events:

1. The individual's own cognitions, behaviors, and emotions regarding family interaction (e.g., the person who notices him- or herself withdrawing from the rest of the family).
2. The actions of individual family members toward him or her.
3. The combined (and not always consistent) reactions that several members have toward him or her.
4. The characteristics of the relationships among other family mem-

bers (e.g., noticing that two other family members usually are supportive of each other's opinions).

Thus, there is a vast array of events occurring during family interactions that serve as stimuli for the family members' cognitive appraisals, emotional reactions, and behavioral responses. The next section describes several types of cognitions that family members may experience concerning each of the four types of events in the preceding list.

TYPES OF COGNITIONS INVOLVED IN FAMILY DYSFUNCTION

As noted, the forms of cognition that have become foci of cognitive-behavioral approaches to marital and family problems have been derived in part from cognitive models of individual psychopathology (e.g., Beck, 1976; Ellis, 1962) and partly from social psychological models of social cognition, such as attribution theory (cf. Arias & Beach, 1987). Five major types of cognitions that have been implicated in marital and family dysfunction are (1) *selective perceptions* about what events have occurred during family interactions, (2) *attributions* about why particular events occur, (3) *expectancies* (predictions) about the probabilities that certain events will occur in the future, (4) *assumptions* about the characteristics of family members and their relationships, and (5) *standards* about the characteristics that family members and their relationships "should" have (Baucom & Epstein, 1990; Baucom, Epstein, Sayers, & Sher, 1989; Epstein & Baucom, 1989, 1993, 2002). The following is a summary of research bearing on the roles that these types of cognitions can play in creating and maintaining conflict in family relationships. It is beyond the scope of this chapter to describe how these cognitive variables can contribute to specific family problems (e.g., communication problems, role conflicts, difficulties with extended family). Table 12.1 presents a matrix with examples of the five types of cognitions associated with each of the four previously described types of family *events* that the individual may observe (own responses, actions of individual members, combined actions of two or more other members, and relationships among other members). The table refers to members of the family in the case example presented later in the chapter.

Selective Perceptions

Theorists such as Kelly (1955) and Heider (1958) stressed that perception is an active rather than a passive process. When in the role of observer, an individual cannot possibly notice all of the information available in a situation, and there is a considerable body of research evidence that people engage in selective attention, noticing some of the available stimuli and over-

TABLE 12.1. Types of Cognitions

Kinds of events	Attributions	Expectancies	Assumptions	Standards	Perceptions
Own thoughts, emotions, and behaviors	Jane: "I'm not as good as Robert."	Frank: "If I don't scream, I'll get an ulcer."	Frank: "My concern about my teenage daughter is no different from any other father's."	Robert: "A good child obeys his parents."	Jane: "I never get to have any fun."
Actions of individual relatives toward him or her	Alice: "Frank doesn't listen to me because he doesn't respect me."	Robert: "If I do what Dad says, he'll give me more privileges."	Alice: "Teenagers can learn to control themselves without their parents' help."	Jane: "Parents have no right to give their children orders."	Frank: "Jane never is nice to me."
Combined reactions of several members toward him or her	Jane: "Dad and Robert treat me like this because they don't understand teenage girls."	Robert: "If I comply, Mom and Dad won't bother me."	Jane: "Parents can't understand kids because of the generation gap."	Alice: "Mothers should be treated as experts in child rearing."	Frank: "The women in the family always gang up on me."
Observations of relationships among other members	Jane: "Robert can do anything he wants because Mom and Dad think he's perfect."	Robert: "If Jane keeps this up, she'll break up our parents' marriage."	Alice: "Fathers don't know how to raise girls."	Frank: "Everybody in a family ought to get along."	Robert: "Jane never has a kind word to say."

Note. Frank, father; Alice, mother; Jane, daughter; Robert, son.

looking others (cf. Nisbett & Ross, 1980). *Selective perceptions* are those aspects of the available information that an individual notices. For example, Morton, Twentyman, and Azar (1988) report that parents who tend to use coercive parenting strategies also tend to attend selectively to their children's negative behaviors.

Both clinical observation and empirical research (e.g., Beck, Rush, Shaw, & Emery, 1979; Fiske & Taylor, 1991; Turk & Speers, 1983; Wessler & Wessler, 1980) suggest that perceptions of events can be influenced by a variety of factors, such as the perceiver's current emotional state (e.g., anger), fatigue, and the basic cognitive structures (schemas) that the individual has available for classifying and understanding experiences. Concerning cognitive structures (which will be described more fully in our discussions of assumptions and standards), Kelly's (1955) seminal writings on "personal constructs" emphasized how the concepts that one has developed through past experience for categorizing people and events determine what one notices in daily life situations. For example, an individual whose life experiences have left him or her sensitive to differences in individuals' levels of power in close relationships may be likely to notice behaviors of family members that might reflect their potential or actual attempts to exert control in family interactions. With this in mind, cognitive-behavioral approaches to family problems commonly include therapeutic interventions designed to improve family members' perceptual accuracy.

Attributions

A large body of empirical work has accumulated focusing on attributions that family members make about the causes of the events in their interactions (Baucom, 1987; Baucom et al., 1989; Bradbury & Fincham, 1990, 1992; Thompson & Snyder, 1986). Clinical and empirical evidence supports the theoretical notion (e.g., Heider, 1958; Kelley, 1967) that people spontaneously draw conclusions about possible causes of events in their lives (Baucom, 1987; Holtzworth-Munroe & Jacobson, 1985). Baucom (1987) has described functions that attributions can serve in a close relationship, such as giving one a sense (accurate or not) of understanding another person and his or her actions, a sense of control over the relationship due to that understanding, and a means for minimizing future disappointments in a dissatisfying relationship by attributing stable negative traits to the other person (e.g., "I don't expect [my relative] to act in a caring manner, because she is a selfish person").

Numerous studies have examined the attributions that distressed and nondistressed spouses make about the determinants of positive and negative events in their relationships (see reviews by Baucom and Epstein, 1990, and by Bradbury and Fincham, 1990). The most consistent findings from these studies are that distressed spouses are more likely than nondistressed spouses to attribute negative partner behavior to trait-like (global, stable) characteristics of the partner, including malicious intent, selfish motivation, and lack of love. Concerning positive partner behaviors, nondistressed spouses are more likely to attribute them to global, stable causes. Furthermore, evidence that physically abusive husbands are more likely than both distressed and nondistressed husbands to attribute their wives' negative behaviors to negative intentions (e.g., trying to hurt the husband's feelings or put him down) suggests that particular types of attributions may be especially common in abusive relationships (Holtzworth-Munroe & Hutchinson, 1993). Longitudinal studies (e.g., Fincham & Bradbury, 1987, 1993; Fincham, Harold, & Gano-Phillips, 2000) have indicated that spouses' attributions about their partners' behaviors influence their subsequent marital satisfaction levels and behaviors toward their partners.

Research also has been conducted concerning attributions that family members other than the marital partners make about other members' behaviors, and the results tend to be consistent with the findings from marital studies. For example, Morton et al. (1988) report that in their clinical work with child-abusing parents, it is common for the abusers to believe that their children misbehave intentionally in order to annoy and spite them. Azar (1986) found that within samples of abusive parents the tendency to make negative trait attributions about children was associated with more negative and less positive parental behavior toward the children. Thus, family therapists need to assess whether or not parents' attributions about their children's behavior are accurate, but in either case they also need to help the parents be aware of (and reward) positive behaviors and changes in negative behaviors.

Expectancies

Based on past experiences, people develop expectancies or predictions about the probabilities that certain events will occur in the future under particular circumstances (Bandura, 1977; Rotter, 1954). An individual continuously makes decisions to act or not act in certain ways due to the outcomes that he or she anticipates from each action. Rotter (1954) made a distinction between *specific expectancies*, which are situation-specific (e.g., "If I ask Mom to help me with my homework right after she gets home from work, she will get angry and refuse"), and *generalized expectancies*, which are more global and stable (e.g., "My children won't cooperate with anything that I might ask of them"). The individual's choices of behaviors toward other family members depend on the predictions that he or she makes about the outcomes *and* the degree to which he or she finds each outcome pleasant or unpleasant.

Bandura notes that expectancies are a normal and efficient aspect of learning from one's experiences. The crucial issue concerning family problems is that often family members' expectancies are accurate, but sometimes they are distorted. An inaccurate expectancy may lead an individual to behave in a dysfunctional manner toward other family members, initiating negative behavioral spirals and blocking conflict resolution (Doherty, 1981). An inaccurate expectancy also can elicit inappropriate emotional responses within the individual who holds it, as when a person predicts an aversive response from another family member and feels anxiety about the anticipated trouble.

Two major types of expectancies described by Bandura (1977) are *outcome expectancies* and *efficacy expectancies*. Outcome expectancies are predictions about the probability that a particular action will lead to a particular outcome. In contrast, efficacy expectancies involve estimates about the likelihood that one will be able to perform those actions successfully, which would lead to a particular outcome. Thus, a father may have an optimistic outcome expectancy, "If we all take turns expressing our opinions about an issue, we are likely to find some common ground for making a decision acceptable to everyone in the family," but he may also have a pessimistic efficacy expectancy such as "It is unlikely that members in this family will stop talking about their own ideas long enough to listen to others' opinions."

Results of preliminary studies (e.g., Fincham et al., 2000; Kurdek & Berg, 1987; Pretzer, Epstein, & Fleming, 1991; Vanzetti, Notarius, & NeeSmith, 1992) indicate that family members' negative expectancies are associated with greater relationship distress. However, there is a need for much more research, particularly investigating the degree to which individuals' expectancies influence their actual behaviors toward other family members.

Assumptions and Standards

Both assumptions and standards are forms of "cognitive structures," "tacit beliefs," "knowledge structures," or "schemas" (Fiske & Taylor, 1991; Nisbett & Ross, 1980; Seiler, 1984; Turk & Speers, 1983). Through experiences beginning early in life, an individual develops concepts about the characteristics of objects (including other people and the self), as well as how these objects relate to each other. Once a cognitive structure has been established, it serves as a "template" by which the individual understands objects and situations in the future. For example, members of a family have developed cognitive structures concerning the characteristics of people who fill particular roles (e.g., father, daughter) and the ways in which people filling particular family roles interact with each other. Assumptions are those cognitive structures concerning characteristics of objects and events that an individual believes *do* exist, whereas standards are the person's conceptions of how objects and events *should* be (Baucom & Epstein, 1990).

Assumptions

An assumption about a person or relationship typically includes a set of "descriptors," or characteristics that are interrelated, and beliefs about the degrees to which those characteristics are correlated. Consequently, once an individual assigns a person or object to a category based on a characteristic that he or she has observed, the individual tends to make inferences about unseen characteristics. For example, a person may assume that a "father" is someone who is kind, works hard to provide for his family, is strict, and is protective. The person also may assume that all of these characteristics are highly correlated with each other. Therefore, when this person meets a man who is identified as a father and who is strict with his children, the observer is likely to conclude that this father is very protective. The inference may be accurate, but it also may be invalid. Perhaps this particular father's strict behavior reflects his irritation about having children and his attempt to stop his children from bothering him. Correlational findings indicate associations between family members' assumptions and both their attributions and expectancies about family interactions (cf. Baucom & Epstein, 1990; Epstein & Baucom, 1993), as well as with members' actual negative behavior toward each other (Bradbury & Fincham, 1993). Further research is needed to determine whether cognitive structures that exist before an individual enters a relationship shape the attributions and expectancies that he or she subsequently makes about events in the relationship.

Standards

Unrealistic or extreme standards have been implicated in a wide variety of family problems, such as child abuse, adjustment difficulties in stepfamilies, poor coping with an addicted family member, and ineffective control of children with conduct disorders. Rational-emotive therapy focuses on the distress that family members experience when (1) events in their relationships do not meet their unrealistic, extreme standards and (2) they evaluate the failure to meet those standards very negatively (e.g., as "awful" or "intolerable") (Dryden, 1984; Ellis, 1962). Beck's cognitive model (Beck, 1976; Beck et al., 1979) also emphasizes the role of extreme standards in producing distress in individuals' lives, viewing these relatively stable schemas as the bases of distortions in inferential processes such as attributions. Rational-emotive therapists have paid considerable attention to standards that specifically affect the quality of family relationships (Dryden, 1985; Ellis et al., 1989).

Standards can be based on experiences that people had in their own families as they were growing up, patterns that they observed in other families, or aspects of their family relationships in adulthood. Whereas some standards represent an individual's wish to re-create the best characteristics that he or she has observed in family relationships, in other cases standards involve attempts at avoiding unpleasant characteristics that one observed or experienced. For example, an individual whose family of origin spent large amounts of leisure time together may have come to believe that in a "good" family the individual members should not pursue independent interests and activities. A person whose family of origin was characterized by frequent aversive hostile arguments may have developed a standard that members of a family should avoid expressing conflict. In addition, people's standards about family relationships commonly are influenced by media representations (e.g., books, popular songs, movies) of intimate relationships that often involve idealized conditions, such as the stepfamily whose members quickly form cohesive relationships.

It is important to distinguish inappropriate, unrealistic standards from more reasonable standards that may guide people's ethical behavior with others. For example, the widely held standard that parents should not act in ways that cause physical or psychological damage to their children is neither unrealistic nor irrational. Unfortunately, individuals commonly are not able to distinguish between their standards that are dysfunctional (harmful to themselves or others) and those that facilitate individual and family functioning, as they experience both types of long-standing beliefs as familiar and appropriate. Consequently, treatment procedures for altering problematic standards involve aiding family members in a careful examination of the appropriateness and consequences of living according to their standards.

There appear to be a variety of ways in which family members' assumptions and standards can influence the quality of family relationships. Robin and Foster (1989), for example, describe a variety of "absolute assumptions" (some of which appear to be standards and some to be assumptions in the taxonomy we are using) commonly held by parents and adolescents that contribute to parent–child conflict. Recurrent themes involve perfectionism (e.g., "Teenagers should always behave responsibly"), ruination (e.g., "If we permit him to stay out late, he will become an irresponsible adult"), fairness (e.g., "My parents should be at least as lenient as my friends' parents"), love/approval (e.g., "If my mother really loved me, she wouldn't question what I do"), obedience (e.g., "Young people have no right to challenge their parents' decisions"), self-blame (e.g., "If he fails at school, I'm a bad mother"), malicious intent (which appears to involve attributions; e.g., "My daughter is trying to drive me crazy"), and autonomy (e.g., "I'm all grown up at 16 and should be able to go out with anyone I like"). Robin and Foster note that such extreme views polarize family members into inflexible positions that impede problem solving and increase anger, which itself interferes with the use of constructive communication skills and increases reciprocal negative exchanges. Similarly, the role of unrealistic standards in stepfamily problems (e.g., emotional bonds developing instantly among members who previously were not related) has been described by family educators and therapists (Leslie & Epstein, 1988; Sager et al., 1983; Stuart & Jacobson, 1985; Visher & Visher, 1988). Clinicians who work with a variety of other family problems also have described how unrealistic standards can interfere with constructive family functioning. For example, Schlesinger (1988) discusses how the beliefs of family members of substance abusers and addicts concerning how a caring relative should treat another family member produce guilt and inertia when the family is faced with the need to set very firm limits (e.g., making it clear to the addict that he or she will not receive support without entering treatment for the addiction).

In contrast, Baucom, Epstein, Rankin, and Burnett (1996) found that, in a sample of community couples, adherence to standards emphasizing investment in one's marriage (e.g., that partners should spend a lot of time sharing leisure activities) was associated with greater marital satisfaction. Spouses' marital satisfaction was only weakly associated with the strength of their adherence to particular standards but strongly correlated with the degree to which spouses reported that they were satisfied with the manner in which their standards were met in their ongoing relationship. In other words, as long as a couple found acceptable ways to meet the two partners' standards, even if their standards were strong and different, the spouses reported satisfaction with their marriage. Thus, strong belief in standards concerning one's intimate relationships is not necessarily dysfunctional, and in fact it can contribute to a positive relationship, depending on the type of standard and the individuals' satisfaction with how their standards are met in their relationship.

BEHAVIORAL FACTORS IN FAMILY DYSFUNCTION

Family therapists who use a cognitive-behavioral approach to understanding and treating close relationships generally focus on behavioral aspects of family interactions as major targets of therapy (cf. Falloon, 1991; Robin & Foster, 1989). These include (1) excesses of negative behaviors and deficits in pleasing behaviors exchanged by family members, (2) expressive and listening skills used in communication, (3) problem-solving skills, and (4) negotiation and behavior change skills. The theoretical models underlying behavioral approaches to family therapy are social learning theory (e.g., Bandura, 1977) and social exchange theory (e.g., Thibaut & Kelley, 1959). Both models assume that family members exert mutual influences over each other's behavior. Social learning theory emphasizes that interpersonal behavior is learned, especially through operant conditioning and through vicarious observation of other people's actions and consequences, and that current behavior is controlled by its actual or expected consequences. Social exchange theory describes an interpersonal relationship as an economic exchange in which each person's satisfaction is a function of the ratio of the benefits received to the costs incurred. It is assumed that in a satisfying relationship the parties exchange rewards in a reciprocal manner and restrain the escalation of negative exchanges. In contrast, relationship distress is associated with relatively uncontrolled reciprocity in exchanges of aversive, coercive behavior (Falloon, 1991).

Social learning theory and social exchange theory have strongly influenced behaviorally oriented research and clinical practice with families. The following are representative findings concerning the four types of behaviors that are foci of cognitive-behavioral assessment and treatment with families.

Pleasing and Displeasing Behavior Exchanges

As noted, social exchange theory postulates that exchanges in a relationship tend to be reciprocal; that is, each party tends to give what he or she receives from the other person. Consistent with a social learning perspective, research by Patterson and his colleagues has demonstrated reciprocal coercion patterns in families, in which each member's behavior both elicits and reinforces aversive behavior in other members (e.g., Patterson, 1982). For example, parents may reinforce their children's negative behavior by selectively paying attention to it and failing to notice and encourage positive behavior. Furthermore, many parents attempt to reduce their children's negative behavior by means of aversive behavior such as insults, threats, and physical punishment. Patterson (1982) notes that at best such parental strategies typically suppress unwanted child behavior only temporarily (while the punisher is present), and that they teach the children that aggression is an acceptable means of expressing anger and dissatisfaction with other people. The behavioral interventions Patterson and his colleagues have developed (e.g., Patterson, 1975; Patterson & Forgatch, 1987) focus on changing the behaviors of both children and parents that contribute to coercive cycles.

Communication Skills Deficits

Research on family communication behavior typically has involved coding family interactions according to a standard system (see Grotevant and Carlson, 1989, and Markman and Notarius, 1987, for reviews). Studies using behavioral coding systems have indicated that distressed families exhibit higher rates of negative communication behaviors and lower rates of positive communication behaviors than those who are nondistressed (Baucom & Adams, 1987; Markman & Notarius, 1987; Patterson, 1982). Furthermore, investigations of behavioral *sequences* between spouses and between parents and children (Gottman, 1994; Margolin & Wampold, 1981; Patterson, 1982; Revenstorf, Hahlweg, Schindler, & Vogel, 1984) have identified interaction patterns common in distressed relationships, particularly escalating aversive exchanges. Such findings emphasize the *mutual* influence process in negative family communication. Given the consistent theoretical and empirical support for the importance of clear and constructive communication in family relationships, the assessment and modification of communication problems is an important component of cognitive-behavioral therapy for family problems.

Some problems in communication among family members involve misinterpretations, wherein messages that one person intends to send are received inaccurately. These discrepancies can result from faulty expression by the person sending the message (e.g., vague messages, frequent topic shifts), or from ineffective listening by the recipient (e.g., formulating responses to the other person rather than attending carefully to what he or she is saying). At other times, family members complain that they cannot communicate, when in fact they receive messages from each other clearly but find them unacceptable, either because the messages are sent in an aversive manner (e.g., a sarcastic tone; threatening words) or because the recipient does not agree with the ideas expressed. When assessing family communication, it is crucial to distinguish among these different kinds of communication problems. When there are real deficits in expressive and listening skills, communication skills training can be used. In contrast, when family members send aversive verbal and nonverbal messages, skills training may also be appropriate, but it also may be important to identify and modify emotions (e.g., strong anger) and cognitions (e.g., an attribution that a child's misbehavior is caused by malicious intent) that can influence an individual's tendency to send aversive messages. Furthermore, when a complaint of poor communication represents conflict among family members' preferences or values, intervention would focus much more on conflict resolution.

Problem-Solving Skills Deficits

Families inevitably are faced with a variety of problems that require them to work as a unit to devise and implement solutions. These problems range from the relatively trivial (e.g., how to coordinate transportation when one of the family cars is inoperable) to major issues affecting family life (e.g., how the family should cope with a parent's unemployment and the associated financial problems). Problem solving is a cognitive-behavioral process that involves the abilities to (1) clearly define the nature of a problem in behavioral terms, (2) identify alternative solutions, (3) evaluate the relative costs and benefits of the alternative solutions, (4) reach family consensus on a solution, (5) implement the solution (with each family member fulfilling his or her specific role), and (6) evaluate the effectiveness of the solution and revise it if necessary (Baucom & Epstein, 1990; Bornstein & Bornstein, 1986; Epstein & Baucom, 2002; Jacobson & Christensen, 1996; Jacobson & Margolin, 1979; Robin & Foster, 1989; Stuart, 1980). Deficits in problem-solving skills have been identified among members of dysfunctional family relationships such as distressed parent–adolescent relationships (Robin & Foster, 1989), distressed couples (Schaap, 1984), abusive parents (Azar, Robinson, Hekimian, & Twentyman, 1984), and families of schizophrenics (Falloon, Boyd, & McGill, 1984). Consequently, training in problem-solving skills is an important focus of behavioral interventions for family conflict (Epstein et al., 1988; Falloon, 1991; Robin & Foster, 1989).

Behavior Change Skills Deficits

Once members of a family have generated promising solutions to problems, the degree to which the solutions are in fact implemented is likely to be due at least in part to the family members' skills for encouraging and reinforcing each other's behavior changes. Coercion (e.g., threats, punishment) and other forms of negative communication have been found to be common dysfunctional ways in which members of distressed family relationships attempt to resolve their conflicts and problems (Patterson, 1982; Robin & Foster, 1989; Schaap, 1984). Cognitive-behavioral family therapists often assist families in constructing behavioral contracts that structure the behavior changes that each family member will make in order to implement a solution, such that "win–lose" orientations are avoided. Contracts range from the highly structured *quid pro quo* form, in which each member of a relationship agrees to behave in certain ways in exchange for particular behavior changes by other members, to *holistic* contracts (Stuart, 1980) in which each individual agrees to behave in some ways requested (in a list) by other family members, with no reinforcements contingent on doing so. Parents often are aided in setting up contracts with children and adolescents in which specific rewards and punishments are provided for specific types of positive and negative behavior, respectively (Falloon, 1991; Patterson & Forgatch, 1987).

Marital Factors in Family Dysfunction

Research on the relationship between the state of a couple's marriage and the emotional and physical well-being of the partners and their offspring seems to establish a clear link between a happy, stable marriage and better physical and emotional health for both parents and children. In contrast, chronic unresolved marital conflict commonly affects the emotional well-being of partners and their children (Burman & Margolin, 1992; Diener, Suh, Lucas, & Smith, 1999; Schmaling & Sher, 2000). It has been associated with child and parent depression, child behavioral problems, academic difficulties, and children's social problems (Amato & Booth, 1997; Amato & Keith, 1991; Cowan & Cowan, 1999; Davies & Cummings, 1994; Forehand, Brody, Long, Slotkin, & Fauber, 1986; Hetherington, Bridges, & Insabella, 1998; Katz & Gottman, 1993; O'Leary, Christian, & Mendell, 1994; Peterson & Zill, 1986). For those children from families in which unresolved marital conflict eventually leads to divorce, the emotional damage begins long before the legal formalities (Hetherington et al., 1998).

COGNITIVE INTERVENTIONS

Cognitive restructuring procedures are intended to help family members test whether their cognitions about aspects of family interaction are appropriate or valid. Because people generally do not question the validity of their thoughts, one of the therapist's major goals is to increase each family member's sensitivity as an *observer* of his or her own cognitions. A second goal is to help each family member become a systematic and relatively objective *evaluator* of those cognitions, developing skills for collecting data concerning their appropriateness and validity. The following are common strategies used in cognitive restructuring work with distressed families.

Building Cognitive Self-Monitoring Skills

Family members can be assisted in increasing their attention to their cognitions by teaching them about the ways in which cognitions can influence one's emotions and behaviors. The therapist can begin by presenting a brief didactic "mini-lecture" describing a cognitive mediation model and concrete examples of how individuals' responses to life events can be influenced by their interpretations of those events. It is important to introduce the concept of "cognitive distortion" gradually and tactfully, in order to minimize defensiveness on the part of family members. Members of distressed relationships tend to blame their partners for relationship problems and can become defensive if a therapist suggests that part of the problem lies in their own thought processes. Perhaps the best way to demonstrate the subjectivity of cognitions is to elicit a cognition from a family member and then elicit information from that person, supplemented by data from other family members, that disconfirms that cognition. In other words, family members are more likely to accept the validity of the cognitive mediation model if the therapist can demonstrate its operation with concrete examples from the clients' daily experiences. This socialization process is also employed in cognitive therapy with individuals (cf. Beck et al., 1979). The presence of other family members in conjoint sessions provides both the advantage of external sources of data concerning an individual's cognitions and the risk that the other members' responses may elicit defensiveness on the part of the individual whose cognitions are being evaluated.

Family members also are introduced to the concept of "automatic thoughts" (Beck et al., 1979) that occur spontaneously, are fleeting, may not be fully conscious, and seem highly plausible to the individual at the time when they occur. In order to help family members to increase their awareness of their cognitions, a therapist can teach them to notice when they have become upset by another family member *during a therapy session* and to ask themselves questions such as "What thoughts popped into my mind as I was getting upset with her?" and "When she acted that way, what did it *mean* to me that upset me?" Family members commonly are assigned the "homework" of recording their automatic thoughts (word for word), associated emotions, and behaviors in written logs such as Beck et al.'s (1979) Daily Record of Dysfunctional Thoughts (DRDT). As in individual cognitive therapy, the therapist reviews these records with each family member during sessions, identifying the specific content of automatic thoughts that is associated with particular emotions. Having family members observe this analysis of each other's situation–cognition–emotion links can increase mutual empathy, and members can give each other feedback that can alter interpretations of each other's behavior.

Another important aspect of improving monitoring skills involves logging *sequences* of interactions between the self and other family members. Cognitive-behavioral family therapists coach family members in avoiding unidirectional causal observations (seeing one's own behavior as caused by behaviors of other family members). Instead, family members are aided in observing how their own behavior elicits responses from other members as well, such that causes of negative family interactions tend to be circular. As noted earlier, members of distressed families are likely to blame each other for problems, so the therapist must exercise care in focusing on circular causality in order to minimize defensiveness.

Altering Selective Perceptions

During therapy sessions it often becomes evident that two or more family members have different perceptions either of a past event or of an event that has occurred as recently as during the session. The therapist can draw this perceptual discrepancy to their attention, emphasizing that it is natural for people to notice different aspects of a complex interaction, but noting that it is important for each family member to avoid assuming that he or she has noticed everything. When a therapist is able to videotape a therapy session, it is possible to first ask each family member for his or her recollections of an interaction that just took place and then to replay the tape in order to examine the accuracy and comprehensiveness of the perceptions.

Family members also can be coached in monitoring and recording their cognitions concerning interactions with other members in daily life. They can be sensitized to selective perception through comparisons of the perceptions that family members recorded concerning the same events. For example, it is common for family members to record different perceptions of who started an argument, with each person commonly perceiving a linear causal process in which his or her negative behaviors were elicited by another person's negative behavior. As is the case when the therapist points out instances of reciprocal causality in family interactions that occur during therapy sessions, the therapist can note possible mutual influences in family members' reports of negative exchanges at home. Also, when an individual's written logs include all-or-nothing perceptions of another family member's behavior, such as "He *always* . . . " or "She *never* . . .," the person can be coached in considering evidence for exceptions to such an absolute view.

Modifying Inaccurate Attributions

There are several skills that family members can be taught for testing the accuracy of the causal inferences that they make about family events. These approaches are similar to those used in individual cognitive therapy (e.g., J. Beck, 1995; A. Beck et al., 1979; A. Beck & Emery, 1985; Leahy, 1996), although the presence of other family members provides additional sources of data that may be lacking in individual treatment.

Using Socratic questioning, a therapist can guide family members in a "logical analysis" of attributions, essentially answering the question "Does it make logical sense that this event was due to the particular cause that you have inferred?" A second form of logical analysis is coaching family members in thinking of "alternative explanations" (attributions) for an event. Consistent with the collaborative empirical approach of cognitive therapy, the therapist notes that an individual's attribution may be accurate, but that it is important to consider other possibilities in order to avoid making a faulty inference that leads to emotional upset and negative behavioral interactions. One of the most powerful ways of demonstrating the negative effects of inaccurate attributions is to "catch" these when they occur during family therapy sessions. Thus, a therapist may observe that one family member has become upset at another member, and it appears to the therapist that the former person's upset may have been due to a faulty attribution about the cause of the second family member's behavior. The therapist can interrupt the interaction, explore the individual's attributions, and use input from all family members to test the accuracy of the attributions. When one family member attributes another's negative behavior to negative causes (e.g., unpleasant personality traits, malicious intent), the latter individual can provide feedback about what he or she sees as the actual cause of the behavior. Although such an explanation may be viewed with skepticism by the family member who made the original negative attribution, especially when it appears to be self-enhancing or a "rationalization," the therapist can stress the importance of considering all possible attributions seriously. At times, family members' feedback concerning alternative explanations for their own behavior can broaden each other's perspective and result in more benign attributions.

Modifying Inaccurate Expectancies

Cognitive restructuring with problematic expectancies is similar in form to the interventions used to modify negative attributions. Logical analysis of an expectancy involves examining whether it makes sense that other family members will react as expected if the individual behaves in a particular manner, as well as identifying other possible outcomes. Other data concerning the validity of an expectancy can be derived from family members' memories of past outcomes and logs of current outcomes in similar situations. *In vivo* behavioral experiments are the most powerful tool for addressing maladaptive expectancies. Although the experiments can be quite anxiety-provoking for the person who expects negative consequences for his or her behavior, these experiments (enacted during therapy sessions and at home) provide vivid, incontrovertible evidence that the outcome is not as predicted.

Modifying Unrealistic or Inappropriate Assumptions and Standards

Several cognitive restructuring methods used to test and alter perceptions, attributions, and expectancies can be applied with assumptions and standards as well. These include logical analysis, examination of alternative assumptions and standards that may be more appropriate for the family's current circumstances, and identification of experiences (including behavioral experiments devised during therapy sessions) that are or are not consistent with the assumptions and standards. In addition, family members can be coached in examining the *utility* of living according to a particular standard (e.g., "Children should never question their parents' rules regarding the children's responsibilities"). This involves generating lists of the advantages and disadvantages of adhering to the standard, deciding whether the balance of disadvantages versus advantages suggests that a revised standard may be appropriate, substituting a more realistic or appropriate standard when that seems prudent, and experimenting with living according to the new standard (Epstein et al., 1988). Therapists should be sensitive to the discomfort that commonly arises when individuals' long-standing assumptions and standards about family relationships are challenged, understanding the need for a supportive environment in which family members can explore alternative beliefs that are palatable to them.

BEHAVIORAL INTERVENTIONS

As noted, dysfunctional behavioral patterns commonly are associated with family problems, regardless of the specific content of the problem (e.g., child abuse, stepfamily conflicts), and they typically involve excessive exchanges of negative behaviors, deficits in exchanges of positive behaviors, communication skill deficits, and problem-solving skill deficits. The following are descriptions of interventions that cognitive-behavioral family therapists commonly use to address each type of behavioral problem.

Altering Behavioral Exchanges

Members of some families are able to increase their exchanges of positive affectional and instrumental behaviors with no guidance other than a therapist stressing to them how much daily exchanges affect the subjective quality of close relationships. Other families, however, have low rates of positive exchanges because they spend little time together. Not only can a lack of shared activities detract from long-standing relationships, but it also can interfere with the establishment of cohesion in newly formed relationships such as those of stepfamilies (Leslie & Epstein, 1988). Consequently, therapists can help family members to identify activities that they could share and to agree to engage in certain activities from the list between therapy sessions. For clients who have difficulty generating lists of potentially pleasurable activities, therapists can provide written lists of activities that other couples and families have tended to enjoy (Baucom & Epstein, 1990).

Similarly, therapists can coach family members in generating lists of aversive behaviors that they exchange. They can then reach agreements that all family members will attempt to decrease particular negative behaviors, in conjunction with their efforts to increase positive exchanges. Sometimes family members' negative cognitions about each other's intentions must be addressed before they will feel motivated to stop behaving negatively toward each other.

Contingency contracting can be used when families have difficulty adhering to informal agreements to change their behaviors. When used with families, contracting sometimes is described as if the parents are trained as therapists who reinforce positive changes in their children's behavior. However, Goldenberg and Goldenberg (1991) note that these procedures in fact change the parents' behavior toward their children as well (e.g., reducing parents' inconsistency and use of aversive behavior to control their children). There are excellent texts (e.g., Barkley & Benton, 1998; Patterson &

Forgatch, 1987) that can be used as instructional aids in teaching clients parenting skills, including the monitoring of children's behaviors and the implementation of reward systems.

Contracts can vary, as such, in their degree of structure, and the degree to which one person's behavior changes are contingent on another person also making desired changes. However, what contracts have in common is that they direct family members to identify specific pleasing and displeasing behaviors that they would like each other to increase or decrease. Furthermore, contracts emphasize collaborative efforts toward making desired behavior changes.

Communication Skills Training

Most commonly, family therapists focus on behavioral skills involved in (1) expressing messages to other family members and (2) listening effectively to messages sent by others. Skills training typically involves giving family members specific instructions about problematic and constructive forms of communication. This may include handouts and other reading material, and is accompanied by specific feedback about the family's own communication behavior. Specific, constructive communication behaviors are then modeled, and the family is coached in communication skills during therapy sessions (Baucom & Epstein, 1990; Epstein et al., 1988; Robin & Foster, 1989). Guerney's (1977) Relationship Enhancement program provides guidelines for expressive and empathic listening skills. For example, a person expressing his or her thoughts and emotions is to be brief and specific, acknowledge the subjectivity of the feelings, note positive as well as negative aspects of situations being described, and convey empathy for the listener's position. The listener's goal is to understand the expresser's subjective experience and convey that understanding to him or her by paraphrasing the message back to the expresser. The listener is to avoid introducing his or her own thoughts and emotions about the topic discussed by the expresser.

In addition to focusing on the expressive and listening skills, therapists commonly conduct individualized assessments of excesses and deficits in a particular family's communication behaviors. For example, in their work with families that include a schizophrenic member, Falloon et al. (1984) look for problems such as deficits in eye contact, confusing body posture and gestures, lack of variation in facial expressions and vocal tone, poverty of content in verbal messages, vagueness, mixed messages, overgeneralized statements, interruptions, and hostile threats. Robin and Foster's (1989) communication training with adolescents and their parents also focuses on teaching constructive alternatives to a variety of negative behaviors (e.g., making "I statements" rather than accusing or blaming, or suggesting alternative solutions rather than threatening the other person).

Problem-Solving Skills Training

Training families in problem-solving skills includes the same components of instruction, feedback, modeling, and coaching in behavioral rehearsal used in the training of expressive and listening skills. The emphasis is on collaborative efforts to define a problem in terms of observable behaviors, "brainstorm" possible solutions, evaluate the costs and benefits of solutions, select a solution that will be implemented, specify who in the family is responsible for enacting each component of the solution, attempt to implement the solution, and evaluate its effectiveness in resolving the problem. Problem-solving skills training is widely used in the treatment of couple and family problems (e.g., Baucom & Epstein, 1990; Bornstein & Bornstein, 1986; Epstein et al., 1988; Falloon et al., 1984; Jacobson & Christensen, 1996; Jacobson & Margolin, 1979; Robin & Foster, 1989).

Marital Interventions

Because the quality of a marriage has significant consequences for family health, a comprehensive approach to family treatment includes evaluating how the couple's marital functioning may contribute to the family dysfunction, and recommending ways for parents to address those marital problems. Although some couples are aware that their marital conflicts are affecting their children, others find the suggestion that they examine their own relationship threatening, and want a family therapist to focus on the child's problems. Consequently, the therapist must use tact and good timing in suggesting to a couple that addressing particular aspects of their own interactions may help in the treatment of their child. One strategy is to focus on the couple's ability to work together effectively as a "team" to help their child overcome his or her difficulties. Even though the therapist may talk to the couple primarily about their relationship as a parental team, the therapeutic interventions (e.g., communication and problem-solving training) will in fact target the basic behavioral and cognitive processes that affect their overall marital quality. It is beyond the scope of this chapter to consider the assessment and treatment of marital difficulties, but several references describe the cognitive and behavioral procedures comprehensively (Baucom & Epstein, 1990; Epstein & Baucom, 1989, 1998, 2002; Epstein & Schlesinger, 1991; Rathus & Sanderson, 1999; Schlesinger & Epstein, 1986). Empirical research has provided support for the effectiveness of cognitive-behavioral marital therapy (Baucom, Shoham, Mueser, Daiuto, & Stickle, 1998).

In addition to considering *therapy* for a couple as a resource to address marital problems, a therapist can refer a couple to one of a number of recently developed couple *education* programs to teach the skills associated with happy and satisfying relationships (Floyd, Markman, Kelly, Blumberg,

& Stanley, 1995; Van Widenfelt, Markman, Guerney, Behrens, & Hosman, 1997). Some couples prefer a nontherapy setting for relationship skill building, and, for all but seriously deteriorated relationships, an educational workshop or seminar may be quite appropriate. Of the many relationship education programs now available, some have been constructed by their founders from a base of research. For example, Prevention and Relationship Enhancement (PREP) stems from the work of Howard Markman, Scott Stanley, and Susan Blumberg at the University of Denver (Markman, Floyd, Stanley, & Jamieson, 1984; Stanley, Blumberg, & Markman, 1999). PREPARE (a program for engaged couples available fairly widely through churches and synagogues) and ENRICH (a program for experienced couples) grew out of the work of David Olson and his colleagues at the University of Minnesota (Fowers & Olson, 1986; Olson & Fowers, 1993). Sherod and Phyllis Miller in Littleton, Colorado, developed their Couple Communication programs in part from earlier research in Minnesota (Miller, Nunnally, Wachman, & Miller, 1991; Russell, Bagarozzi, Atilanao, & Morris, 1984).

The variety of available couple education programs is represented in the self-help literature and on the Internet. Berger and Hannah's (1999) edited volume is a collection of program descriptions prepared by each program's founders and includes further citations to their work. A listing of couple education resources is included in the reference section of this chapter. Although outcome research on brief, educational skills training for couples is far less plentiful than research on couple therapy, the available results suggest that couple education programs effectively increase communication skills, reduce negative aspects of couple conflict (including the incidence of violent acting out), increase relationship satisfaction, and stem the attrition of quality over time normally found in marriages (see, e.g., Halford & Moore, 2002; Markman, Floyd, Stanley, & Storaasli, 1988; Hahlweg, Markman, Thurmaier, Engl, & Eckert, 1998; Wampler, 1990). A prudent interpretation of data from studies of couple education programs must take into account the samples upon which conclusions were drawn. Study couples tended to have relatively high pretreatment functioning, and the effectiveness of these programs for poorly functioning couples has yet to be tested. As the level of marital dysfunction increases for a couple, so too may their need for the greater intensity of couple therapy.

CASE EXAMPLE

Frank and Alice (ages 40 and 38, respectively) sought assistance at an agency providing child and family mental health services because of their 13-year-old daughter Jane's behavior problems. Jane had been getting into trouble at school for smoking and truancy, and at home she was uncooperative with parental requests, stayed out beyond her curfew, and used disrespectful language with both parents. Diagnostically, Jane appeared to meet criteria for oppositional defiant disorder as defined in the *Diagnostic and Statistical Manual of Mental Disorders*, fourth edition (DSM-IV; American Psychiatric Association, 1994). Frank and Alice's 15-year-old son Robert also accompanied them to the first session, and both parents noted that he had no history of behavior problems at home or at school. During the therapist's initial interview with the family, Jane alternated between arguing with her parents and withdrawing from them. Robert was fairly quiet and responded to questions by his parents and the therapist in a polite manner.

The therapist conducted a systematic inquiry about (1) the family members' definitions of the problem for which they had sought help; (2) the history of the problem, including its development over time and the ways in which the family had attempted to solve it up to this point; and (3) the family's overall developmental history, including any significant positive and negative life events that had occurred since the time when the parents first met and established their relationship. The therapist tried to identify any events that affected the parents' own relationship and bore on the family problems. Generally, it is important to curtail this type of inquiry if parents become defensive, in order to preserve the option of pursuing remedies during treatment. This information was collected in order to help the therapist understand the nature of the presenting problem within its family context. In other words, the therapist took it at face value that Jane's behavior was problematic for her parents (and for school officials) but also began to look for characteristics of family interactions that may have contributed to the development and/or maintenance of the aversive behavior. Thus, the therapist's evaluation of the family during the initial interview and subsequent sessions was based not only on what they described during the interview, but also on how they interacted with each other in the therapist's office.

Although Frank and Alice had presented their problem as "Jane's nasty, defiant behavior, caused by her poor attitude about taking on responsibilities in life," the therapist's systematic assessment revealed that the family's problems were more complex than that. The following were some of the salient patterns observed by the therapist:

1. The father–daughter relationship had been close until Jane reached adolescence and sought greater independence from the family. As Jane spent less time talking with her father or accompanying her parents on family outings, and more time visiting her friends, Frank increasingly attempted to restrict her independence. Jane responded to her father's restrictive behavior by arguing with him and disobeying him.

2. The mother–daughter relationship was strained, but not to the same extent as the father–daughter relationship. In fact, Alice was more ac-

cepting of Jane's becoming independent than was Frank. Alice related to the therapist that she remembered her own need to be independent during adolescence, and her own struggles with her parents. At times she sided with Frank concerning Jane's negative behavior, but on other occasions she expressed disagreement with him in front of Jane. During one heated exchange between Frank and Jane in the therapist's office, Alice interrupted Frank, telling him that he was too strict and that Jane needed to develop friendships apart from the family.

3. Jane complained that her parents, particularly her father, applied a double standard for her behavior versus her brother Robert's behavior, and this appeared to the therapist to be true. Neither parent questioned Robert about his activities outside the home to the extent that they inquired about Jane's plans and activities. Alice told the therapist that her husband seemed especially protective of Jane, and Frank agreed that this was so, because he did not think that a young girl could handle "difficult situations" that might come up in dealing with other people.

4. The parents appeared to have had some chronic conflict in their marital relationship, particularly concerning their roles as parents, and their philosophies about child rearing. Alice tended to base her child rearing practices on her belief that children need to have opportunities to learn from their own mistakes, whereas Frank acted on his belief that it is the parents' responsibility to protect their children from misfortune, even if it means restricting the children's freedom. It also was clear to the therapist that the couple lacked emotional intimacy in their relationship. The relative lack of close feelings seemed to create chronic tension, so it took little to set off an argument. The couple often had loud verbal fights about parenting issues, which rarely proceeded to resolution. Jane described their fights to the therapist and said that she found them very upsetting, especially when her parents made comparisons between herself and Robert. Robert said that he did not like to hear his parents fighting, but that it really was not any of his business.

5. One area in which the parents were united in their concern about Jane involved her academic problems. They both restricted her social activities when they received negative reports from school officials, which Jane felt was "unfair."

The initial assessment of this family revealed that although Jane's negative behavior at home and at school was problematic in itself, the interactions among the members of her family exacerbated her "acting out." Further assessment was focused on identifying cognitive and behavioral factors that contributed to the escalation of conflict in the family.

One of Jane's *perceptions* about her family was revealed when she stated, "I *never* get to have any fun." Although she truly believed this to be an accurate perception, when she was asked to describe her activities over the course of a week she was able to identify a number of experiences (particularly time spent with friends) that had been pleasurable. Similarly, Alice's statement about her husband's relationship with their children, "He's so rigid with the rules and doesn't give of himself to the children," failed to take into account instances of flexible and nurturant behavior that he exhibited.

Interviews revealed a variety of *attributions* that family members were making related to Jane's behavior. For example, Alice stated that Frank was especially restrictive with Jane "because he has old-fashioned values, a double standard for boys and girls." When the therapist asked Jane for her thoughts about her parents' reasons for allowing Robert more independence, she said, "They love him more than me; they trust him more than me." It was important for the therapist to help the family examine the validity of each of these distressing attributions.

Concerning *expectancies* that were associated with problematic family interaction, Frank expressed the idea that "If I don't scream at Jane to let out my frustration, I'll develop an ulcer. I know it's unhealthy to keep your feelings bottled up." Unfortunately, the actual outcome of his screaming was to elicit anger, screaming, and withdrawal from Jane (which frustrated Frank further). When discussing parental conflict about childrearing practices, Alice expressed the expectancy, "If I try to negotiate with Frank about child rearing, it will be futile." Not only did this turn out to be an inaccurate overgeneralization, but it was a thought that made Alice angry on many occasions.

Jane expressed an *assumption* she held that parents cannot understand their children because of the age difference between them. This assumption clearly reduced her willingness to listen to her own parents' views about her behavior. Frank revealed that although he readily argued with Jane, he avoided open conflict with his wife, because he assumed that disagreements are a sign of marital problems. He also held an assumption that his concerns about his daughter were "no different from any father's concerns." Frank was not aware that his restrictiveness had reached an unreasonably high level. As is generally the case with basic cognitive structures, the members of the family did not consider questioning their long standing assumptions about family relationships; they took the validity of their cognitions for granted.

The therapist uncovered a variety of *standards* held by the family members that appeared to influence their interactions. For example, Robert expressed the belief that "A good child always obeys his or her parents." As a consequence, he was excessively conforming to his parents' requests and became very angry at his sister whenever she questioned their parents' authority. Frank held a standard that "Mothers should *always* support fathers when the fathers are attempting to discipline their children." Consequently, Frank became angry at Alice whenever she disagreed with his strict discipline of Jane. Frank also believed that children should adopt the values, beliefs, and preferences of their parents. Whenever there was evidence that the family did not share a common worldview, Frank became quite upset.

There was clear evidence of a marked drop in *positive affectional and instrumental behaviors* exchanged by the family members, particularly between father and daughter, but also between the spouses. The family members spent little time together, and when they were together their interactions focused on problems concerning Jane. It was not surprising that none of the family members felt much satisfaction about their relationships.

Frank and Jane perceived each other as inflexible, so neither listened carefully to the other's opinions, and both began any discussion with defensive and attacking messages. In contrast, each of them expressed feelings and listened well when talking individually with the therapist. Another communication problem identified was a high rate of coercive messages (threats, criticism, insults) between father and daughter, and between the spouses. Furthermore, samples of the family's conversations indicated that they used vague terms when attempting to express their concerns and requests to each other. Finally, they typically became caught in escalating cycles of negative exchange that they were only able to interrupt when one of the involved family members escaped the interaction (e.g., Jane running out of the house).

The therapist learned that both parents used effective problem-solving skills in their jobs, but not at home. As a group, the family tended to criticize each other's suggested solutions to problems, and when the parents felt pressured, they tended to try to implement the first solution that came to mind.

Frank and Alice had tried to institute their own version of a *quid pro quo* behavioral contract, specifying positive actions that they would take if Jane exhibited particular positive behaviors. Unfortunately, as soon as Jane failed to comply with any aspect of the contract, her father withdrew all of his positive behavior toward her. She responded to his punitiveness with oppositional behavior (creating a new negative escalation).

As noted, Jane attributed her father's restrictive behavior to a lack of love for her. The therapist helped her to modify this inaccurate and maladaptive attribution by generating alternative explanations, such as "He is very worried about some harm possibly coming to me" and "He is very attached to me and finds it hard to have me leave home." When she described past occasions when she shared leisure activities with her father and kept a log of similar events for 2 weeks, there were several instances in which Frank had expressed his caring for Jane. Furthermore, during a family therapy session the therapist was able to elicit Frank's fears that his daughter could be harmed in what he saw as an increasingly dangerous world. The therapist also helped the family to plan and conduct a behavioral experiment in which Jane calmly proposed an outing for herself with her friends, describing to her father the precautions she would take to protect her well-being. She listened calmly while her father expressed his concerns to her, and then made sure that she was home on time. After the family had conducted the experiment, all expressed satisfaction with the outcome. Jane remarked that she could see that her father's restrictiveness was more likely due to worry than to a lack of caring.

The therapist helped Alice modify her expectancy that any attempts to negotiate with Frank would be futile. Her expectancy shifted when the therapist coached the couple in problem solving about ways of dealing with Jane's oppositional behavior, and Frank agreed to a compromise that was acceptable to Alice. It was clear to the therapist that Frank and Alice were uncomfortable with the idea of focusing on their marital relationship. It was equally clear that interventions that improved their functioning as a "parental team" would improve the overall health and functioning of both the marriage and the family. Consequently, the therapist expressed empathy for the couple's frustration about Jane's behavior, and then suggested that the couple would most likely be more effective in dealing with her if they consistently worked as a parenting team. The therapist noted that when parents present a united front, children and adolescents quickly learn that they need to take parental direction seriously. The therapist pointed out some recent incidents in which Jane had used a parental argument as an opportunity to do what she pleased. Alice and Frank readily acknowledged this pattern, and the therapist then proposed to them that a few couple sessions focused on communication and joint problem solving could decrease the chance of similar situations in the future.

The therapist then worked on communication and problem-solving skills with Frank and Alice during several couple sessions. In order to maintain the momentum of the family therapy as well, the therapist scheduled one couple session and one family session per week. Frank and Alice recognized that their poor conflict resolution skills were interfering with their parenting, and they decided that their marriage and family would benefit from some additional intervention. Consequently, as a supplement to the family treatment, the therapist referred Frank and Alice to a skill-building couples' educational program to bolster their ability to talk about and resolve problems, and to improve their ability to maintain an emotionally intimate marriage. As the couple addressed their own relationship problems, their ability to resolve parent–child issues improved.

Frank held the standard that children should adopt the values and preferences of their parents. Consistent with the rational-emotive therapy concept of an "irrational belief," Frank concluded that it would be "awful" if his children did not conform to his values and standards. The therapist attempted, as a consequence, to help Frank modify his standard. When the therapist explored the logic of the standard with Frank, he could see that it was unrealistic to expect children to become replicas of their parents. Frank acknowledged that no two people are exactly alike, due to a complex inter-action of innate temperament and unique life experiences. Furthermore, when asked to review what he had observed about other families whom he knew, he described some families in which the children clearly had devel-oped some values and preferences that were different from those of their parents, with no apparent ill effects on the children or the parent–child re-lationships.

In spite of these interventions, Frank continued to cling to his belief that his children should share his values and preferences. When the thera-pist coached him in listing advantages and disadvantages of the standard, it became clear that, from Frank's perspective, there were some compelling advantages to maintain it. For example, Frank noted that in a home where everyone agreed about everything, there would be no conflict (which was important to him, because he was very uncomfortable with overt conflict). He also noted that having his children mirror his views was comforting and bolstered his self-esteem. Finally, having such predictable children mini-mized a parent's need to worry about the children's welfare, another issue quite salient to Frank.

On the other hand, Frank was able to see that pressuring children to conform could impair their personal development, leaving them with lower self-confidence and little ability to think for themselves. He saw this as a se-rious deficit, because he viewed the world as a difficult place in which to live that demanded self-confidence and an ability to make decisions in the face of potentially harmful outside pressures. Another disadvantage that Frank saw in his standard was that a household in which everyone was the same actually could become boring.

Frank concluded that although there were advantages to his standard, the disadvantages pointed to a need to soften his views. With the help of the therapist and his family, he devised a more tolerant revised standard: "Parents should share with their children the knowledge that they have gained through their experiences of living in the world, including informa-tion about opportunities and dangers; however, they also should encourage each child to develop a healthy identity and self-esteem, which at times is likely to involve the child's testing him- or herself against the world, includ-ing the parents." Frank found the revised standard acceptable and agreed to devise behavioral experiments consistent with the alternative philosophy that he, Jane, and Robert could enact. After repeated successful experi-ments, Frank began to *believe* the alternative philosophy.

The therapist helped the family plan some shared leisure time during which there would be no discussion of problems. Given Jane's emerging need for independence, the therapist attempted to structure just enough joint activity to increase cohesion but not so much as to threaten Jane's de-veloping sense of autonomy. Furthermore, communication training was used to decrease the aversive messages, interruptions, and other dysfunctional behaviors common in this family. All of the family members felt more respect from each other when they were able to use expressive and listening skills effectively. The therapist also taught the family problem-solving skills, which they applied to responsibilities for household chores, independent activities by the children, and decision making about family leisure activities. Finally, the therapist helped the parents enact a contract with Jane, in which she received specific rewards that she desired in return for completing her chores and being home on time.

REFERENCES

Amato, P. R., & Booth, A. (1997). *A generation at risk*. Cambridge, MA: Harvard University Press.

Amato, P. R., & Keith, B. (1991). Parental divorce and the well-being of children: A meta-analysis. *Psychological Bulletin, 110,* 26–46.

American Psychiatric Association. (1994). *Diagnostic and statistical manual of mental disorders* (4th ed.). Washington, DC: Author.

Arias, I., & Beach, S. R. H. (1987). Assessment of social cognition in the context of marriage. In K. D. O'Leary (Ed.), *Assessment of marital discord: An integration for research and clinical practice* (pp. 109–137). Hillsdale, NJ: Erlbaum.

Azar, S. T. (1986, November). *Identifying at-risk populations: A research strategy for developing more specific risk indicators and screening devices*. Paper presented at the annual meeting of the Association for Advancement of Behavior Therapy, Chicago.

Azar, S. T., Robinson, D., Hekimian, E., & Twentyman, C. T. (1984). Unrealistic expectations and problem solving ability in maltreating and comparison mothers. *Journal of Consulting and Clinical Psychology, 52,* 687–691.

Bandura, A. (1977). *Social learning theory*, Englewood Cliffs, NJ: Prentice-Hall.

Barkley, R. A., & Benton, C. M. (1998). *Your defiant child: Eight steps to better behavior*. New York: Guilford Press.

Baucom, D. H. (1987). Attributions in distressed relations: How can we explain them? In S. Duck & D. Perlman (Eds.), *Heterosexual relations, marriage and divorce* (pp. 177–206). London: Sage.

Baucom, D. H., & Adams, A. (1987). Assessing communication in marital interaction. In K. D. O'Leary (Ed.), *Assessment of marital discord* (pp. 139–182). Hillsdale, NJ: Erlbaum.

Baucom, D. H., & Epstein, N. (1990). *Cognitive-behavioral marital therapy*. New York: Brunner/Mazel.

Baucom, D. H., Epstein, N., Rankin, L. A., & Burnett, C. K. (1996). Assessing relationship standards: The Inventory of Specific Relationship Standards. *Journal of Family Psychology, 10,* 72–88.

Baucom, D. H., Epstein, N., Sayers, S., & Sher, T. G. (1989). The role of cognitions in marital relationships: Definitional, methodological, and conceptual issues. *Journal of Consulting and Clinical Psychology, 57,* 31–38.

Baucom, D. H., Shoham, V., Mueser, K. T., Daiuto, A. D., & Stickle, T. R. (1998). Empirically supported couple and family interventions for marital distress and adult mental health problems. *Journal of Consulting and Clinical Psychology, 66,* 53–88.

Beck, A. T. (1976). *Cognitive therapy and the emotional disorders.* New York: International Universities Press.

Beck, A. T. (1988). *Love is never enough.* New York: Harper & Row.

Beck, A. T., & Emery, G. (1985). *Anxiety disorders and phobias: A cognitive perspective.* New York: Basic Books.

Beck, A. T., Rush, A. J., Shaw, B. F., & Emery, G. (1979). *Cognitive therapy of depression.* New York: Guilford Press.

Beck, J. S. (1995). *Cognitive therapy: Basics and beyond.* New York: Guilford Press.

Berger, R., & Hannah, M. T. (1999). *Preventive approaches in couples therapy.* Philadelphia: Brunner/Mazel.

Bornstein, P. H., & Bornstein, M. T. (1986). *Marital therapy: A behavioral-communications approach.* New York: Pergamon Press.

Bradbury, T. N., & Fincham, F. D. (1990). Attributions in marriage: Review and critique. *Psychological Bulletin, 107,* 3–33.

Bradbury, T. N., & Fincham, F. D. (1992). Attributions and behavior in marital interaction. *Journal of Personality and Social Psychology, 63,* 613–628.

Bradbury, T. N., & Fincham, F. D. (1993). Assessing dysfunctional cognition in marriage: A reconsideration of the Relationship Belief Inventory. *Psychological Assessment, 5,* 92–101.

Burman, N., & Margolin, G. (1992). Analysis of the association between marital relationships and health problems: An interactional perspective. *Psychological Bulletin, 112,* 39–63.

Cowan, P., & Cowan, C. P. (1999). *When partners become parents.* Hillsdale, NJ: Erlbaum.

Dattilio, F. M. (1994). Families in crisis. In F. M. Dattilio & A. Freeman (Eds.), *Cognitive-behavioral strategies in crisis intervention* (pp. 278–301). New York: Guilford Press.

Dattilio, F. M. (1998). Cognitive-behavioral family therapy. In F. M. Dattilio (Ed.), *Case studies in couple and family therapy: Systemic and cognitive perspectives* (pp. 62–84). New York: Guilford Press.

Dattilio, F. M., & Padesky, C. A. (1990). *Cognitive therapy with couples.* Sarasota, FL: Professional Resource Exchange.

Davies, P. T., & Cummings, E. M. (1994). Marital conflict and child adjustment: An emotional security hypothesis. *Psychological Bulletin, 116,* 387–411.

Diener, E., Suh, E. M., Lucas, R. E., & Smith, H. L. (1999). Subjective well-being: Three decades of progress. *Psychological Bulletin, 125,* 276–302.

Doherty, W. J. (1981). Cognitive processes in intimate conflict: II. Efficacy and learned helplessness. *American Journal of Family Therapy, 9*(2), 35–44.

Dryden, W. (1984). *Rational-emotive therapy: Fundamentals and innovations.* Beckenham, Kent, UK: Croom-Helm.

Dryden, W. (1985). Marital therapy: The rational-emotive approach. In W. Dryden (Ed.), *Marital therapy in Britain* (Vol. 1, pp. 195–221). London: Harper & Row.

Ellis, A. (1962). *Reason and emotion in psychotherapy.* New York: Lyle Stuart.

Ellis, A., Sichel, J. L., Yeager, R. J., DiMattia, D. J., & DiGiuseppe, R. (1989). *Rational-emotive couples therapy.* New York: Pergamon Press.

Epstein, N. (1982). Cognitive therapy with couples. *American Journal of Family Therapy*, 10(1), 5–16.

Epstein, N., & Baucom, D. H. (1989). Cognitive-behavioral marital therapy. In A. Freeman, K. M. Simon, H. Arkowitz, & L. Beutler (Eds.), *Comprehensive handbook of cognitive therapy* (pp. 491–513). New York: Plenum Press.

Epstein, N., & Baucom, D. H. (1993). Cognitive factors in marital disturbance. In K. S. Dobson & P. C. Kendall (Eds.), *Psychopathology and cognition* (pp. 351–385). San Diego, CA: Academic Press.

Epstein, N., & Baucom, D. H. (1998). Cognitive-behavioral couple therapy. In F. M. Dattilio (Ed.), *Case studies in couple and family therapy: Systemic and cognitive perspectives* (pp. 37–61). New York: Guilford Press.

Epstein, N., & Baucom, D. H. (2002). *Enhanced cognitive-behavioral therapy for couples: A contextual approach.* Washington, DC: American Psychological Association.

Epstein, N., & Schlesinger, S. E. (1991). Marital and family problems. In W. Dryden & R. Rentoul (Eds.), *Adult clinical problems: A cognitive-behavioural approach* (pp. 288–317). London: Routledge.

Epstein, N., Schlesinger, S. E., & Dryden, W. (Eds.). (1988). *Cognitive-behavioral therapy with families.* New York: Brunner/Mazel.

Falloon, I. R. H. (1991). Behavioral family therapy. In A. S. Gurman & D. P. Kniskern (Eds.), *Handbook of family therapy* (Vol. 2, pp. 65–95). New York: Brunner/Mazel.

Falloon, I. R. H., Boyd, J. L., & McGill, C. W. (1984). *Family care of schizophrenia.* New York: Guilford Press.

Fincham, F. D., & Bradbury, T. N. (1987). The impact of attributions in marriage: A longitudinal analysis. *Journal of Personality and Social Psychology*, 53, 510–517.

Fincham, F. D., & Bradbury, T. N. (1993). Marital satisfaction, depression, and attributions: A longitudinal analysis. *Journal of Personality and Social Psychology*, 64, 442–452.

Fincham, F. D., Harold, G. T., & Gano-Phillips, S. (2000). The longitudinal association between attributions and marital satisfaction: Direction of effects and role of efficacy expectations. *Journal of Family Psychology*, 14, 267–285.

Fiske, S. T., & Taylor, S. E. (1991). *Social cognition* (2nd ed.). New York: McGraw-Hill.

Floyd, F., Markman, H., Kelly, S., Blumberg, S. L., & Stanley, S. (1995). Preventive intervention and relationship enhancement. In N. S. Jacobson & A. S. Gurman (Eds.), *Clinical handbook of couple therapy* (pp. 212–226). New York: Guilford Press.

Forehand, R., Brody, G., Long, N., Slotkin, J., & Fauber, R. (1986). Divorce/divorce potential and interparental conflict: The relationship to early adolescent social and cognitive functioning. *Journal of Adolescent Research*, 1, 389–397.

Fowers, B. J., & Olson, D. H. (1986). Predicting marital success with PREPARE: A predictive validity study. *Journal of Marital and Family Therapy*, 12, 403–413.

Goldenberg, I., & Goldenberg, H. (1991). *Family therapy: An overview* (3rd ed.). Pacific Grove, CA: Brooks/Cole.

Gottman, J. M. (1994). *What predicts divorce? The relationship between marital processes and marital outcomes.* Hillsdale, NJ: Erlbaum.

Grotevant, H. D., & Carlson, C. I. (1989). *Family assessment: A guide to methods and measures*. New York: Guilford Press.

Guerney, B. G., Jr. (1977). *Relationship enhancement*. San Francisco: Jossey-Bass.

Hahlweg, K., Markman, H. J., Thurmaier, F., Engl, J., & Eckert, V. (1998). Prevention of marital distress: Results of a German prospective longitudinal study. *Journal of Family Psychology, 12*, 543–556.

Halford, W. K., Moore, E. N. (2002). Relationship education and the prevention of couple relationship problems. In A. S. Gurman & N. S. Jacobson (Eds.), *Clinical handbook of couple therapy* (3rd ed., pp. 400–419). New York: Guilford Press.

Heider, F. (1958). *The psychology of interpersonal relations*. New York: Wiley.

Hetherington, E. M., Bridges, M., & Insabella, G. M. (1998). What matters? What does not?: Five perspectives on the association between marital transitions and children's adjustment. *American Psychologist, 53*, 167–184.

Holtzworth-Munroe, A., & Hutchinson, G. (1993). Attributing negative intent to wife behavior: The attributions of maritally violent versus nonviolent men. *Journal of Abnormal Psychology, 102*, 206–211.

Holtzworth-Munroe, A., & Jacobson, N. S. (1985). Causal attributions of married couples: When do they search for causes? What do they conclude when they do? *Journal of Personality and Social Psychology, 48*, 1398–1412.

Huber, C. H., & Baruth, L. G. (1989). *Rational-emotive family therapy: A systems perspective*. New York: Springer.

Jacobson, N. S. (1984). The modification of cognitive processes in behavioral marital therapy: Integrating cognitive and behavioral intervention strategies. In K. Hahlweg & N. S. Jacobson (Eds.), *Marital interaction: Analysis and modification* (pp. 285–308). New York: Guilford Press.

Jacobson, N. S., & Christensen, A. (1996). *Integrative couple therapy: Promoting acceptance and change*. New York: Norton.

Jacobson, N. S., & Margolin, G. (1979). *Marital therapy: Strategies based on social learning and behavior exchange principles*. New York: Brunner/Mazel.

Katz, L. F., & Gottman, J. F. (1993). Patterns of marital conflict predict children's internalizing and externalizing behaviors. *Developmental Psychology, 29*, 940–950.

Kelley, H. H. (1967). Attribution theory in social psychology. In D. Levine (Ed.), *Nebraska symposium on motivation* (Vol. 15, pp. 192–238). Lincoln: University of Nebraska Press.

Kelly, G. A. (1955). *The psychology of personal constructs*. New York: Norton.

Kurdek, L. A. (1993). Predicting marital dissolution: A 5-year prospective longitudinal study of newlywed couples. *Journal of Personality and Social Psychology, 64*, 221–242.

Kurdek, L. A., & Berg, B. (1987). Children's beliefs about parental divorce scale: Psychometric characteristics and concurrent validity. *Journal of Consulting and Clinical Psychology, 55*, 712–718.

Leahy, R. (1996). *Cognitive therapy: Basic principles and applications*. Northvale, NJ: Aronson.

Leslie, L. A., & Epstein, N. (1988). Cognitive-behavioral treatment of remarried families. In N. Epstein, S. E. Schlesinger, & W. Dryden (Eds.), *Cognitive-behavioral therapy with families* (pp. 151–182). New York: Brunner/Mazel.

Margolin, G., & Wampold, B. E. (1981). Sequential analysis of conflict and accord in distressed and nondistressed marital partners. *Journal of Consulting and Clinical Psychology, 49,* 554–567.

Markman, H., Floyd, F., Stanley, S., & Jamieson, K. (1984). A cognitive-behavioral program for the prevention of marital and family distress: Issues in program development and delivery. In K. Hahlweg & N. S. Jacobson (Eds.), *Marital interaction: Analysis and modification* (pp. 396–428). New York: Guilford Press.

Markman, H., Floyd, F., Stanley, S., & Storaasli, R. (1988). The prevention of marital distress: A longitudinal investigation. *Journal of Consulting and Clinical Psychology, 56,* 210–217.

Markman, H. J., & Notarius, C. I. (1987). Coding marital and family interaction: Current status. In T. Jacob (Ed.), *Family interaction and psychopathology: Theories, methods, and findings* (pp. 329–390). New York: Plenum Press.

Miller, S. L., Nunnally, E. W., Wachman, D. B., & Miller, P. A. (1991). *Talking and listening together.* Denver-Littleton, CO: Interpersonal Communication Programs.

Morton, T. L., Twentyman, C. T., & Azar, S. T. (1988). Cognitive-behavioral assessment and treatment of child abuse. In N. Epstein, S. E. Schlesinger, & W. Dryden (Eds.), *Cognitive-behavioral therapy with families* (pp. 87–117). New York: Brunner/Mazel.

Nisbett, R., & Ross, L. (1980). *Human inference: Strategies and shortcomings of social judgment.* Englewood Cliffs, NJ: Prentice-Hall.

O'Leary, K., Christian, J., & Mendell, N. (1994). A closer look at the link between marital discord and depressive symptomatology. *Journal of Social and Clinical Psychology, 13,* 33–41.

Olson, D. H., & Fowers, B. J. (1993). Five types of marriage: An empirical typology based on ENRICH. *The Family Journal: Counseling and Therapy for Couples and Families, 1,* 196–207.

Patterson, G. R. (1975). *Families.* Champaign, IL: Research Press.

Patterson, G. R. (1982). *Coercive family process.* Eugene, OR: Castalia.

Patterson, G. R., & Forgatch, M. S. (1987). *Parents and adolescents living together: Part 1. The basics.* Eugene, OR: Castalia.

Peterson, J. L., & Zill, N. (1986). Marital disruption, parent–child relationships, and behavior problems in children. *Journal of Marriage and the Family, 48,* 295–307.

Pretzer, J., Epstein, N., & Fleming, B. (1991). The Marital Attitude Survey: A measure of dysfunctional attributions and expectancies. *Journal of Cognitive Psychotherapy: An International Quarterly, 5,* 131–148.

Rathus, J. H., & Sanderson, W. C. (1999). *Marital distress: Cognitive behavioral interventions for couples.* Northvale, NJ: Aronson.

Revenstorf, D., Hahlweg, K., Schindler, L., & Vogel, B. (1984). Interaction analysis of marital conflict. In K. Hahlweg & N. S. Jacobson (Eds.), *Marital interaction: Analysis and modification* (pp. 159–181). New York: Guilford Press.

Robin, A. L., & Foster, S. L. (1989). *Negotiating parent–adolescent conflict: A behavioral–family systems approach.* New York: Guilford Press.

Rotter, J. B. (1954). *Social learning and clinical psychology.* Englewood Cliffs, NJ: Prentice-Hall.

Russell, C. S., Bagarozzi, D. A., Atilanao, R. B., & Morris, J. E. (1984). A comparison of two approaches to marital enrichment and conjugal skills training: Minnesota

Couples Communication Program and Structured Behavioral Exchange Contracting. *American Journal of Family Therapy, 12*, 13–25.

Sager, C. J., Brown, H. S., Crohn, H., Engel, T., Rodstein, E., & Walker, L. (1983). *Treating the remarried family.* New York: Brunner/ Mazel.

Schaap, C. (1984). A comparison of the interaction of distressed and nondistressed married couples in a laboratory situation: Literature survey, methodological issues, and an empirical investigation. In K. Hahlweg & N. S. Jacobson (Eds.), *Marital interaction: Analysis and modification* (pp. 133–158). New York: Guilford Press.

Schlesinger, S. E. (1988). Cognitive-behavioral approaches to family treatment of addictions. In N. Epstein, S. E. Schlesinger, & W. Dryden (Eds.), *Cognitive-behavioral therapy with families* (pp. 254–291). New York: Brunner/Mazel.

Schlesinger, S. E., & Epstein, N. (1986). Cognitive-behavioral techniques in marital therapy. In P. A. Keller and L. G. Ritt (Eds.), *Innovations in clinical practice: A source book* (Vol. 5, pp. 137–156). Sarasota, FL: Professional Resource Exchange.

Schmaling, K. B., & Sher, T. G. (2000). *The psychology of couples and illness.* Washington, DC: American Psychological Association.

Schwebel, A. I., & Fine, M. A. (1994). *Understanding and helping families: A cognitive-behavioral approach.* Hillsdale, NJ: Erlbaum.

Seiler, T. B. (1984). Development of cognitive theory, personality, and therapy. In N. Hoffman (Ed.), *Foundations of cognitive therapy: Theoretical methods and practical applications* (pp. 11–49). New York: Plenum Press.

Stanley, S. M., Blumberg, S. L., & Markman, H. J. (1999). Helping couples fight for their marriages: The PREP approach. In R. Berger & M. Hannah (Eds.), *Handbook of preventive approaches in couples therapy* (pp. 279–303). New York: Brunner/Mazel.

Stuart, R. B. (1980). *Helping couples change: A social learning approach to marital therapy.* New York: Guilford Press.

Stuart, R. B., & Jacobson, B. (1985). *Second marriage: Make it happy! Make it last!* New York: Norton.

Thibaut, J. W., & Kelley, H. H. (1959). *The social psychology of groups.* New York: Wiley.

Thompson, J. S., & Snyder, D. K. (1986). Attribution theory in intimate relationships: A methodological review. *American Journal of Family Therapy, 14*, 123–138.

Turk, D. C., & Speers, M. A. (1983). Cognitive schemata and cognitive processes in cognitive-behavioral interventions: Going beyond the information given. In P. C. Kendall (Ed.), *Advances in cognitive-behavioral research and therapy* (Vol. 2, pp. 1–31). New York: Academic Press.

Van Widenfelt, B., Markman, H. J., Guerney, B., Behrens, B. C., & Hosman, C. (1997). Prevention of relationship problems. In W. K. Halford & H. J. Markman (Eds.), *Clinical handbook of marriage and couple interventions* (pp. 651–678). Chichester, UK: Wiley.

Vanzetti, N. A., Notarius, C. I., & NeeSmith, D. (1992). Specific and generalized expectancies in marital interaction. *Journal of Family Psychology, 6*, 171–183.

Visher, E. B., & Visher, J. S. (1988). *Old loyalties, new ties: Therapeutic strategies with stepfamilies.* New York: Brunner/Mazel.

Wampler, K. S. (1990). An update of research on the Couple Communication Program. *Family Science Review, 3,* 21–40.
Watzlawick, P., Beavin, J. H., & Jackson, D. D. (1967). *Pragmatics of human communication.* New York: Norton.
Wessler, R. A., & Wessler, R. L. (1980). *The principles and practice of rational-emotive therapy.* San Francisco: Jossey-Bass.

SUGGESTED READINGS

Cognitive-Behavioral Marital and Family Therapy

Baucom, D. H., & Epstein, N. (1990). *Cognitive-behavioral marital therapy.* New York: Brunner/Mazel.
Dattilio, F. M. (Ed.). (1998). *Case studies in couple and family therapy: Systemic and cognitive perspectives.* New York: Guilford Press.
Dattilio, F. M., & Padesky, C. A. (1990). *Cognitive therapy with couples.* Sarasota, FL: Professional Resource Exchange.
Epstein, N. B., & Baucom, D. H. (2002). *Enhanced cognitive-behavioral therapy for couples: A contextual approach.* Washington, DC: American Psychological Association.
Epstein, N., Schlesinger, S. E., & Dryden, W. (Eds.). (1988). *Cognitive–behavioral therapy with families.* New York: Brunner/Mazel.
Rathus, J. H., & Sanderson, W. C. (1999). *Marital distress: Cognitive behavioral interventions for couples.* Northvale, NJ: Aronson.
Schwebel, A. I., & Fine, M. A. (1994). *Understanding and helping families: A cognitive-behavioral approach.* Hillsdale, NJ: Erlbaum.

Couple Education

Beck, A. T. (1988). *Love is never enough.* New York: Harper & Row.
Gottman, J. M. (1994). *Why marriages succeed or fail.* New York: Simon & Schuster.
Gottman, J. M. (1999). *The marriage clinic.* New York: Norton.
Markman, H., Stanley, S., & Blumberg, S. (1994). *Fighting for your marriage: Positive steps for preventing divorce and preserving a lasting love.* San Francisco, CA: Jossey-Bass.
Miller, S., Miller, P., Nunnally, E., & Wachman, D. (1991). *Talking and listening together.* Littleton, CO: Interpersonal Communication Programs.
Notarius, C., & Markman, H. (1993). *We can work it out.* New York: Putnam.

The website *www.smartmarriages.com* is devoted to marriage education, with descriptions of many couple education programs and links to their websites.

13

Play Therapy with a Sexually Abused Child

SUSAN M. KNELL
CHRISTINE D. RUMA

Cognitive-behavioral play therapy (CBPT) incorporates cognitive and be-havioral interventions within a play therapy paradigm. It uses verbal as well as nonverbal communication, and incorporates both cognitive and behavioral interventions. However, cognitive-behavioral play therapy is more than the use of specific techniques. It provides a theoretical frame-work that is based on cognitive-behavioral principles and applies those principles in a developmentally sensitive way (Knell, 1993a, 1993b, 1994, 1999, 2000).

CBPT is designed specifically for preschool and school-age children, and emphasizes the child's involvement in treatment by addressing issues of control, mastery, and responsibility for one's own change in behavior. By incorporating attention to cognitive variables in treatment, the child is en-abled to become an active participant in the change process (Knell, 1993a). When children identify and modify potentially maladaptive beliefs, for ex-ample, they may increase their capacity to experience a sense of personal understanding and empowerment.

The literature on cognitive-behavioral interventions with young chil-dren is relatively sparse. This may be due, in part, to the belief that such in-terventions are not applicable with young children. Some researchers have argued that cognitive-behavioral interventions are beyond the cognitive ca-pabilities of young children (e.g., Campbell, 1990). In contrast, Knell (1993a, 1993b, 1994) contends that with minor modifications the princi-ples of cognitive therapy can be applied to youth. Among the most important differences are that the principles of collaborative empiricism, the reliance on the inductive and Socratic methods, and the use of homework assignments, as delineated by Beck and Emery (1985), do not play a major role in CBPT.

Despite the paucity of research on the use of cognitive-behavioral therapy with very young children, there are several reasons why applying cognitive-behavioral interventions in play therapy makes sense. The properties of CBPT, as outlined by Knell (1993a), are as follows:

1. CBPT involves the child in treatment via play.
2. CBPT focuses on the child's thoughts, feelings, fantasies, and environment.
3. It provides strategies for developing more adaptive thoughts and behaviors.
4. It is structured, directive, and goal-oriented, rather than open-ended.
5. It incorporates empirically supported techniques.
6. It allows for an empirical examination of treatment outcome.

DEVELOPMENTAL ISSUES

Psychotherapy with children and adolescents presents unique challenges not necessarily present with adults. Preschool-age children exhibit certain abilities and limitations, such that principles related to working with school-age children, adolescents, and adults cannot merely be extrapolated to apply to younger children. Among the most critical issues in work with young children in therapy are those involving their cognitive functioning. Cognitive distortions, misperceptions, misattributions, negativistic automatic thoughts, maladaptive schemas, and limitations in social problem solving—the focus of treatment in cognitive-behavioral therapy with adults—may not readily be apparent in children's play. Moreover, young children typically manifest difficulties describing their experiences, labeling emotions, and identifying relationships between thoughts and feelings. Cognitive issues in child therapy are often obscured by play activity, which may lead the child therapist to focus more on nonverbal rather than verbal communications (Shirk, 1988). Shirk further argues that conceptual underpinnings of alternative treatment approaches influence the relative importance paid to cognitive issues. If, for example, abreaction or emotional release is considered to be the basis of change, then cognitive differences may be ignored insofar as play substitutes for words as a mechanism of therapeutic change. Although cognitive skills change over the course of development, they nonetheless exist for individuals of all ages (from infancy on), and are seen as mediating individuals' reactions to life events. Cognitive-behavioral formulations, derived from contemporary social learning theory, may reasonably be used in understanding and treating behavioral and emotional difficulties experienced by young children.

The work of Piaget (1926, 1928, 1930) has influenced much of our thinking about children's cognitive development. For children in the preoperational stage of development (ages 2–7 years), thinking is concrete and egocentric. Although more recent work suggests that these theories may underestimate young children's abilities (Gelman & Baillargeon, 1983), there are striking limitations in aspects of the preoperational child's thinking processes, which may interfere with his or her ability to benefit from more verbally focused forms of psychotherapy, such as cognitive-behavioral therapy.

Piagetian principles have been extrapolated by Harter (1977, 1983) and applied to affective spheres. The same cognitive limitations that lead a child to faulty logic and errors in understanding can be adapted to describe the child's understanding of social phenomena, such as social relationships and perspective taking. As young children typically can attend to only one of two opposite affective dimensions at a time, their understanding of affective material is often characterized by "all-or-nothing" thinking. Such a phenomenon, akin to conservation of affect, greatly influences the way in which the young child understands experiences and the feelings and emotions elicited by them.

Cognitive-behavioral therapy with adults assumes that an individual has the cognitive capacity to differentiate between thoughts that are rational or irrational, logical or illogical, and adaptive or maladaptive. Although an adult may need help in identifying and labeling such thoughts, once they are delineated the individual can understand these inconsistencies. Adults often, for example, experience thoughts and feelings that appear to be "all-or-nothing" in nature. Through cognitive therapy, however, the individual may come to understand the limitations such thinking offers. Such assumptions are not necessarily true with children. In fact, what may appear to be irrational from an adult's perspective often seems quite sensible to a young child.

Despite such significant differences in the cognitive abilities of children and adults, cognitive-behavioral therapy with children and adolescents is receiving increased attention (Emery, Bedrosian, & Garber, 1983; Kendall, 1991; Piacentini, Bergman, & Aikins, in press; Spence & Reinecke, in press; Wilkes, Belsher, Rush, Frank, & Associates, 1994; Zarb, 1992). However, much of the literature deals with school-age children and adolescents, with little attention devoted to preschoolers. Knell (1993a) contends that cognitive therapy can be used with young children, although the treatment must be communicated in indirect ways, such as through play. The therapist must be aware of developmental issues and adapt therapeutic strategies accordingly.

APPLICATIONS OF COGNITIVE-BEHAVIORAL PLAY THERAPY

In order for young children to benefit from CBPT, interventions need to be presented in a format that is accessible to them. The most common method is modeling, learning that occurs as a function of observing the behavior of others and the consequences of that behavior (Bandura, 1969). Among the characteristics shown to improve the efficacy of vicarious learning procedures is the use of coping models in which the individual gradually acquires new skills, in contrast to a mastery model, which presents a confident, flawless performance (Bandura & Menlove, 1968; Meichenbaum, 1971). Utilizing a coping-model approach, modeling in CBPT often involves a puppet or doll that demonstrates acquisition of adaptive coping skills. The model may verbalize problem-solving skills or solutions to particular problems that parallel the difficulties faced by the child. Thus, the child is exposed to a model demonstrating behaviors that the therapist wants the child to learn. Although puppets and dolls are used most frequently to model behaviors, other forms may include drawings, films, and books.

Another commonly used method is that of role playing, in which the puppets (dolls) practice tasks and receive feedback from the therapist. Through role playing, children practice skills with their therapist and receive ongoing feedback regarding their progress. For children who may be too young to benefit from direct role playing, it is possible to use a modeling technique so that dolls or puppets complete the role play, and the child observes and learns from watching the models practice particular skills. For example, maltreated children can be taught skills to help deal with any future abuse, with the therapist role playing both an offender and a child who is trying to say "no," get the perpetrator away, and seek help. The child can listen as the therapist has the puppet practice and receive feedback.

GENERALIZATION AND RELAPSE PREVENTION IN COGNITIVE-BEHAVIORAL PLAY THERAPY

One important goal of therapy is for the child to maintain adaptive behaviors after the treatment has ended and to generalize these behaviors to the natural environment. It is important for the therapist to incorporate efforts to promote and facilitate generalization into treatment, rather than assume that it will occur naturally (Meichenbaum, 1977). It may be necessary to deal directly with issues of generalization by using real-life situations in modeling and role plays, involving significant adults in the child's life in the treatment process, teaching self-management skills, and continuing even past the initial acquisition of skills to ensure that adequate learning occurs.

Therapy should also be geared toward helping the child and family prevent relapse. This is done primarily by preparing the parent and child not only for what to expect, but also for what to do when certain events occur. By doing so, high-risk situations that present a threat to the child's sense of control can be identified. It is important to "inoculate" individuals against failure through preparation, in part to avoid "panic" when there are roadblocks (Marlatt & Gordon, 1985; Meichenbaum, 1985). A child and family can be taught, for example, to use previously learned skills if a particular stressful event occurs, or if specific symptoms or problems recur.

IMPACT OF SEXUAL ABUSE ON CHILDREN

Victims of sexual abuse are often left with distorted perceptions and beliefs about both the incident and themselves. Finkelhor and Browne (1986) have identified four traumagenic dynamics (trauma-causing factors) related to sexual abuse. These can be used to provide a framework for conceptualizing children's reactions to the abuse. These factors are traumatic sexualization, betrayal, powerlessness, and stigmatization. Within this framework one may identify the primary ways in which a child has been affected by maltreatment and direct treatment specifically to these areas.

Porter, Blick, and Sgroi (1982) identified 10 impact issues common to victims of child sexual abuse:

1. A perception that they are "damaged goods"
2. Guilt
3. Fear
4. Depression
5. Low self-esteem and poor social skills
6. Repressed anger and hostility
7. Impaired ability to trust
8. Blurred role boundaries and role confusion
9. Pseudomaturity and failure to accomplish developmental tasks
10. Problems of self-mastery and control

The first five issues are thought to be present for all victims; the last five are considered to be specific to incest victims.

Both of these models describe common outcomes of child sexual abuse, based on the child's cognitions and beliefs regarding the sexual behavior. Another critical factor related to a child's response to the sexual abuse is the attribution of blame for the event. Although it may appear that children who do not blame themselves for the abuse have the healthier belief, it has been suggested that this mode of thinking is related to a sense of helplessness (Shapiro, 1989). Similarly, Janoff-Bulman (1979) distinguished between behavioral self-blame and characterological self-blame. The former involves attribution to a particular behavior or mistake; the latter, attribution to enduring personal qualities. Studies suggest that individuals who have behavioral rather than characterological self-blame tend to have better adjustment, perhaps because they believe they can avoid further victimization by changing their behavior (Janoff-Bulman, 1979; Major, Mueller, & Hildebrandt, 1985).

A young child's beliefs are influenced by many factors, including the beliefs, attitudes, attributions, and behavior of their parents. In the case of sexual abuse, parental response to the child's disclosure of abuse is critical in shaping the child's cognitions and beliefs about the abuse and about themselves. A parent who reacts with blame, horror, or anger toward the child gives a different message than one who responds with support for the child (Friedrich, 1990).

Although there may be common sequelae of abuse, the impact may manifest itself differently with each child. Symptoms that occur frequently in very young children include sleep disturbances, regression in toileting and other skills, expressions of anger and fear, depression, anxiety, and sexualized behaviors (Beitchman, Zucker, Hood, da Costa, & Akman, 1991; Browne and Finkelhor, 1986; Finkelhor, 1990; Green, 1993; Kendall-Tackett, Williams, & Finkelhor, 1993). Additionally, several factors are commonly believed to affect the severity of the child's reaction to sexual abuse. A less severe reaction may be the result of factors such as shorter duration and less frequent sexual contact, less intrusive sexual acts, the absence of force or threat of force, and the perpetrator's being an individual other than the child's parent (Browne & Finkelhor, 1986). Improved adjustment is also predicted for a child with good coping skills and maternal support upon disclosure (Kendall-Tackett et al., 1993). The latter findings with regard to maternal support uphold the notion that positive parental response may be a critical factor in better outcome.

PSYCHOTHERAPY WITH SEXUALLY ABUSED CHILDREN

The literature regarding treatment for sexually abused children generally recommends some combination of individual, group, and family treatment. The role of family therapy in treating sexually abused children has generated a good deal of controversy among therapists. Two schools of thought have evolved: The first emphasizes the importance of individual therapy as a means of restoring victims to mental health and protecting them from further abuse, whereas the second views family issues as critical for conceptualizing and treating the abused child (Friedrich, 1990). Despite differences of opinion regarding whether family treatment should be part of a comprehensive treatment plan, there is little argument that family issues are pertinent, regardless of whether the abuse is intra- or extrafamilial. Treatment approaches will differ significantly, of course, depending on whether the abuse was intra- or extra-familial. Even when individual psychotherapy is indicated, work with the family is often included and, according to Friedrich (1990), should have well-articulated goals.

In regard to individual treatment, much of the literature relates to the treatment of incest victims and overlooks the needs of children maltreated by a known and trusted, although not biologically related, perpetrator. The large majority of research in this area has focused upon older children and adolescents; less has been written about treating preschool-age children who have been sexually abused. In a review of the sex abuse treatment literature, Finkelhor and Berliner (1995) argue that "abuse-specific" therapy is a preferred approach. The common elements of such treatment usually include the following:

1. Encouraging expression of abuse-related feelings
2. Correcting distorted abuse related beliefs
3. Teaching abuse prevention skills
4. Decreasing the sense of stigma and isolation

In some of the earliest references to specific treatment approaches for the preschool-age victim (Deblinger, McLeer, & Henry, 1990; Ruma, 1993), the cognitive-behavioral treatment of young children who have been molested is discussed. More recent clinical descriptions of such treatment come from Deblinger and her colleagues (Deblinger & Heflin, 1996), with empirical evidence for the efficacy of such treatment coming from several studies (Cohen & Mannarino, 1996a, 1996b, 1997, 1998a; Deblinger, Lippmann, & Steer, 1996; Deblinger, Steer, & Lippmann, 1999; Stauffer & Deblinger, 1996).

Traditional play therapy has been adapted for use with children who have been sexually abused, although the focus of these approaches is often on the relationship between child and therapist (e.g., Gil, 1991; Walker & Bolkovatz, 1988). Gil captures the essence of this approach in her statement that "there is an attempt to demonstrate to the child through therapeutic intervention the potentially rewarding nature of human interaction. . . . If given a nurturing, safe environment, the child will inevitably gravitate toward the reparative experience" (pp. 51–52).

The importance of a positive therapeutic relationship, possibly reparative in nature, is stressed in much of the literature on psychotherapy with sexually abused children (e.g., Friedrich, 1990; Gil, 1991). However, recent literature highlights the importance of a more directive, structured approach to working with sexually abused individuals (e.g., Friedrich, 1990). This is consistent with cognitive-behavioral therapy, which is, by definition, structured, directive, and goal-oriented.

COGNITIVE-BEHAVIORAL PLAY THERAPY
WITH SEXUALLY ABUSED CHILDREN

Recent literature has described the use of cognitive behavior therapy with sexually abused children (Cohen & Mannarino, 1996a, 1996b, 1997, 1998a, 1998b; Deblinger & Heflin, 1996; Deblinger et al., 1990, 1999; Farrell, Haines, & Davies, 1998; Ruma, 1993; Stauffer & Deblinger, 1996). CBPT is directive, yet allows the child to develop a sense of control within a structure set by the therapist. This is advantageous, since many sexually abused children avoid matters related to the abuse, perhaps in an effort to avoid the anxiety, guilt, and negative feelings associated with their maltreatment experiences. However, the structure of CBPT allows the child to maintain a sense of trust and control, which is a central issue in the treatment of most sexually abused children (Sgroi, 1982). The experience of sexual abuse often is a betrayal of the child's relationship with the perpetrator (assuming that this person is not a stranger). Because their trust has been betrayed, sexually abused children often test the therapeutic relationship in ways that youth with other problems do not. Sexually abused children may, for example, behave provocatively toward their therapist to see if the therapist will harm them. Additionally, control is taken away from the child. Furthermore, many molested children have difficulty expressing negative feelings. Incestuous families are often typified by their lack of expression of feelings (Friedrich, 1990; Sgroi, 1982). By encouraging the development of communication skills and including families in some sessions, CBPT provides a venue within which family members may express a range of emotions and concerns.

Knell (1993a) outlined ways in which CBPT may be well suited for work with very young children, and Ruma (1993) highlighted its usefulness in work with sexually abused youth. She noted that it is directive, but allows control within the structure set by the therapist. Allowing children to maintain some sense of control in therapy may be beneficial because many children avoid matters related to abuse in order to avoid negative feelings associated with it. Further, Ruma (1993) points out that CBPT can be particularly helpful in providing children with more appropriate ways of expressing their thoughts and feelings related to the abuse experience. Additional ways in which cognitive-behavioral approaches may be applicable for young sexually abused children are reviewed by Deblinger and Heflin (1996). They describe a range of interventions that can be used with various problems. An emphasis is placed on collaborative efforts between therapist and client, on maintaining a therapeutic structure, and of providing a rationale for cognitive-behavioral interventions to the parents.

A variety of treatment techniques are used in CBPT with sexually abused children. Given the relatively limited cognitive abilities of young children and the anxiety that discussing sexual abuse may arouse, play provides sexually molested children with a comfortable and familiar means of expressing their thoughts and feelings. Attention to emotions experienced by the child, environmental cues that elicit these feelings, and the ways in which the child copes with them plays a prominent role in CBPT. This is particularly important given the frequent concern that cognitive-behavioral therapies do not attend to the affective experiences of the child. Our goal is to attend simultaneously to emotions experienced by the child, meanings attached to their experiences, the development of adaptive and maladaptive coping strategies, and the family system in which the child is developing. Some of the most important treatment techniques in CBPT with sexually abused children are bibliotherapy, drawings, art, and puppet and doll play.

Bibliotherapy

Bibliotherapy is commonly used with sexually abused children. There are a number of benefits of reading stories to children about sexual abuse. First, hearing a story about another child who was sexually abused helps children understand that they are not the only ones who have been maltreated. Second, it allows them to see that they are not alone in their feelings, particularly in regard to feelings about the perpetrator. Through modeling, a child may see how others learn to cope with conflicting feelings, such as both love and fear of the perpetrator, particularly if he or she was a known and trusted individual in the child's life. Third, the stories help the child to see that others have learned to gain control over similar situations. This is useful, for example, when the child is reluctant to disclose specific aspects of the abuse. Finally, stories may provide a means of desensitizing the child to the anxiety related to the abuse, and therefore help him or her begin to deal with feelings about the experience.

The therapist will want to select or adapt a story so that some of the variables are similar to that of the child's experience (e.g., relationship to or gender of the perpetrator). Bibliotherapy stories typically are vague in many respects (e.g., type of sexual touching not clearly specified). As a consequence, these stories are not likely to color a child's recall of the actual abuse. The stories focus on more common issues surrounding sexual abuse, such as confused feelings and thoughts, and the positive results of disclosure.

In addition to books that directly address sexual abuse situations, therapists often rely on more indirect stories. One example, *Once Upon a Time: Therapeutic Stories for Children* (Davis, 1988), is a collection of short stories that use metaphors to address issues of abuse. These stories may be particularly useful for children who are too anxious to listen to stories that directly discuss abusive situations. Finally, even when a metaphorical approach is too anxiety provoking, stories may be read in a child's presence but not directly to the child (e.g., reading a story to a puppet with the child in the room).

Sometimes bibliotherapy may take the form of self-created books. With sexually abused children, these books may deal directly with the abuse experience (e.g., McCarthy, 1990; Ruma, 1993).

Drawings and Art

Self-created picture books may be used to help children disclose their own personal history of abuse (L. Hartman-Makovec, personal communication, March 1990). Children are encouraged to tell their story of abuse in small steps through their drawings. They begin with the least threatening aspect of the abuse, and, as they are able to cope with their anxiety, they gradually portray more threatening aspects of the maltreatment. By drawing the abuse experience, the child can disclose through art what happened. Deblinger and Heflin (1996) also refer to the use of gradual exposure through writing and discussion, as well as drawing and art. Whereas cognitive techniques such as cognitive processing and imagery rescripting (e.g., Chard, Weaver, & Resick, 1997; Resick & Schnicke, 1992; Smucker & Niederee, 1995) have been successfully employed with adult survivors of sexual abuse, these may be too anxiety provoking for use with young children. Modifications of these techniques, if applied in a developmentally sensitive way, might be appropriate.

Through their pictures, children may express their cognitive distortions about the abuse in ways that they could not in words. For example, children who have been sexually abused frequently exaggerate the difference in size between the perpetrator and themselves, making the perpetrator much larger and/or themselves much smaller than in reality. Children may also leave out features or extremities when they draw themselves, and may depict the perpetrator in a grotesque way by exaggerating body or facial features. The therapist can then identify and help the child correct these distortions. As the pictures portray more threatening material, the therapist can help desensitize the child to the details related to the abuse.

Other Art Media

Another approach that can be useful with young children who have been sexually abused is the use of play with clay as a medium. This activity can be structured so that the child depicts different aspects of the abuse by sculpting with the clay. Some children feel a sense of control when modeling clay figures depicting themselves as bigger than the perpetrator. Others may feel a sense of mastery and control by destroying a clay model of the perpetrator or saying things to the model that they could not say to the actual person. As with other modalities, the therapist can address distorted beliefs through the child's clay representations.

Puppet and Doll Play

As noted, puppets, dolls, or other figures can be used in CBPT in both assessment (e.g., Knell & Beck, 2000) and treatment (Knell, 1993b, 1997, 1999). In therapy, puppets can be used in several different ways. The therapist can structure play scenarios around the specific issues with which the child is struggling (e.g., mistrust, sadness). First, if the child cannot tolerate the anxiety that might be evoked by structured play around the abuse, the play scenarios might involve "another child," similar to the child being treated but with a different name. Second, a sequence similar to the drawing technique can be used, and is particularly helpful for children who have difficulty expressing themselves through art. With either of these techniques, the therapist can correct the child's distortions by modeling corrective thoughts or experiences via the dolls or puppets. In addition, children can practice, or the therapist can model, prevention skills through doll or puppet play.

In sum, CBPT is similar in many essential ways to cognitive therapy procedures used in treating traumatized or abused adolescents and adults. As in cognitive-behavioral therapy with adults, CBPT is active, collaborative, problem focused, strategic, and structured. Through the use of bibliotherapy, storytelling and play, CBPT attempts to identify and change maladaptive beliefs, attitudes, thoughts and attributions that may be contributing to the child's distress. It attempts to develop cognitive and behavioral coping skills and provides parents with ways of understanding their child's distress and a rationale for treatment procedures. The latter point is quite important given recent work suggesting that it can be helpful to include parents in the treatment of children with anxiety disorders (Silverman, Ginsburg, & Kurtines, 1995; Silverman & Kurtines, 1996). CBPT is developmentally sensitive and, by emphasizing the use of play and storytelling, allows children to address a range of anxiety provoking events.

CASE EXAMPLE

Background Information

Julie, a 5-year-old female, was referred for psychotherapy due to allegations of sexual abuse. She was seen in CBPT for a total of 13 sessions over a 3½-month period. This section gives a brief history of Julie, a description of her presenting features, and a discussion of the course of her treatment.

Julie is the middle of three children living with both biological parents. Her parents are professionals who live in a middle-class neighborhood.

Prior to the disclosure of sexual abuse, the family, including Julie, was not experiencing any unusual stresses or difficulties. Julie had made a good adjustment to the beginning of kindergarten several months before the onset of treatment.

Julie's disclosure of sexual abuse was prompted by her mother's questioning of her after some suspicious behavior by an adult male in their neighborhood. Upon questioning, Julie disclosed that Mike, a neighbor, had "pee-peed" and "touched her" that day. She also disclosed that on a previous occasion he had shown her his "privates" and told her it was a squirt gun. Both incidents occurred at Mike's house. The first incident occurred in a bathroom; the second, upstairs, while her family was elsewhere in the house. Upon hearing this, the parents contacted the child protective services and filed criminal charges against Mike.

Approximately 6 weeks after the disclosure, the parents sought therapy for Julie. Since the incidents of sexual abuse and subsequent disclosure and investigation, she had begun displaying several symptoms that are characteristic of sexually abused children. Julie had become concerned about the need to urinate and consequently felt the need to frequent the bathroom; however, she was also afraid to go into the bathroom alone. She also became fearful of attending school because of the possible need to use the rest room while at school or on the school bus. Finally, Julie became afraid of being alone on one floor of the house while other family members were on another level.

Initial Assessment

During the initial appointment, Julie's mother was interviewed, providing a history of the abuse as she understood it, as well as a complete developmental history of Julie. Julie's parents were concerned about her current symptoms, as well as the effect the abuse might have on their daughter in the future. They had taken Julie to see another therapist for one or two sessions, but had discontinued therapy due to dissatisfaction with the therapist's availability. The mother also completed the Child Behavior Checklist (CBCL; Achenbach, 1991). Figure 13.1 contains the initial CBCL profile. Although there were no clinically significant elevations, there were several significant items that were endorsed as being somewhat or sometimes true. These items included Withdrawn, Fearful, Acts Young, Can't Get Mind Off of Certain Thoughts, and Fears School. The scale of Social Problems registered at the 87th percentile and that of Thought Problems was at the 80th percentile. All other scores were recorded at the 63rd percentile or lower. Although not used in this case, other objective rating scales, such as the Child Symptom Inventory, the Children's Depression Inventory, and the Multidimensional Anxiety Scale for Children, can be useful in identifying specific symptoms and for monitoring therapeutic improvement.

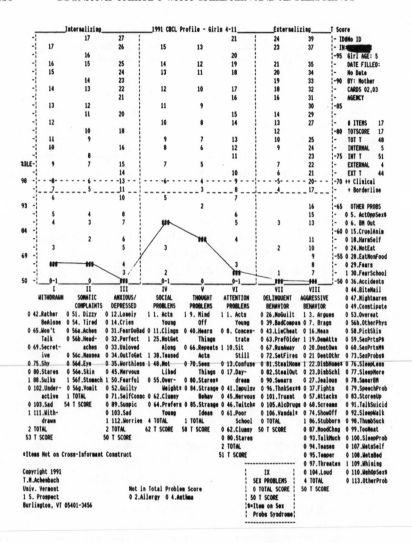

FIGURE 13.1. Initial CBCL completed by Julie's mother.

Case Conceptualization

At the time Julie was referred for treatment, she had already disclosed information about the abuse to her mother. According to Julie's statements, the maltreatment had occurred only two times, had been committed by a non-family member, and did not include penetration or violence. Her family believed her disclosure and supported her. Additionally, they were not experiencing any other stressors which might have been significant factors in treatment.

Julie's symptoms, including a need to urinate frequently and fear of being separated from family members in the house, seemed to be related to the context in which she had been abused. Although neither incident occurred in Julie's home, the anxiety and fear caused by the trauma of being maltreated generalized to her own home. The fear of using the bathroom was likely related to being touched in her genital area by the perpetrator, as well as the fact that one incident of abuse occurred in a bathroom. Her fears related to using the bathroom generalized to school as well. It is significant that although the incident of abuse in the bathroom had occurred at least several weeks prior to disclosure, the symptoms did not manifest themselves until after she disclosed the abuse to her parents. This would suggest that the disclosure served as a trigger for these memories. Similarly, her fear of separation from her family manifested itself after disclosure. It seems that once she was aware that it was "safe" to tell her parents what had happened, and that the perpetrator could do no further harm, Julie clung to her parents in an effort to be totally safe.

Diagnostically, Julie appeared to meet criteria for posttraumatic stress disorder not otherwise specified, according to the *Diagnostic and Statistical Manual of Mental Disorders* fourth edition (DSM-IV; American Psychiatric Association, 1994). Her family was supportive, and she had no reported history of prior psychiatric illness or comorbid disorder. The therapist's perception was that Julie's prognosis was positive. Given Julie's age, play therapy was chosen as the primary treatment modality. Her family was included in treatment in an effort to help them understand the effects of the abuse and to provide them with practical recommendations for how they might best help their daughter. Given their level of support and motivation, and the fact that communication among family members was strong, family psychotherapy was not indicated. Specific play activities were selected based on Julie's interests, her ability to use them as a means of communication, and their usefulness in meeting the main treatment goals of encouraging disclosure, correcting maladaptive cognitions about the abuse, and decreasing symptomatology.

Course of Treatment

Although Julie was not included in the first session, she was seen at each subsequent appointment. Either one or both of Julie's parents were also seen for at least a portion of each session to discuss her progress and to answer any questions they had. On two separate occasions, the entire family was included in a session. Several different play modalities were employed, including bibliotherapy, drawing techniques, puppet play, and clay modeling. Because there was a criminal case in process against the alleged perpetrator, the therapist was especially mindful of being nonleading regarding the abuse experiences while still directing the course of therapy. The following is a summary of each of the remaining 12 play therapy sessions after the initial assessment appointment.

Session 1

After some brief introductory work, the therapist questioned Julie as to her understanding of the reason for therapy. Julie quickly stated that she was there to talk about what Mike had done to her. Following a discussion of the purpose of meeting, the therapist read "The Hidden Boxes" (Davis, 1988). This is a story about a princess who was given a box, but told that she must not let anyone know about it. The more the princess kept this secret, the more upset she became. When the princess finally told an adult about her secret, she felt a great sense of relief. Julie then said she felt sad when she thought of Mike. She also said that since she told her mom about the abuse it had helped her feel better.

Sessions 2–6

The primary task during these five sessions was to make a book of drawings about what had happened with Mike (see Figure 13.2, pictures a–i).

Since Julie was initially very anxious to disclose the abuse, she jumped directly to drawing the abuse after completing the first picture of the home where the abuse occurred. After Julie drew each picture, she dictated the story to the therapist. The first three pictures (pictures a, b, and c) were done during Session 2 and depict the first incident of abuse. During the week after drawing the first three pictures, her parents reported that Julie had become more fearful of using the bathroom alone. Although this increase in symptoms persisted for a brief time, it appeared to be an appropriate and expected reaction to her recalling in therapy this incident of abuse.

The next three drawings (pictures d, e, and f), done during Session 3, depict the second incident of abuse. After each picture and story was completed, the therapist would simply ask Julie to draw a picture of what happened next. Pictures d, e, and f are essentially the same and do not disclose any abuse, but simply the setting where the abuse occurred. Each time Julie was asked to draw a picture of what happened next, she simply repeated what she had just drawn. It appeared that she was uncomfortable with describing the remainder of the incidents.

The final three pictures (pictures g, h, and i) were drawn during the three subsequent appointments. Julie was reluctant to continue working on her picture book, which resulted in the pace of drawing being decreased. After reviewing the previous drawings, Julie was again asked to draw what had happened next. She continued, however, to draw the same picture and

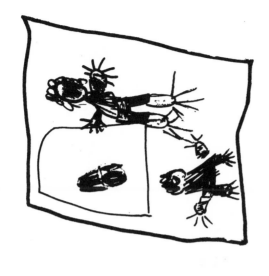

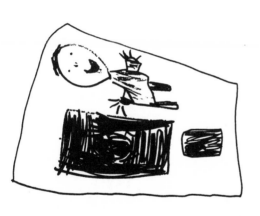

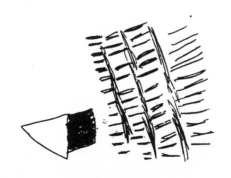

FIGURE 13.2a. "Matthew's house. It was a great big birthday party for Matthew." [Mike is a neighbor and friend of Matthew's family.]

FIGURE 13.2b. "Mike was in the bathroom. The door was closed. I knocked on the door and he said, 'come in.'"

FIGURE 13.2c. "I came in. He stared at me and stuck his private out. I ran out the door. Mike said nothing."

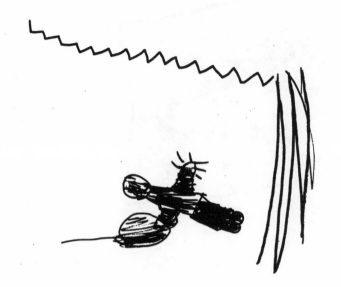

FIGURE 13.2e. "First I was down there and I got mad. Then I punched the punching bag and I got really angry because Mike was still down there."

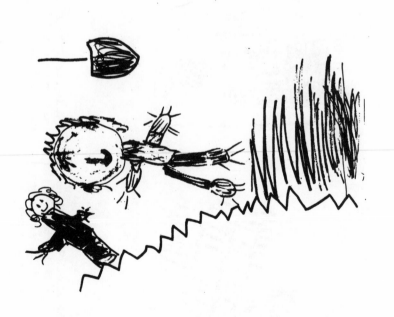

FIGURE 13.2d. "I was going downstairs to punch the punching bag. Mike was still down there."

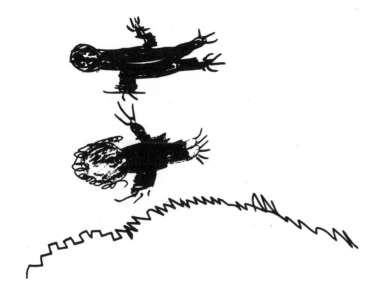

FIGURE 13.2g. "I got real mad. I wished I could punch him in the belly. Mike was really mean. He stuck his private out. It looked really scary."

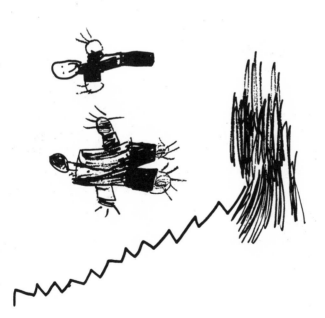

FIGURE 13.2f. "He came back downstairs and I got real mad. I said, 'Mike get out of here.' He stayed there."

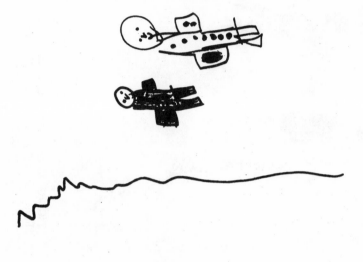

FIGURE 13.2i. [No caption.]

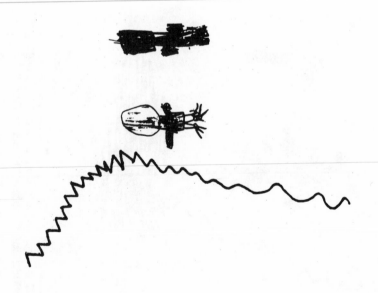

FIGURE 13.2h. "Mike stuck out his private and she [Julie] was real scared."

356

declined to tell a story to accompany it. At this point, the therapist introduced the use of puppets. Julie's puppet then told the therapist's puppet a story to go with the picture. It was with this technique that Julie disclosed that "Mike had shown her his privates."

Session 5 was similar in that Julie drew the same picture and did not wish to tell a story. This time, however, Julie used the puppet to say that she was afraid to tell the story for fear that Mike might hurt her. Although the therapist's puppet attempted to correct this belief, Julie remained reluctant to go further (during Session 7 Julie disclosed that Mike had threatened her and told her not to tell anyone what they had been doing). During Session 6, before starting work on Julie's book, the therapist read her the story of "Taffy and the Invisible Magic Bandage" (Davis, 1988). This story is about a dog who has a fear of telling a secret, but finds that when she does her fears do not come true and she feels much better. Julie's mother was given a copy of this story to take home and read to her daughter.

This intervention, however, did not lead to further disclosure. After reading the story, Julie drew a picture that was similar to her previous ones, and again declined to tell a story to accompany it. It was clear at this point that Julie was not willing to elaborate upon her drawings or her story. During the previous sessions as well as this one, Julie had become anxious and stopped her disclosure at the same point. In Julie's initial disclosure to her mother, and later in therapy, she reported that this was when Mike had touched her in her genital area. It appeared that this aspect of the abuse was more anxiety provoking than the rest.

Session 7

The focus of this session was for Julie to share her story with her family. The purpose of this was to desensitize the child and family about the abuse and to address any concerns or "secrets" that might be held by the family. Julie showed her family each of the pictures she had drawn while the therapist read the story. At the conclusion of the story, Julie's mother asked her about other aspects of the abuse that she had originally disclosed. Julie said that she did not know what words to use to tell about it. Julie was willing, however, to act it out with puppets and asked her father to play the puppet of the perpetrator. By whispering to her father, Julie was finally able to disclose details of the abuse. Julie revealed that, in addition to exposing himself to her, Mike had touched her in her genital area and threatened her not to tell. It is significant that Julie was able to reveal the most threatening aspects of the abuse with her family present and her father playing the role of the perpetrator. Julie appeared to feel safe and protected in the family setting.

Session 8

Julie had not presented any significant distortions or misperceptions related to sexual abuse through her drawings. It remained possible, however, that cognitive distortions and maladaptive attributions might exist that had not been detected. To assess this, the therapist and Julie engaged in puppet play involving incidents of sexual abuse between adult and child puppets. During the puppet play, Julie consistently stated that it was not the child's fault. She displayed no sense of damage to the child and repeatedly said that the child should tell an adult because she would feel better.

Session 9

Due to scheduling problems, there was a 3-week gap between Sessions 8 and 9. The parents reported that during this time Julie had begun having nightmares as frequently as four to five times per week. When Julie was asked to draw a picture of one of her nightmares, she drew a picture of a girl who was scared. The therapist then asked Julie to draw another picture depicting a good ending to her nightmare. She drew a picture of herself yelling for her "huge" dad, and her dad coming for her. Cognitive restructuring was accomplished, as such, by encouraging Julie to develop another, more adaptive outcome for her picture. This procedure is similar to that used in cognitive-behavioral storytelling with depressed youth (Reinecke, 1992).

Session 10

The parents reported no further nightmares after this intervention. They also reported that for several weeks Julie had not displayed any symptoms related to use of the bathroom or fear of being in a room alone. Based on the decrease in symptoms, the lack of any apparent distorted perceptions related to the abuse, and Julie's ability to disclose, we began to prepare for termination.

During the play therapy portion of this session, Julie requested to play with modeling clay. The therapist allowed this, suggesting that Julie make a figure of Mike. Julie quickly agreed and also made a figure of herself. The figure of herself was proportionately smaller than that of Mike. The therapist stood the two figures up face to face and asked Julie what she would like to say to Mike. Julie began laughing at Mike and said that she wanted him to go to jail because he was bad. She repeated different variations of this several times, appearing to enjoy herself fully when laughing at Mike. She eventually punched the figure of Mike, knocked him over and smashed him. This play sequence provided Julie with an opportunity to feel in control of Mike and to express her feelings to him. This was important to do through play as the perpetrator had not admitted to the offenses or received any treatment. It was unlikely, then, that Julie would have an opportunity to confront him directly.

Session 11

During our last therapy session prior to termination, the therapist and Julie discussed the reasons for termination and their feelings about the abuse and her treatment. In preparation for termination, a decision was made with Julie and her family to mark the end of treatment with a "party." This would serve to mark the conclusion of Julie's treatment and to help her view the end of therapy as a positive event. Together they planned a termination party that, at Julie's request, would include her entire family. Julie felt that she was ready to end therapy. She stated that she had come here to talk about Mike so that it didn't make her feel so bad. She also said that she used to think about Mike all the time, but now she only thinks about him "a little." In order to better assess the change in Julie's thoughts and feelings related to Mike, the therapist drew a measuring line from 0–100 on a chalkboard. The therapist asked Julie to mark on the line how strongly she felt "mad," "sad," or "scared" when she thought about Mike, both before therapy and now. For mad, Julie marked 100 for both, before and now. For sad, she marked 100 before and 0 now. For scared, she marked 7 before and 0 now. Julie then included "happy" to this list and rated 0 for both before and now.

Although Julie seemed quite certain of her ability to talk to her family if she were ever to be exposed to sexual abuse again, the therapist engaged her in puppet play to reinforce this skill. In this play, the therapist's puppet (Gramps) attempted to trick Julie's puppet (Jimmy) into sexual touching. Despite several attempts at threats and manipulations, Jimmy went immediately and told his mother. Although Jimmy's mother did not believe him immediately, he insisted and the mother finally responded appropriately. Julie then put on the police puppet and arrested Gramps and put him in jail. Next, Julie sent a therapist puppet to the jail to talk to Gramps. The therapist (played by Julie) told Gramps that he should apologize to Jimmy, and said that Jimmy would "get better." Through this play, not only did Julie practice her disclosure skills, she again demonstrated that she understood that responsibility for the abuse rested with the adult, not the child, and that it is possible to be abused but learn to "get better."

Termination

As a means of objectively assessing treatment gains, Julie's mother was asked to complete the CBCL at termination (see Figure 13.3). As can be

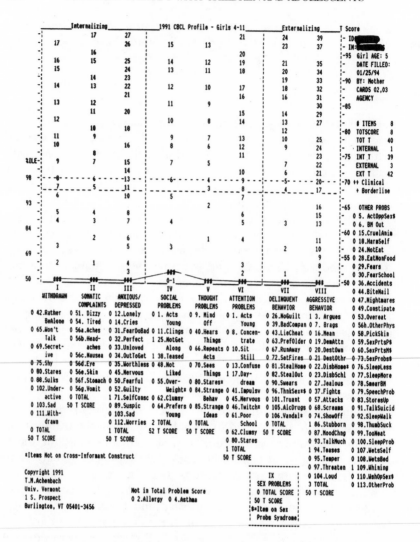

FIGURE 13.3. Termination CBCL completed by Julie's mother.

seen, all of the subscales of the CBCL were within the normal range. The significant items mentioned previously all had decreased from 1 to 0.

Session 12

Before starting the termination party, the therapist met with Julie's parents to discuss issues related to the conclusion of treatment. Julie's gains over the course of treatment were discussed, and parenting techniques that might be helpful in their work with her were reviewed. Their thoughts and feelings about the abuse, Julie's treatment, and the termination process were also discussed. Julie's parents were given information regarding normative child sexual behavior in order to help them react appropriately to any sexual play that Julie may engage in. The potential recurrence of symptomatology related to the sexual abuse at various developmental milestones was discussed. The family was encouraged to continue to openly discuss abuse-related issues with all of their children whenever the need arose. The therapist met briefly with Julie to discuss her feelings related to termination. However, Julie was so excited about the party that she was only able to focus on termination-related issues for a very limited amount of time. The entire family then joined in the party.

Follow-Up

Follow-up data was obtained from Julie's mother 8 months after the termination of treatment. At that time, she reported that Julie was continuing to do well. Her mother did not report any further concerns regarding Julie's emotional or behavioral functioning. Julie's mother completed a follow-up CBCL at this point (see Figure 13.4). In comparing this profile with the initial CBCL, it should be noted that it was also a nonclinical profile, with all scales at the 5th percentile, with the exception of the Anxious/Depressed scale, which was at the 55th percentile. The scales of Social Problems and Thought Problems, which had been elevated at the initial assessment, were now at the 50th percentile. As was true with the termination CBCL, each of the positively endorsed significant items on the initial CBCL had again decreased from 1 to 0. Julie's treatment gains, then, appeared to have been maintained.

DISCUSSION

The present case provides an example of the successful use of CBPT with a sexually abused child. There are a number of ways in which children are sexually molested, and the range of emotional and behavioral sequelae of the abuse is wide. It is important that we not consider an act of sexual abuse as a distinct entity, or expect that all sexually abused children will manifest the same reactions to their maltreatment. If sexual abuse and its effects on children can be viewed on continua with regard to severity, duration, adaptive resources, and availability of social support, then Julie might be considered to fall at the less severe end. Her maltreatment was not incestuous, although her neighbor was a known and trusted individual; the abuse occurred two times, rather than frequently; no penetration of any kind had occurred, although she was fondled by the perpetrator; and her parents believed her as soon as she told them what had happened. Consequently, she presented with relatively few symptoms compared with many

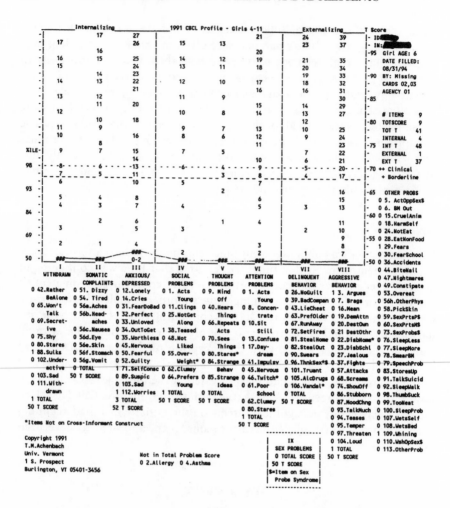

FIGURE 13.4. Follow-up CBCL completed by Julie's mother.

sexually abused children. She did not, for example, manifest encopresis, sexual acting out, severe depression, social withdrawal, or blunted affect. Julie and her family appeared to have been functioning well prior to the incident of abuse. Because of this, and the fact that attention was paid to her disclosure relatively soon after the abuse, her symptoms may not have had a chance to become more serious, and thus more difficult to treat. Our treatment of Julie's nightmares, fear of the bathroom, and fear of being alone was both brief and successful.

For CBPT to be effective, it must provide structured, goal-directed activities, as well as allow time for the child to spontaneously bring material to the session. By allowing the child the opportunity for unstructured play, he or she may convey information that might not arise if sessions are entirely structured and therapist-directed. An example from the present case occurred when Julie desired to play with the clay. The therapist permitted her to do this, but at some point focused Julie's play by requesting that she make a clay figure of the perpetrator. Through her clay representations of herself and the perpetrator, Julie conveyed angry feelings toward the perpetrator, along with her perception that he had deprived her of any control. The play structured by the therapist allowed Julie to express her feelings and gather a sense of control.

Our experience suggests that CBPT can be effective with a wide range of sexually abused children (Ruma, 1993). The past few years have witnessed an increase in cognitive-behavioral therapy with preschool-age children (e.g., Deblinger & Heflin, 1996), as well as some preliminary, but very encouraging, empirical studies that have highlighted the effectiveness of cognitive-behavioral interventions for sexually abused children (Cohen & Mannario, 1996a, 1996b, 1997; Deblinger et al., 1999; Stauffer & Deblinger, 1996). The 2-year follow up from the Deblinger et al. (1999) study, indicating that pre- to posttreatment improvements held at follow-up, is particularly encouraging.

One cannot generalize from our work with Julie to the treatment of children who have suffered more extensive abuse. Although the general principles and techniques of CBPT would not differ, the duration of treatment would likely be increased for a child who had been more severely abused over a longer period of time. Additional issues may influence both the type and duration of treatment. For example, a child whose disclosure is not believed by his or her parents will likely bring additional issues of mistrust to therapy that will need to be addressed as part of the treatment. Similarly, abuse by a family member may present problems, often related to the division of family loyalties.

A range of techniques and approaches can be incorporated into CBPT. The approaches utilized most successfully in CBPT with sexually abused children include bibliotherapy, drawings, art, and puppet play. With Julie, all of these approaches were used to desensitize her to feelings associated with the abuse, give her the courage to disclose details of the abuse, show how others learn to cope with their feelings, help to identify and correct maladaptive beliefs about the abuse and about herself, and reinstate a sense of control over her life. Although not used this way with Julie, drawings and bibliotherapy can also be used to convey to an abused child he or she is not alone in these experiences—other children have also been maltreated and experience similar feelings—and to teach prevention skills.

In using CBPT, one must be flexible and able to change modalities as needed. For instance, when it was clear that Julie was not able to tell the story of abuse on her own, puppets were incorporated into the drawing techniques. When using CBPT with sexually abused children, the therapist needs to estimate the child's readiness to disclose the details of the abuse through the drawing technique. If the therapist finds that the child is not yet able to tolerate this level of anxiety, it will be necessary to first introduce less-threatening modalities. Whether or not a perpetrator overtly threatens a child not to disclose what has happened, there is often a covert or perceived threat that makes disclosure difficult, especially for very young children.

As in cognitive-behavioral therapy with adults, generalization and maintenance of gains are important concerns. Explicit attempts are made to generalize skills the child has acquired in therapy to the natural environment and to maintain adaptive behaviors learned after the treatment has ended. The therapist must incorporate these goals into treatment and not assume they will occur naturally. In the present case, generalization and response prevention were addressed in a number of ways, including teaching and reinforcement of self-protection skills and using puppet play to teach Julie how to disclose any future abuse. Additionally, the parents were provided guidelines for what to expect in regard to normal sexual development, so that they could be aware of any problems that might arise. Finally, open communication and discussion were modeled for the family and encouraged in an effort to prevent future problems. In CBPT with sexually abused children, it is important for the therapist to handle termination in a way that does not contribute to difficulties with trust or feelings of abandonment on the part of the child. It is often helpful to hold a celebration to mark the child's achievements at the termination of therapy. This occasion can be used to reinforce the child's sense of self-control, as well as to help him or her see what has been accomplished through his or her own efforts in treatment.

REFERENCES

Achenbach, T. M. (1991). *Manual for the Child Behavior Checklist 4–18 and 1991 profile*. Burlington: Department of Psychiatry, University of Vermont.

Bandura, A. (1969). *Principles of behavior modification*. New York: Holt, Rinehart, & Winston.

Bandura, A., & Menlove, F. L. (1968). Factors determining vicarious extinction of avoidance behavior through symbolic modeling. *Journal of Personality and Social Psychology, 8*, 99–108.

Beck, A. T., & Emery, G. (1985). *Anxiety disorders and phobias: A cognitive perspective*. New York: Basic Books.

Beitchman, J. H., Zucker, K. J., Hood, J. E., da Costa, G. A., & Akman, D. (1991). A review of the short-term effects of child sexual abuse. *Child Abuse and Neglect, 15*, 537–556.

Browne, A., & Finkelhor, D. (1986). Initial and long-term effects: A review of the research. In D. Finkelhor, S. Araji, L. Baron, A. Browne, S. Doyle Peters, & G. Wyatt (Eds.), *A sourcebook on child sexual abuse* (pp. 143–179). Beverly Hills, CA: Sage.

Campbell, S. (1990). *Behavior problems in preschool children.* New York: Guilford Press.

Chard, K. M., Weaver, T. L., & Resick, P. A. (1997). Adapting cognitive processing therapy for child sexual abuse survivors. *Cognitive and Behavioral Practice, 4,* 31–52.

Cohen, J. A., & Mannarino, A. P. (1996a) Factors that mediate treatment outcome in sexually abused preschool children. *Journal of the American Academy of Child and Adolescent Psychiatry, 35,* 1402–1410.

Cohen, J. A., & Mannarino, A. P. (1996b) A treatment outcome study for sexually abused children: Initial findings. *Journal of the American Academy of Child and Adolescent Psychiatry, 35,* 1402–1410.

Cohen, J. A., & Mannarino, A. P. (1997). A treatment study for sexually abused preschool children: Outcome during a one-year follow-up. *Journal of the American Academy of Child and Adolescent Psychiatry, 36,* 1228–1235.

Cohen, J. A., & Mannario, A. P. (1998a). Factors that mediate treatment outcome of sexually abused preschool children: Six and 12 month follow-up. *Journal of the American Academy of Child and Adolescent Psychiatry, 37,* 44–51.

Cohen, J. A., & Mannarino, A. P. (1998b). Interventions for sexually abused children: Initial treatment outcome findings. *Child Maltreatment, 3,* 17–26.

Davis, N. (1988). *Once upon a time: Therapeutic stories.* Oxon Hill, MD: Nancy Davis.

Deblinger, E., & Heflin, A. H. (1996) *Treating sexually abused children and their nonoffending parents: A cognitive behavioral approach.* Thousand Oaks, CA: Sage.

Deblinger, E., Lippmann, J., & Steer, R. (1996). Sexually abused children suffering posttraumatic stress symptoms: Initial treatment outcome findings. *Child Maltreatment, 1,* 310–321.

Deblinger, E., McLeer, S. V., & Henry, D. (1990). Cognitive behavioral treatment for sexually abused children suffering post-traumatic stress: Preliminary findings. *The American Academy of Child and Adolescent Psychiatry, 29,* 747–752.

Deblinger, E., Steer, R. A., & Lippmann, J. (1999). Two-year follow-up study of cognitive behavioral therapy for sexually abused children suffering post-traumatic stress symptoms. *Child Abuse and Neglect, 23,* 1371–1378.

Emery, G., Bedrosian, R., & Garber, J. (1983). Cognitive therapy with depressed children and adolescents. In D. P. Cantwell & G. A. Carlson (Eds.), *Affective disorders in childhood and adolescence: An update* (pp. 445–471). New York: Spectrum.

Farrell, S. P., Hains, A. A., & Davies, W. H. (1998). Cognitive behavioral interventions for sexually abused children exhibiting PTSD symptomatology. *Behavior Therapy, 29,* 241–255.

Finkelhor, D. (1990). Early and long-term effects of child sexual abuse: An update. *Professional Psychology: Research and Practice, 21,* 325–330.

Finkelhor, D., & Berliner, L. (1995). Research on the treatment of sexually abused children: A review and recommendations. *Journal of the American Academy of Child and Adolescent Psychiatry, 34,* 1408–1423.

Finkelhor, D., & Browne, A. (1986). Initial and long-term effects: A conceptual framework. In D. Finkelhor, S. Araji, L. Baron, A. Browne, S. Doyle Peters, & G. Wyatt (Eds.), *A sourcebook on child sexual abuse* (pp. 180–198). Beverly Hills, CA: Sage.

Friedrich, W. N. (1990). *Psychotherapy of sexually abused children and their families.* New York: Norton.

Gelman, R., & Baillargeon, R. (1983). A review of some Piagetian concepts. In J. H. Flavell & E. M. Markman (Eds.), *Handbook of child psychology: Vol. 3. Cognitive development* (pp. 167–230). New York: Wiley.

Gil, E. (1991). *The healing power of play.* New York: Guilford Press.

Green, A. H. (1993). Child sexual abuse: Immediate and long-term effects and intervention. *Journal of the American Academy of Child and Adolescent Psychiatry, 32,* 890–902.

Harter, S. (1977). A cognitive-developmental approach to children's expression of conflicting feelings and a technique to facilitate such expression in play therapy. *Journal of Consulting and Clinical Psychology, 45,* 417–432.

Harter, S. (1983). Cognitive-developmental considerations in the conduct of play therapy. In C. Schaefer & K. O'Connor (Eds.), *Handbook of play therapy* (pp. 95–127). New York: Wiley.

Janoff-Bulman, R. (1979). Characterological versus behavioral self-blame: Inquiries into depression and rape. *Journal of Personality and Social Psychology, 37,* 1798–1809.

Kendall, P. C. (Ed.). (1991). *Child and adolescent therapy.* New York: Guilford Press.

Kendall-Tackett, K. A., Williams, L. M., & Finkelhor, D. (1993). Impact of sexual abuse on children: A review and synthesis of recent empirical studies. *Psychological Bulletin, 113,* 164–180.

Knell, S. M. (1993a). *Cognitive-behavioral play therapy.* Northvale, NJ: Aronson.

Knell, S. M. (1993b). To show and not tell: Cognitive-behavioral play therapy. In T. Kottman & C. Schaefer (Eds.), *Play therapy in action* (pp. 169–208). Northvale, NJ: Aronson.

Knell, S. M. (1994). Cognitive-behavioral play therapy. In K. O'Connor & C. Schaefer (Eds.), *Handbook of play therapy: Vol. 2* (pp. 111–142). New York: Wiley.

Knell, S. M. (1997). Cognitive-behavioral play therapy. In K. O'Connor & L. Mages (Eds.), *Play therapy theory and practice: A comparative presentation* (pp. 79–99). New York: Wiley.

Knell, S. M. (1999). Cognitive behavioral play therapy. In S. W. Russ & T. Ollendick (Eds.), *Handbook of psychotherapies with children and families* (pp. 385–404). New York: Plenum Press.

Knell, S. M. (2000). Cognitive behavioral play therapy with children with fears and phobias. In H. G. Kaduson & C. E. Schaefer (Eds.), *Short-term play therapy for children* (pp. 3–27). New York: Guilford Press.

Knell, S. M., & Beck, K. W. (2000). Puppet sentence completion task. In K Gitlin-Weiner, A. Sandgrund, & C. E. Schaefer (Eds.), *Play diagnosis and assessment* (2nd ed., pp. 704–721). New York: Wiley.

Major, B., Mueller, P., & Hildebrandt, K. (1985). Attributions, expectations, and coping with abortion. *Journal of Personality and Social Psychology, 48,* 585–599.

Marlatt, G. A., & Gordon, J. R. (Eds.). (1985). *Relapse prevention: Maintenance strategies in the treatment of addictive disorders.* New York: Guilford Press.

McCarthy, B. W. (1990). Treatment of incest families: A cognitive-behavioral model. *Journal of Sex Education and Therapy, 16,* 101–114.

Meichenbaum, D. (1971). Examination of model characteristics in reducing avoidance behavior. *Journal of Personality and Social Psychology, 17,* 298–307.

Meichenbaum, D. (1977). *Cognitive-behavior modification: An integrative approach.* New York: Plenum Press.

Meichenbaum, D. (1985). *Stress inoculation training.* New York: Pergamon Press.

Piacentini, J., Bergman, R., & Aikins, J. (in press). Cognitive-behavioral interventions in childhood anxiety disorders. In M. Reinecke & D. Clark (Eds.), *Cognitive therapy across the lifespan: Prospects and challenges.* Cambridge, UK: Cambridge University Press.

Piaget, J. (1926). *The language and thought of the child.* London: Routledge & Kegan Paul.

Piaget, J. (1928). *Judgment and reasoning in the child.* London: Routledge & Kegan Paul.

Piaget, J. (1930). *The child's conception of physical causality.* New York: Harcourt, Brace.

Porter, F. S., Blick, L. C., & Sgroi, S. M. (1982). Treatment of the sexually abused child. In S. M. Sgroi (Ed.), *Handbook of clinical intervention in child sexual abuse* (pp. 109–146). Lexington, KY: Lexington Books.

Reinecke, M. (1992). Childhood depression. In A. Freeman & F. Dattilio (Eds.), *Comprehensive casebook of cognitive therapy* (pp. 147–158). New York: Plenum Press.

Resick, P. A., & Schnicke, M. K. (1992). Cognitive processing therapy for sexual assault victims. *Journal of Consulting and Clinical Psychology, 60,* 748–756.

Ruma, C. (1993). Cognitive-behavioral play therapy with sexually abused children. In S. M. Knell (Ed.), *Cognitive-behavioral play therapy* (pp. 199–230). Northvale, NJ: Aronson.

Sgroi, S. (1982). *Handbook of clinical intervention in child sexual abuse.* Lexington KY: Lexington Books.

Shapiro, J. P. (1989). Self-blame versus helplessness in sexually abused children: An attributional analysis with treatment recommendations. *Journal of Social and Clinical Psychology, 8,* 442–455.

Shirk, S. R. (1988). Introduction: A cognitive-developmental perspective on child psychotherapy. In S. R. Shirk (Ed.), *Cognitive development and child psychotherapy* (pp. 1–16). New York: Plenum Press.

Silverman, W., Ginsburg, G., & Kurtines, W. (1995). Clinical issues in treating children with anxiety and phobic disorders. *Cognitive and Behavioral Practice, 2,* 93–117.

Silverman, W., & Kurtines, W. (1996). *Anxiety and phobic disorders: A pragmatic approach.* New York: Plenum Press.

Smucker, M. R., & Niederee, J. (1995). Treating incest-related PTSD and pathogenic schemas through imaginal exposure and rescripting. *Cognitive and Behavioral Practice, 2,* 63–93.

Spence, S., & Reinecke, M. (in press). Cognitive approaches to understanding, preventing, and treating child and adolescent depression. In: M. Reinecke & D.

Clark (Eds.), *Cognitive therapy across the lifespan: Prospects and challenges.* Cambridge, UK: Cambridge University Press.

Stauffer, L., & Deblinger, E. (1996). Cognitive behavioral groups for nonoffending mothers and their young sexually abused children: A preliminary treatment outcome study. *Child Maltreatment, 1,* 65–76.

Walker, L. E., & Bolkovatz, M. S. (1988). Play therapy with children who have experienced sexual assault. In L. Walker (Ed.), *Handbook of sexual abuse of children* (pp. 249–269). New York: Springer.

Wilkes, T. C. R., Belsher, G., Rush, A. J., Frank, E., & Associates. (1994). *Cognitive therapy for depressed adolescents.* New York: Guilford Press.

Zarb, J. (1992). *Cognitive-behavioral assessment and therapy with adolescents.* New York: Brunner/Mazel.

SUGGESTED READINGS

Deblinger, E., & Heflin, A. H. (1996) *Treating sexually abused children and their nonoffending parents: A cognitive behavioral approach.* Thousand Oaks, CA: Sage.

Finkelhor, D., & Berliner, L. (1995). Research on the treatment of sexually abused children: A review and recommendations. *Journal of the American Academy of Child and Adolescent Psychiatry, 34,* 1408–1423.

King, N., Tonge, B. J., Mullen, P., Myerson, N., Heyne, D., & Ollendick, T. H. (1999). Cognitive-behavioural treatment of sexually abused children: A review of research. *Behavioural and Cognitive Psychotherapy, 27,* 295–309.

Knell, S. M. (1994). Cognitive-behavioral play therapy. In K. O'Connor & C. Schaefer (Eds.), *Handbook of play therapy: Vol. 2* (pp. 111–142). New York: Wiley.

Ruma, C. (1993). Cognitive-behavioral play therapy with sexually abused children. In S. M. Knell (Ed.), *Cognitive-behavioral play therapy* (pp. 199–230). Northvale, NJ: Aronson.

Sgroi, S. (1982). *Handbook of clinical intervention in child sexual abuse.* Lexington, KY: Lexington Books.

14

Treatment of Adolescents and Young Adults with High-Functioning Autism or Asperger Syndrome

DEAN W. BEEBE
SUSAN RISI

Autism is a pervasive developmental disorder that is characterized by the childhood onset of qualitative impairments in social interaction, qualitative impairments in communication, and restricted repetitive and stereotyped patterns of behaviors, interests, and activities (American Psychiatric Association, 1994; World Health Organization, 1992). Its prevalence is roughly 4–31 per 10,000, depending on the diagnostic criteria used (Filipek et al., 1999). Roughly 75–80% of cases display intellectual abilities below 70 (in the mentally retarded range; Lord & Rutter, 1994). The remaining 20–25%, referred to as "high functioning" by many within the autism community, have attracted increased interest in recent years because of their somewhat unique symptom expression, relatively stronger adaptive potential, and amenability to a variety of research and clinical tools (e.g., Howlin, 1999; Kunce & Mesibov, 1998; Mesibov, Shea, & Adams, 2001; Wing, 1989). Recent interest has also emerged around a related syndrome, Asperger disorder (American Psychiatric Association, 1994) or Asperger syndrome (World Health Organization, 1992). Currently distinguished from autism only by a lack of specific language delay and lack of mental retardation, there is some controversy as to whether Asperger syndrome represents a disorder distinct from high-functioning autism (e.g., Mesibov et al., 2001; Schopler, Mesibov, & Kunce, 1998).

The etiology of autism and Asperger syndrome remains unclear. Early psychoanalytic explanations have not withstood empirical test (Smith, 1993). Strong evidence of a genetic component to autism, coupled with numerous but difficult to replicate medical findings, have led to the currently dominant theory that autism and Asperger syndrome are neurodevelopmentally based disorders (e.g., Tsai, 1999). However, no specific biological cause or sets of causes has emerged that can account for more than a small minority of cases, and multiple "breakthroughs" over the years have failed to make good on their treatment promises. Heflin and Simpson (1998) recently reviewed a number of empirically discounted interventions for autism, including holding therapy, gentle teaching, facilitated communication, dietary interventions, and optical lenses. Pharmacological interventions, though yielding symptomatic change in some individuals, have also failed to show consistent benefits across cases (Martin, Patzer, & Volkmar, 2000).

Neither the failure of these treatments nor the neurodevelopmental model rules out effective behavior change. Behavioral treatment techniques have been demonstrated to be efficacious, even for very impaired children with autism (Heflin & Simpson, 1998). Individuals with high-functioning autism (HFA) and Asperger syndrome (AS), by virtue of their increased cognitive and verbal capacity, are candidates for cognitive-behavioral approaches (Heflin & Simpson, 1998). As discussed later, the cognitive-behavioral therapeutic stance is in some ways well suited for dealing with adolescents and adults with HFA or AS. In other cases, adaptations can be made to established cognitive-behavioral techniques, or unique interventions have been described that nonetheless fit within a cognitive-behavioral framework.

Even so, cognitive-behavioral treatment (CBT) may not be appropriate for young children with HFA or AS because of their social immaturity, possible language delays, and difficulties with higher-order reasoning and problem solving. Indeed, the need for CBT may increase with age. During adolescence, social demands increase, there is a greater societal push for major life transitions (e.g., career choices; Tantam, 2000), and the individual's increasing cognitive sophistication often leads him or her to become more aware of interpersonal and work failures (Stoddart, 1998). As a result, this chapter is focused on CBT for adolescents and young adults with HFA or AS.

The goal of this chapter is to provide an overview of the symptoms and treatment of HFA and AS in adolescents and young adults. Because there is considerable overlap in the symptoms, outcomes, and potential treatments of HFA and AS, we address both disorders in this chapter. We begin by summarizing the most commonly described features of individuals with HFA or AS, highlighting how these may impact upon psychotherapy. Integrated into this discussion are potential benefits of, and suggested modifications to, the CBT approach. We then discuss issues of clinical assessment, followed by a number of potential treatment techniques. Finally we present a treatment case that illustrates the use of CBT in an older adolescent with HFA.

SUMMARY OF KEY FEATURES OF HFA/AS

Terms such as "high functioning" should not obscure the marked adaptive impairments shown by individuals with HFA/AS (Klin, Volkmar, & Sparrow, 2000; Schopler et al., 1998). Indeed, as noted by Howlin (1999), "because of their relatively high cognitive ability, and their *apparently* competent communication skills, this group of children is often least well served or understood [of children with pervasive developmental disorders]" (p. 176). The following is a brief summary of key features of HFA/AS, particularly as they relate to outpatient CBT.

Social Deficits

Adolescents and adults with HFA/AS display markedly disrupted social interaction skills, as evidenced in poor use of nonverbal communication, lack of social or emotional reciprocity, poor use of time and space in social interactions, limited social play and recreational skills, and generally poorly developed social relationships. Multiple core deficits have been proposed for these poor social skills. These include an underdeveloped "theory of mind" or "mindblindedness" (e.g., Howlin, Baron-Cohen, & Hadwin, 1999). The argument is that individuals with HFA/AS have an impaired ability to "infer other people's mental states (their thoughts, beliefs, desires, intentions, etc.) . . . [and] use this information to interpret what they say, make sense of their behavior and predict what they will do next" (Howlin et al., 1999, p. 2). Neuropsychologists have further suggested that these individuals have extremely poor "executive functioning" (e.g., Ozonoff, 1998). Despite having seemingly intact basic perceptual and expressive skills, they lack the planning, organization, cognitive integration, attentional regulation, and flexibility to appropriately use these basic skills. Others have proposed a lack of "central coherence" (Frith, 1989), in which specific details of social events are selectively attended to, without a sense of their connected meaning—the extreme of "not seeing the forest for the trees" (Mesibov, 1992).

By adolescence, individuals with HFA/AS often have an emerging awareness of their social difficulties (Stoddart, 1998). Though stereotyped as being socially uninterested, many of these individuals have some desire for social contact or at least social acceptance (Eliasoph & Donnellan, 1995), but lack the skills to reach these goals. Instead, they have experienced repeated relationship failures, peer rejection, and even exploitation

(Howlin, 1999). Particularly during adolescence and young adulthood, many also desire formal aspects of relationships (e.g., having a "boyfriend" or "girlfriend"), but have a limited understanding of the nature of these relationships (Gillberg & Schaumann, 1989). Many young adults with HFA/AS are frustrated by an inability to obtain or keep a job that is commensurate with their intellectual or academic skills. Depression may follow repeated but poorly informed and unsuccessful attempts to remediate what they perceive as "the problem." Anxiety is also common in unstructured, rapidly changing, emotionally loaded, or socially challenging situations (e.g., lunch periods), compounding social reasoning deficits and potentially resulting in maladaptive behaviors (e.g., abrupt withdrawal, increased stereotypies, verbal or physical aggression).

The clinician should expect to be faced with social difficulties within the therapeutic context. Eye contact may be fleeting or inconsistent. The client may make poor use of social space (too much or too little). He or she may draw surprisingly inaccurate conclusions regarding the therapist's intentions. The client may take a rather self-absorbed stance toward therapy not out of narcissism, but rather due to social incompetence. There may be a fragmented understanding of time and space, such that cause–effect relationships are distorted or unrecognized. To the client, an occupied and active waiting room may be torturous, and unstructured periods in psychotherapy may be anxiety-provoking and disorganizing. He or she may have both a poor understanding of others' intentions and emotions and a rather poorly developed and fragmented sense of his or her own. Under these circumstances, the task of developing a supportive, empathic working relationship is particularly challenging.

Communication Impairments

By definition, individuals with HFA display early language impairments that are not present in AS. However, individuals with both HFA and AS can perform within the normal range on the language tests typically administered by psychologists. In these cases, communication may most accurately be described as deviant, rather than delayed (though both may be present in the same individual). Diane Twachtman-Cullen (1998) summarized the deviant communication patterns often seen in HFA/AS. These include paralinguistic aspects of speech (e.g., prosody, rhythm, timing), nonverbal paralinguistic communication features (e.g., gestures, facial expression, eye gaze) and communication pragmatics (e.g., dealing with nonliteral communication such as analogies or figures of speech, and understanding the needed communication quantity, quality, relevance, and level of clarity/detail for a given situation). Echolalic speech may be present, but less obvious than in lower-functioning autism (Howlin, 1999). Individuals with HFA/AS may echo whole phrases or sentences from a variety of sources (e.g., film, television) and may use them in reasonably appropriate situations.

The theories regarding mindblindedness (i.e., theory of mind), executive dysfunction, and central coherence described earlier also are applicable in explaining the language impairments seen in HFA/AS. In addition, neurological explanations have been evoked based upon symptom similarities with individuals with right hemispheric (especially right temporal lobe) injuries (e.g., Robbins, 1997). However, neuroimaging and autopsy data have yet to confirm any consistent or specific neuropathological process in autism or AS (Filipek, 1999).

Therapists working with individuals with HFA/AS should be careful in their own expressive communication and in their interpretations of their clients' communications. The therapist should use concrete, literal language, and should not assume that his or her tone of voice, posture, or other verbal or nonverbal paralinguistic aspects of speech have been attended to or interpreted accurately by the client. Paralinguistic markers for emotion or intention may be absent or odd in the client's communication, but the therapist must withhold judgment on the meaning of this. For example, a "pained" facial expression and apparently flat affect may not be associated with depression, yet the absence of sad facial features and sing-song intonation may accompany a subjective sense of sadness in the client. In general, it should not be assumed that the therapist understands the workings of the client's mind any more than the client with "mindblindedness" understands the therapist's (Gray, 1998; Mesibov, 1992). Individuals with HFA/AS have described their own mental processing as being quite different from that of their unaffected peers (e.g., "thinking in pictures"; Grandin, 1995). Thus, the therapist's empathic skills are often put to a greater test than his or her technical skills (Morgan, 1996). This is especially important in cognitive-behavioral case conceptualization, in which the emphasis is on the mental processes that underlie behaviors, rather than the behaviors alone.

Restricted Repetitive and Stereotypied Behavior, Interests, and Activities

Adolescents and adults with HFA/AS are often cognitively and behaviorally rigid. They cling to routine and deal poorly with unexpected change. Transitions between activities can be anxiety-provoking and disorganizing. In contrast to the stereotyped and repetitive motor mannerisms that are common in lower-functioning individuals with autism, the stereotypies involved in HFA/AS are more complex and involve increased cognitive sophistication (Howlin, 1999). However, without explicit training and a supportive environment, this sophistication is rarely functional in daily life. Individuals with HFA/AS may amass tremendous factual knowledge about a circumscribed area of interest at the expense of other potential interests, and without an understanding of how these facts interrelate on a higher, meaning-related level. For example, they may focus excessively on baseball statistics without true comprehension of, appreciation of, or enjoyment of the sport itself. Some extreme interests may have superficially age-appropriate content (e.g., computers to a 16-year-old), but remain maladaptive in quality and intensity. Verbal routines, which can take the form of incessant repetitive questions, can move beyond the individual to involve larger systems, such as the family (Howlin, 1999). One parent with whom we worked was exhausted by what she called "jukebox mommy," in which her daughter repeatedly demanded that she recite a series of songs while driving.

Research on executive dysfunction has indicated that mental flexibility is particularly weak for individuals with HFA/AS (Ozonoff, 1998), suggesting one possible explanation for this rigidity and stereotyped interests and behaviors. In addition to this impairment-based explanation, it has been suggested that these stereotypies serve to reduce anxiety by imposing structure and order upon otherwise overwhelming and confusing situations (Jordan & Powell, 1996; Tantam, 2000).

The individual with HFA/AS may attempt to engage the therapist in his or her routines. This can be frustrating, especially when it appears to interfere with other planned activities. Though it is important that the therapist not become locked into a repetitive pattern of interaction around a client's particular area of interest, this pattern should be addressed therapeutically. A functional analysis of the situation should be undertaken to determine what function, if any, the stereotypy might serve for the client. It may be possible to minimize sources of anxiety (e.g., unstructured time) or other environmental antecedents or maintaining factors for the behaviors. Suggesting alternative courses of behavior, even if these courses are themselves scripted, may be helpful. It may also be helpful to work with the client to place limits upon when and under what circumstances it is acceptable to engage in discussions about his or her specific interests or routines. For example, the last 5 minutes of each session could be devoted to such a discussion. As described later, a therapist may also use these special interests to increase motivation for gains in other areas, or may facilitate the more adaptive use of these interests.

Cognitive and Developmental Variability

Aside from the definitional requirement that individuals with HFA/AS not fall within the mentally retarded range, there is little homogeneity across individuals in specific cognitive skills or developmental level. There is some research to suggest relatively stronger nonverbal than verbal skills in HFA and the reverse pattern in AS (Gillberg, 1998). However, such a pattern is not truly modal to either diagnosis, and tends to be an oversimplification even when it is found for a given case (Ozonoff & Griffith, 2000). Even within a seemingly unitary measure, such as the subtests that enter into Verbal IQ, there is often considerable variability in subtest scores. This variability also holds true on other developmental issues that lend themselves less to formal psychometric measurement. For example, some aspects of social discourse may be more challenging than others for any given individual. Little research has been devoted to other developmental issues, such as moral reasoning, but clinical experience suggests that areas of delay or deviance may be present to some degree in individuals with HFA/AS.

The client's functional use of these cognitive and other developmentally driven skills may vary depending on the situation. The maximal use of these skills often occurs in familiar, structured, routine, and emotionally neutral situations. To the degree that the situation deviates from this "ideal"—and most social, educational, and occupational situations deviate substantially—the client will probably have greater difficulty applying these skills in an adaptive manner (Matthews, 1996).

The therapist should be prepared to work with individuals who have tremendous variability in their abilities. He or she should not make assumptions about a person's adaptive ability in a given context based upon observations or measurements in a different context. The behaviors displayed in the therapy room may be quite discrepant from those seen in daily life. Even more than with most clients, generalization of treatment effects is a particular challenge when working with individuals with HFA/AS. Koegel, Koegel, and Parks (1995) and Schreibman (1994) presented concrete suggestions for improving treatment generalization. These include intervening in multiple applied contexts, teaching "pivotal behaviors" (described later), using intermittent reinforcement schedules, and taking advantage of naturally occurring behavioral contingencies.

THE APPLICABILITY OF COGNITIVE-BEHAVIORAL THERAPY TO INDIVIDUALS WITH HFA/AS

There has been little empirical examination of the efficacy of CBT techniques in the treatment of individuals with HFA/AS. However, the cognitive-behavioral model and therapeutic stance have clear application. CBT takes into account the cognitive mechanisms that cause and maintain maladaptive behaviors (Kendall, Marrs, & Chu, 1998). This provides an opportunity to get beyond the "tip of the iceberg" to understand not only environment–behavior contingencies in HFA/AS, but also the underlying cognitive mechanisms that can cut across situations (Schopler, 1989). Cognition is seen as multifaceted in CBT (Kendall, 1993). Individuals with HFA/AS do not simply have maladaptive cognitive content and products (i.e., self-talk, thoughts, and attributions); first-hand accounts from these individuals describe idiosyncratic cognitive processes (i.e., unusual perceptual, memory, and interpretive processes; e.g., Grandin, 1995). The therapist using a CBT model appreciates and seeks to understand the client's unique worldview so that appropriate interventions can be put into place.

In CBT, developmental variables are taken into account as well. Emphasis is placed upon breaking down environmental demands into the subskills required under a given set of motivation and task characteristics (Kimball, Nelson, & Politano, 1993). This has particular applicability with individuals diagnosed with HFA/AS, whose skills and adaptive behaviors can be highly variable. CBT is skill-driven and focused on the here and now, rather than insight-driven and based upon historical causes (Ronen, 1998). The abysmal history of psychotherapies based upon "intrapsychic insight" in the treatment of autism attests to the difficulties using the latter strategy (e.g., Smith, 1993). In contrast, there is accumulating evidence that here-and-now skill-driven programs can lead to lasting positive effects (Heflin & Simpson, 1998).

In the therapy room, CBT therapists are active and provide structure as needed (Kendall, Panichelli-Mindel, & Gerow, 1995). Appropriately applied, this stance tends to minimize the anxiety and disorganization that can result when an individual with HFA/AS is placed in an unstructured social situation. CBT also recognizes the need to understand and access situations outside of the therapy office (Ronen, 1998). When working with individuals with HFA/AS, it is essential to assess and intervene (or coordinate interventions) in the applied environment because of their behavioral variability and difficulties generalizing treatment effects across situations.

Despite this applicability of CBT to clinical work with individuals with HFA/AS, some deviations from CBT as traditionally practiced are also required. Though CBT is typically time-limited (Kendall et al., 1998), the lifelong developmental nature of HFA/AS may dictate longer-term treatment, or at least planned long-term follow-up with intermittent periods of more intensive interventions. This raises the issue of therapeutic goals. CBT recognizes that treatment is often not curative, but rather is focused on building coping skills (Kendall et al., 1998). Even so, treatment for some syndromes, such as enuresis and school phobia, is essentially curative. However, no treatment has proven to be curative for HFA/AS. Rather, the CBT "coping skill" model is taken to its most intensive level with individuals with HFA/AS; realistic goals are typically framed around maximizing adaptive functioning in a given area, realizing that the core dysfunction(s) in HFA/AS will remain. Thus, a goal of employment or vocational training may be reached as much by environmental accommodations as it is by building the client's skills or by modifying his or her interpretive style (Schopler, 1989).

Because of executive dysfunction and of delayed psychosocial development, adolescents and adults with HFA/AS may also require the use of techniques that are often applied when working with younger children. This may include using verbal labeling and rational self-talk, reducing abstract concepts to concrete examples, using visual supports (e.g., blackboards, "feeling" scales and charts, "thought bubbles"), and, when modeling or role playing behaviors, simplifying the behavior sequences and explicitly drawing attention to important cues in the model or situation (Bernard & Joyce, 1993; Kimball et al., 1993).

Finally, the therapist must be cautious around issues of client confidentiality with young adults with HFA/AS (Tantam, 2000). Despite being beyond the age of legal independence, many of these individuals remain dependent on others for their basic needs, including coverage of mental health care costs. Moreover, successful treatment typically hinges upon the involvement of individuals in the client's natural environment, such as parents, instructors, and employers. We advise a thorough discussion of these issues with the client and those working with him or her, with additional legal consultation as needed, so that the nature and limitations of confidentiality are clear from the start.

ASSESSMENT

Individuals with suspected HFA/AS should undergo a thorough initial assessment to (1) clarify diagnostic issues; (2) characterize the individual's functioning across multiple contexts; (3) identify targets for intervention; (4) characterize cognitive, functional, or behavioral issues that cause or maintain maladaptive behaviors; (5) identify personal and environmental resources and needs; and (6) develop an initial treatment plan.

Though diagnostic issues are given quick consideration with some disorders, HFA/AS requires more thorough attention. Many individuals with HFA/AS have endured multiple misdiagnoses, resulting in inadequate or counterproductive interventions. The accurate diagnosis of an individual with HFA/AS can lead to a fundamental "paradigm shift" in the conceptualizations of those working with him or her. Behaviors that were at one time thought to be volitional can be reframed as the results of skill deficits and idiosyncratic cognitive processes that stem from neurodevelopmental anomalies. This requires careful diagnostic analysis and documentation. At the time of this writing, the diagnostic "gold standards" were the Revised Autism Diagnostic Interview (ADI-R; Lord, Rutter, & Le Couteur, 1994) and Autism Diagnostic Observation Schedule (ADOS; Lord et al., 2000; Lord, Rutter, DiLavore, & Risi, 1999). The ADI-R is a detailed clinical interview covering key diagnostic (including differential diagnostic) issues and associated features of autism. The ADOS is a semistructured observation schedule in which the examiner creates situations, varying according to the child's developmental level, which tend to elicit autistic symptoms. Both the ADI-R and ADOS have clinically validated diagnostic algorithms and yield a wealth of qualitative information to guide treatment planning. Unfortunately, both also require extensive training, and the ADOS, though commercially available, is prohibitively costly for practitioners who do not focus on individuals with pervasive developmental disorders. Other formal instruments, such as the Childhood Autism Rating Scale (CARS; Schopler, Reichler, & Rochen-Renner, 1988) and the Autistic Spectrum Screening Questionnaire (ASSQ; Ehlers, Gillberg, & Wing, 1999) can be helpful. However, each has weaknesses. For example, the CARS, which yields a composite severity index, may tend to underdiagnose individuals of normal intelligence, such as those with HFA/AS (Klin, Sparrow, Marans, Carter, & Volkmar, 2000). The reader is referred to Filipek and colleagues (1999) for a thorough discussion of diagnostic issues.

As summarized by Klin, Sparrow, and colleagues (2000), the assessment process often requires the involvement of multiple disciplines, including speech and language therapy (focused on language pragmatics rather than mechanics), neuropsychology, psychiatry, and educational or vocational specialists. It typically involves multiple interviews, potentially including the client, family members, educators, other treating clinicians, and employers. *In vivo* observations and videotapes of the client in the natural environment often yield a wealth of information that is unavailable in the structured office environment. Though adding unique information, unidimensional evaluations such as neuropsychological testing should never take place in isolation (Ozonoff, 1998). It is imperative to develop a truly integrative perspective, using specialty input as needed, and placing the findings in a cognitive-behavioral therapeutic framework.

Case Formulation

Beyond diagnosis, we agree with Klin, Sparrow, and colleagues' (2000) assertion that the goal of a comprehensive assessment of individuals with HFA/AS "is not to stop at a simple list of standardized test results but to attempt to capture the disability as it affects the individual in his or her day-to-day life" (pp. 309-310). The foundation of this is an awareness of the maladaptive behaviors displayed by the client, including dimensions such as frequency, severity, duration, and pervasiveness across situations. A well-built case formulation then explores how these behaviors affect the child's adaptive functioning at home, school, work, and in the community. For example, though it is important to know the amount of time a child invests in a preoccupation with baseball statistics, it is even more important to take the next step to understand how this limits his or her ability to function socially, disrupts family life, and prevents effective education. The therapist should also understand how the client's environment might be modified to accommodate the unique worldview and developmental strengths and weaknesses of the client. This environmental accommodation model, which has been promoted extensively through North Carolina's TEACCH program (e.g., Mesibov, 1992), contrasts with many traditional behavioral and CBT approaches, which focus on client changes.

Supplementing this behavioral and contextual information, the cognitive-behavioral case formulation attempts to characterize the "meaning" of a behavior (Jordan & Powell, 1996; Mesibov, 1992). This meaning refers to the behavior's foundation in cognitive processes (e.g., poor social perception) and contents (e.g., specific erroneous beliefs about a social situation). In CBT, it is not an examination of "symbolic" aspects of the behavior (Kendall et al., 1998). For example, a boy who uses a racial slur may be echoing it from a movie or television show in which it was used as a term of familiarity or endearment. Prior to exploring the racist undertones of the slur, or trying to interpret the slur in terms of a symbolic expression of personal power, it may be more productive to determine the "meaning" of this behavior. It would be instructive to learn that, despite the negative emotional load of the slur, the boy may have been attempting to connect socially, but using a terribly misguided sense as to when such language is appropriate.

Thus, a complete case formulation has multiple facets, including diagnostic information, a functional behavioral analysis, characterization of the client's adaptive functioning across multiple contexts, understanding of both client and environmental resources, and characterization of the client's cognitive processes and cognitive contents/interpretations. This case formulation then acts as a guide for the choice and implementation of treatment strategies.

TREATMENT STRATEGIES

In this section we provide a summary of potential treatment strategies. Though some of these have been formally researched in samples of lower-functioning individuals with autism, few of these studies have been well controlled (Heflin & Simpson, 1998). The research literature on HFA/AS has been focused almost exclusively on descriptive, diagnostic, and medical and neuropathological issues – controlled intervention research with these individuals is conspicuously limited in the current literature. Thus, the treatment options in the following list are based upon reasonable theoretical or clinical grounds and are therefore considered promising, but not yet empirically supported. This list is neither prescriptive nor comprehensive, but is intended to give the clinician a sense of the strategies that may be adapted for any given case. Citations are provided for reader follow-up. Pragmatic communication skills are addressed in many of these interventions, but we recommend that more intensive language interventions, if needed, be directed by a speech and language therapist who has specialty training in pragmatic communication work (see Twachtman, 1996, for guidance).

Strategies for Treating Social Skills Deficits

A number of social skill promotion programs have been developed for children with non-autistic psychiatric issues and are commercially available. Unfortunately, the severity of deficit, unique cluster of difficulties, and particular problems with cross-contextual treatment generalization found with HFA/AS generally preclude the use of these programs with clients with HFA/AS (Klin & Volkmar, 2000). Instead, it may be helpful to begin with concrete rules of conduct (Howlin, 1999). These rote rules and sequences are not adequate substitutes for fluid social problem solving. However, developing fluid social skills may not be a reasonable goal for many individuals with HFA/AS, and well-formulated rules can help clients through a number of challenging situations that allow for greater exposure to natural contingencies (Mesibov, 1992). General guidelines for developing interventions were laid out by Attwood (1998) and Mesibov and colleagues (2001). Faherty (2000) also provided helpful "workbook" materials that can be used to supplement treatment. What follows are summaries of selected specific approaches.

The concepts of "mindblindedness" and theory of mind, as explanations for autistic behaviors, remain controversial. Even so, interventions based upon this model may be useful in effecting symptomatic change. Howlin and colleagues (1999) published a manual of interventions to improve recognition of emotional states in others, perspective taking, and prediction of others' behaviors. Though preliminary research cited in the manual is supportive, the manualized tasks were designed for young children, and therefore require adaptation for use with adolescents and young adults with HFA/AS.

Carol Gray (e.g., 1998) has developed two interventions to aid the social interaction of individuals with autism: "social stories" and "comic strip conversations." These are visually based strategies for helping individuals with autism to comprehend social situations. In social stories, text is coordinated with pictures in a documentary-like fashion to make situations that are difficult to "read" more predictable and meaningful. Comic strip conversations combine simple drawings, text embedded in dialogue "bubbles," symbols to visually represent paralinguistic aspects of conversation (e.g., upper-case letters for loud words), and colors to symbolize the motivation behind actions or statements. In creating the comic strip sequence, the therapist helps focus the client's attention on relevant information from a given social situation and problem solves appropriate courses of action with the client.

Video feedback, coupled with problem-solving and role-playing alternative behaviors, can also be helpful (Howlin, 1999). Videotapes take advantage of the visual strengths of many individuals with HFA. They also slow down social situations to allow the therapist to draw attention to salient contextual information and to points at which social miscommunication occurred. Videotapes may further help clients gain awareness of the relationship between their actions and the situational outcome (Quinn, Swaggart, & Myles, 1994). Role playing, which can be an effective CBT technique for a variety of conditions (Kendall et al., 1995), may not only encourage problem-solving skills, but also help bridge the gap between the artificial therapy environment and *in vivo* community situations.

The dependency and isolation experienced by individuals with HFA/ AS tends to be self-perpetuating. The absence of graduated opportunities for independence and socialization prevents the development of social skills that normally rise from natural environmental feedback (Hurley-Geffner, 1995). To counteract this, young adults may be encouraged to develop daily routines that are relatively predictable and that bring them into consistent positive social contact with others (e.g., a daily trip to a coffee shop or store). Well-supervised groups centered around structured activities (e.g., computer club, scouting programs) can also be helpful, especially when they are well matched to the client's interests and skills (Howlin, 1999). However, it is important to educate leaders of these programs about the child's specific symptoms and needs, to assist them in developing appropriate activities, and to closely monitor the activities to ensure that they remain therapeutic. Lord (1995) and Mesibov (1992) provided guidelines for building social skills interaction groups that integrate both affected and typically-developing individuals.

Though unstructured play therapy with individuals with pervasive developmental disorders is generally contraindicated, the development of *play skills* may be a reasonable goal for CBT. If generalized, such skills provide the opportunity for increased learning and independence in the community. Hurren (1994) and Stahmer (1999) described systematic techniques to build play skills.

Individuals with HFA/AS may feel more comfortable interacting online than in person, and may turn to the Internet for information, support, and acceptance. Such computer-mediated discourse has a number of potential advantages, including slowing down social interactions and the use of explicit visual symbols to denote communication nuances (e.g., accompanying a joke with a smiley face). However, because the Internet, e-mail, and chat rooms are often minimally regulated, the therapist should be alert to the client's interactions online and be prepared to intervene as appropriate (e.g., to protect the client from possible exploitation). Charman (1999) and Klin, Volkmar, and Sparrow (2000) reviewed some potentially useful Internet sites.

Therapists often misguidedly avoid issues of sexuality when working with individuals with autism (Tantam, 2000). Ford (1987) noted that therapists often have extreme views regarding the capability of these individuals to establish and maintain mutually pleasurable intimate relationships without exploiting others or themselves becoming exploited. She described techniques for structuring social opportunities and for implementing sex educational programming. In the absence of appropriate structured services in the area, the therapist may need to meet these educational goals to protect his or her client and to build relationship skills.

Strategies for Treating Restricted and Stereotyped Interests and Behaviors

Howlin (1999) suggested a "graded change" approach to stereotyped and ritualistic behaviors. She recommended systematic gradual restriction of the situations in which these behaviors are allowed. For example, verbal rituals can be systematically limited in terms of when, where, with whom, and for how long the ritual is allowed. The goal is not elimination of the stereotypy, but rather gradual change so that the stereotyped interests and behaviors interfere less with daily life and become more under the control of parents or of the child him- or herself. The process is slow, systematic, and involves breaking down the target behaviors into their component parts so that each can be approached in turn.

The therapist should also consider possible functional aspects of restricted or stereotyped behaviors, as well as skill weaknesses that might underlie these behaviors. For example, individuals with HFA/AS often experience temporal disorganization and confusion, which may result in anxious questioning about the sequence of upcoming events, difficulty navigating transitions, and increased dependency upon others. Visual schedules are a simple intervention to help individuals with HFA/AS "identify the sequence and time of various daily and weekly activities and events ... thereby making more concrete time and activity concepts" (Heflin & Simpson, 1998, p. 199). Similarly, assisting clients to organize recurring aspects of their daily lives into explicit routines can reduce anxiety and promote more efficient and reliable task completion (Kunce & Mesibov, 1998). Other strategies for reducing anxiety, such as visual organizers, increased use of clear and unambiguous social cues, relaxation, distraction, relaxing music, and exercise may also be helpful in minimizing investment in restricted or stereotyped behaviors (Howlin, 1999; Jordan & Powell, 1996).

Prior to targeting a client's special interest, however, therapists are urged to make a realistic appraisal of whether an interest can be molded into a functional vocation. For example, Dr. Temple Grandin, who has HFA, has become an internationally recognized expert on livestock handling, having built upon an early preoccupation with farm animals (Grandin, 1995). Individuals with HFA and AS who achieve independence often do so based upon their ability to apply their specialized knowledge in a vocationally functional way (Wing, 1989).

Rituals and obsessions can also be used as powerful reinforcers in behavior modification programs designed to build other skills. As noted by Howlin (1999), such use of these rituals and obsessions has been empirically demonstrated to be effective, taps into the child's idiosyncratic motivational system, has few if any negative side effects, is less prone to suffer from habituation or satiation effects than the use of other reinforcers such as food, and avoids the need for punishment-based treatments.

Unrealistic, extremely narrow, or ill-defined personal goals may be addressed in therapy using a procedure described by Fullerton and Coyne (1999). In this procedure, clients are guided through a series of visually based activities to help them "create a 'picture' of their life now and in 5 years, set personal goals, identify and prioritize steps needed to accomplish a goal, and sequence those steps into an action plan" (p. 43). Of particular appeal in working with adolescents and young adults with autism, this procedure facilitates the client's own problem solving, planning, and participation in self-determination.

General Intervention Strategies for Behavior Management and Emotional Disruption

Though the majority of the techniques summarized here were drawn from the pervasive developmental disorder literature, a variety of interventions drawn from other areas are potentially applicable. However, the unique social, communication, behavioral, cognitive, and developmental features of clients with HFA/AS must be taken into account. A volume edited by Koegel and Koegel (1995) and a chapter by Schreibman (1994) provide practical suggestions for improving the motivation of individuals with autism to work within behavioral, CBT, and educational frameworks, as well as strategies for improving treatment generalization.

R. L. and L. K. Koegel (1995; Koegel, Koegel, & McNerney, 2001) suggested targeting "pivotal behaviors"—skills that can be used to facilitate generalized learning across a number of contexts. In particular, they highlighted self-management intervention. This involves five steps: operationally defining a target behavior, identifying functional reinforcers, choosing a self-management method (e.g., notebook, stickers, wrist counter), teaching the individual to use the method, and teaching self-management independence. Quinn, Swaggart, and Myles (1994) elaborated on the self-management technique, providing specific guidance for working with individuals with HFA/AS. Other pivotal behaviors may include instruction in metacognitive strategies, such as designing a rote series of steps to follow when approaching a work assignment, or the use of calendars and checklists (Ozonoff, 1998). Self-management intervention is grounded in the tradition of operant behavioral techniques, which play a major role in CBT for a variety of disorders (Kendall et al., 1995) and which have been successful in effecting change with even low-functioning children with autism (Heflin & Simpson, 1998).

Emotional crises are best managed through prevention (Greene, 1998; Kunce & Mesibov, 1998; Myles & Southwick, 1999). This involves (1) using other strategies summarized here (e.g., strategies for reducing anxiety); (2) identifying the specific triggers and signs of an impending emotional "meltdown"; (3) intervening to minimize the occurrence of, or to prepare the individual for, these triggers; (4) finding ways for the individual or those around him or her to diffuse the situation upon identification of pre-meltdown signs; and (5) using calm periods to problem solve an appropriate course of action. Morgan (1996) listed a number of therapist responses that can help diffuse emotional crises in the moment. These include decreasing the vulnerability of the therapist and client; removing others from the situation; maintaining a calm, nonthreatening demeanor; avoiding physical contact and continuous eye contact; using distraction; continuing to listen for salient information the client may be relating; and cueing relaxation techniques. For example, if a client has an angry "meltdown" in a waiting room, it may be more prudent to calmly ask others to leave the room for a few minutes than try to relocate the client. Prior to follow-up in the therapy room, this immediate intervention would allow the therapist to limit the number of "eyes" upon the client, to reduce the situational uncertainty associated with social circumstances, to minimize external sources of anxiety for the client (e.g., by calmly reassuring the client that he or she is safe and need not leave but can if he or she wants to), to observe and listen for information the client may provide (e.g., about a trigger for the meltdown), to model relaxation techniques (e.g., slow breathing), and perhaps to distract the client by initiating a discussion on the topic of the client's preoccupation.

Clinical anxiety disorders and depression can be treated using traditional CBT techniques with some modifications. For example, a client can be taught Beck's (Beck, Rush, Shaw, & Emery, 1979) multiple column technique to analyze antecendent events, automatic thoughts, emotional reactions, rational thoughts, and self-statements, as well as the resulting emotional changes. Given their particular difficulties interpreting others' mental states, individuals with HFA/AS may benefit from the cognitive strategy of separating facts from assumptions (Bernard & Joyce, 1993). Teaching the individual to be his or her own "scientist" or "empiricist" (Beck et al., 1979) can capitalize upon the individual's preference for facts. In each case, the therapist must be aware of the difficulties with problem solving and organization that are often present with individuals with HFA/AS. Often, the therapist will need to guide the client to see the relationships between events, focusing on the salient features and outcomes. Basic emotion recognition and a varied emotion vocabulary may need to be taught before launching into more complex cognitive-behavioral techniques (Mesibov, 1992). Written and visual techniques, such as cartoon-like emotion cards and emotion "thermometers," can be teaching tools to help clients characterize the nature and intensity of their emotions (Bernard & Joyce, 1993).

External Resource Management

It can be difficult to obtain appropriate educational and vocational assistance for individuals with HFA/AS because they look "normal" and have reasonably developed rote verbal skills. The therapist may need to educate school or work staff, to advocate for the needs of the client, and to provide ongoing consultation with a school or employers (Volkmar, Klin, Schultz, & Cohen, 1998). Typically, the greatest success is achieved through a combination of behavior and skill changes in the client with modifications in his or her school or work environment (Ozonoff, 1998; Schopler, 1989). Therapists who are not themselves well versed in the educational and vocational training of individuals with HFA/AS should seek out the consultation of someone who is (Stoddart, 1998). Resources to assist the therapist and parents in this education, advocacy, and consultation process include Howlin (1999), Klin and Volkmar (2000), and Kunce and Mesibov (1998).[1]

   In the process of calling upon parents to provide interventions, to coordinate community services, and to act as their child's advocate, therapists often overlook the mental health needs of the family members of individuals with HFA/AS. Parents and siblings may require their own supports, which may come in the form of individual psychotherapy or support groups. Cutler and Kozloff (1987) listed a number of needs that the child's psychotherapist can coordinate. These include educational and vocational advocacy, respite care, home training skills, and basic advocacy skills. Ultimately, the support needs of any given family are unique, and interventions are based upon the specific match of available support services with the needs of the family (Albanese, San Muguel, & Koegel, 1995).

CASE EXAMPLE

Case History and Initial Diagnostic Evaluation

We will use the case of Randy to illustrate a cognitive-behavioral approach with an individual with HFA. Randy was 19 when he was first seen for a

---

[1]An excellent resource for families and professionals is the Autism Society of America (1-800-3-AUTISM, *www.autism-society.org*), which supports education, advocacy, and research regarding autism. They also have a number of local chapters that can provide support and referral services.

diagnostic evaluation through a developmental disorders clinic (DDC). Prior to that time, he had seen several physicians, psychologists, and educational specialists in an effort to understand his speech delays, poor social skills, emotional lability, and explosive temper. He had been diagnosed with a language disorder, attention-deficit/hyperactivity disorder, oppositional defiant disorder, and even bipolar disorder. However, speech therapy focused on semantic language skills, mood-stabilizing medications, and psychodynamic therapies were of limited efficacy. At the time of his referral to the DDC, his parents had become increasingly concerned because, following graduation from high school, Randy had become extremely isolated, seemed depressed, was unable to obtain a job, had become immersed in skateboarding, and had become increasingly difficult to motivate without the structure and routine of school. Based upon parental report of his history, a psychiatry intake worker suspected a possible pervasive developmental disorder, and referred him to the DDC for evaluation and follow-up.

The diagnostic evaluation included a parent interview (ADI-R) and an observational measure (a preliminary version of the ADOS). On both measures, Randy's scores met standard criteria for a diagnosis autism. On the ADI-R, his parents reported significant speech delays. He progressed by integrating stereotyped words and phrases into his developing speech. Over time this echolalia was less obvious, but his speech remained limited to specific topics of his interest, was characterized by poor speech prosody, and was rarely reciprocal in nature. Despite displaying an interest in developing friendships, he did not have close friends throughout his childhood. His social behaviors seemed scripted, awkward, and were often inappropriate. He spent most of his free time skateboarding or in related activities (e.g., reading magazines and surfing websites related to skateboarding). He had displayed a strong interest in skateboards and skateboarding since he was a young child, to the point that he had accumulated an expensive collection of skateboards and skateboard paraphernalia. He was not a particularly talented skateboarder, but he spent hours daily at a nearby skateboarding park. He was prone to "mood swings" that, upon closer examination, typically consisted of anger outbursts that followed changes in routine, entry into complex or rapidly changing social situations, or interference with his ability to pursue activities related to skateboarding. Not surprisingly, these mood swings contributed to his social isolation.

Randy's parents related that, during his elementary school years, others in his environment seemed more concerned than he was. He had seemed largely unaware of his social difficulties and performed reasonably well in school. However, once he started middle school, his slowness in completing assignments and difficulty organizing himself, coupled with the demand of transitioning from class to class (as well has having several different teachers), presented formidable obstacles. Also, middle school was much less structured and his routines were often violated without much warning, leading to repeated "meltdowns" that required Randy to leave school early. He also became increasingly aware of his deficits and difficulties in establishing friendships and negotiating daily social encounters at school.

At the time of his referral to the DDC, Randy lived with his parents and a younger sister. He was attending a local community college part-time, taking a computer course. His parents reported that he had periods of time with few overt difficulties. However, these were punctuated by periods during which his mood fluctuated from being silent and sad to belligerent in situations that would easily be tolerated by others (e.g., having to wait in line at the grocery store).

During the interview with Randy, the ADOS was used to obtain a standardized assessment of his social and communicative behavior. During the observation, his preoccupations and poor pragmatic and social communication skills were obvious. He rarely made eye contact, had unusual speech intonation, talked incessantly about skateboarding, and did not pick up on subtle to moderately obvious social cues to change the topic of conversation. He described a desire to have more friends, and even to have a girlfriend. However, he had difficulty describing what constituted a friendship or romantic relationship. He stated that he spent his time skateboarding, surfing the Web for skateboarding information, and watching television. He was uncertain as to whether he wanted to complete a course of studies at the community college or to obtain gainful employment, as it would interfere with the routine he had established over the past year since his graduation from high school (see Figure 14.1). He was unwilling to enroll in more than one class at a time because he was concerned that he would be unable to negotiate the demands of going to school full-time, and because it might interfere with his skateboarding practice. He stated that he wanted to win a major skateboard competition, showing little recognition of his objective lack of skill (he had won only consolation prizes in multiple local competitions) and the increasingly developmentally inappropriate nature of this aspiration.

An extensive psychometric evaluation was not undertaken during the DDC evaluation because educational testing had previously been conducted several times, on each occasion yielding similar findings: average to high average verbal, nonverbal, and overall intellectual functioning and no formal learning disability. However, during the DDC evaluation, his skills were briefly screened via a picture vocabulary test and a matrix reasoning task, on which he obtained average and high average scores, respectively. Even so, and despite average scores in the Communication domain of the Vineland Adaptive Behavior Scales (Sparrow, Balla, & Cicchetti, 1984), he obtained scores in the borderline to mildly impaired range in both the Daily Living Skills and Socialization domains. Based upon results from the overall diagnostic process, Randy was diagnosed with autism. His relatively

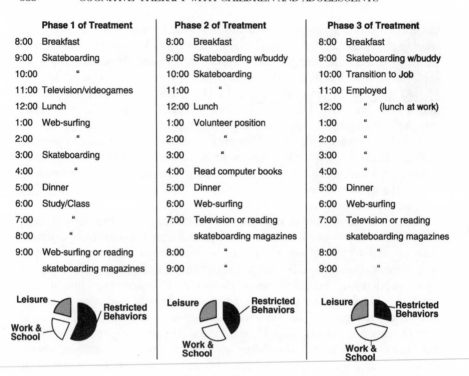

Phase 1 of Treatment	Phase 2 of Treatment	Phase 3 of Treatment
8:00 Breakfast	8:00 Breakfast	8:00 Breakfast
9:00 Skateboarding	9:00 Skateboarding w/buddy	9:00 Skateboarding w/buddy
10:00 "	10:00 Skateboarding	10:00 Transition to Job
11:00 Television/videogames	11:00 "	11:00 Employed
12:00 Lunch	12:00 Lunch	12:00 " (lunch at work)
1:00 Web-surfing	1:00 Volunteer position	1:00 "
2:00 "	2:00 "	2:00 "
3:00 Skateboarding	3:00 "	3:00 "
4:00 "	4:00 Read computer books	4:00 "
5:00 Dinner	5:00 Dinner	5:00 Dinner
6:00 Study/Class	6:00 Web-surfing	6:00 Web-surfing
7:00 "	7:00 Television or reading	7:00 Television or reading
8:00 "	skateboarding magazines	skateboarding magazines
9:00 Web-surfing or reading	8:00 "	8:00 "
skateboarding magazines	9:00 "	9:00 "

FIGURE 14.1. Change in Randy's daily schedule according to phase of treatment.

strong scores on measures of cognitive ability indicated that he might be labeled "high functioning."

Beyond this diagnostic label, the initial diagnostic process allowed for a functional analysis of a number of problematic behaviors (e.g., his "mood swings"). Moreover, it revealed the extreme degree to which his functional adaptation was limited by his preoccupation with skateboarding and poor social skills. Figure 14.1 illustrates how his rigid schedule allowed little room for age-appropriate and fulfilling educational, occupational, or social activities. Some environmental resources, such as his family, were readily noted during the diagnostic process, while others, such as an understanding supervisor, were explored later in therapy.

In terms of underlying cognitive mechanisms, comparison of parental and self-report of key events indicated a clear discrepancy between Randy's interpretation of what happened and the interpretations of those around him, highlighting distorted cognitive contents. For example, whereas Randy interpreted a fellow skateboarder's advice during a competition as "rubbing it in," his parents perceived that the other skateboarder clearly had benevolent intentions, and had in fact taken Randy somewhat under his wing. Randy's cognitive distortions had foundations in atypical cognitive processes. As is common with individuals with autism, all three of the cognitive processing deficit models described earlier were applicable to Randy. Based upon his history and our personal interactions with him, he displayed a poor understanding of what others might be thinking and the impact his behaviors had upon them (i.e., poor theory of mind). Consistent with the executive functioning hypothesis, his on-the-fly problem-solving skills were weak, and he tended to cling rigidly to repetitive routines rather than flexibly meet the needs of changing situations, even though he had solid basic cognitive skills (e.g., average IQ). Finally, consistent with Frith's (1989) central coherence model, he tended to focus on details at the expense of how they were connected on a higher level. For example, he seemed focused on the outward trappings of what it meant to have a "normal" romantic relationship, without a greater sense of romantic love or even interpersonal attraction.

This comprehensive understanding of his behaviors, contextual factors, and cognitive factors allowed for better-informed treatment planning. Importantly, treatment was not designed to be curative, but rather to help him and those around him to better cope with the biological and cognitive features central to autism. The overarching goal was to increase his quality of life, including healthier emotional functioning and increased age-appropriate and future-oriented adaptive functioning.

Treatment

At the time of diagnosis, Randy had multiple potential targets for intervention. However, both he and his parents identified deepening depression as a primary concern, with his social isolation and lack of occupational and independent living skills in the background. It was recommended that he attend weekly individual psychotherapy sessions to address his mood disturbance and to promote his movement toward interpersonal and life adjustment goals (e.g., completing school, obtaining employment, and increasing his level of independence). Concurrently, he was offered the opportunity to become involved in bimonthly social group sessions for autistic adolescents and adults. Though he initially attended group sessions reluctantly, they quickly became part of his routine. These sessions focused on skills needed for group interaction, including negotiating and conversing with others during shared activities and participating in a range of age-appropriate social activities. As suggested by Lord (1995), typical young adult volunteers were integrated into the group sessions. Clear rules of social conduct were established, and scheduled social activities allowed Randy to experience some comfort and sense of acceptance and personal value in a group setting, while at the same time increasing the opportunities for constructive feedback regarding social interactions.

Further discussion of the cognitive-behavioral intervention techniques used in Randy's case will focus only on his individual therapeutic work, which could be divided into three distinct phases. Initial sessions were focused on alleviating immediate symptoms. Next, sessions focused on setting and obtaining reasonable and achievable goals. Third, continuing at the time of this writing, less frequent sessions have focused on maintaining and extending his earlier gains. A therapeutic alliance with Randy was established through careful explanation of what was expected during the individual sessions. A routine was established such that Randy was expected to negotiate an agenda with the therapist at the beginning of each session, maintain a willingness to participate in therapy, and complete homework as it was assigned. After two sessions that were dominated by his interest in skateboarding, he agreed to limit this discussion to the last 10, then 5, minutes of each session. Also, Randy agreed to involve in therapy significant people in his life, including his parents, teachers, and supervisors, if necessary.

Initial sessions focused on alleviating immediate depressive symptoms and initiating coping and problem-solving strategies. Randy described feelings of emptiness, hopelessness, and isolation. He reported that he recognized that he was different in many ways from other people, in that others his same age were involved in school or their jobs, and most were active socially and had romantic relationships. He had less understanding of the skills he needed to be successful in these areas. Moreover, he appeared not to have questioned whether these things would, in fact, make him happy. Consider the following example, prompted by a discussion of frustrations at the skateboarding park:

RANDY: And there are all these couples running around, in the way.

THERAPIST: They get in the way?

RANDY: Well, not exactly in the way. They're not on the ramps or anything. It's just that they're always walking around, holding hands and making out and stuff.

THERAPIST: That bothers you.

RANDY: Yeah. It's like, all the other guys have girlfriends and stuff, and here I've *never* had one. It's not right, you know?

THERAPIST: You wish you had one?

RANDY: Yeah!

THERAPIST: Well, this might sound silly, because the guys you notice seem to be running around with girlfriends, but how would your life be different if you had one?

RANDY: (*Pause*) I don't know. Just spend time together. She could bring me lunch or something. I could say, "This is my girlfriend, Jackie."

THERAPIST: Anything else?

RANDY: I don't know. I'm not really into holding hands or anything.

THERAPIST: How else might your life change?

RANDY: Not much, I don't think.

THERAPIST: Oh, I'm not so sure. You mentioned things that she could do for you. Do you think that she might want some things from you?

RANDY: If you mean going out and stuff, forget it. That would mess up my schedule. I *hate* that.

Upon further examination, Randy stated that he was unsure that he wanted to spend that much time with another person, particularly if it meant disrupting his routine and training. This led to a specific intervention: When Randy began to feel "abnormal," he routinely wrote down what would be needed to be "normal" and five pros and cons of attaining that goal. These were then reviewed in session, with the therapist helping to cue him to consider all sides of the situation. As Randy did so, his views toward the goals tended to become less extreme, and he seemed to enjoy the sense that he had some choice in whether to pursue these goals.

Several other techniques were used during sessions to address Randy's symptoms of depression. First, because he had difficulty recognizing the presence and degree of his emotional experience, he was directed to use "emotion thermometers" to monitor his levels of depression and anger (Figure 14.2). Coupled with this intervention, he and the therapist developed a modified version of Beck's (Beck et al., 1979) multiple-column technique, in which he associated his initial feelings with immediate (automatic) thoughts about daily events, identified more rational ways of thinking about the situation, and then re-rated his emotional response. The expressed purpose was to "train" his thinking skills just as he trained for skateboarding competitions. Second, he was assigned homework to increase routine activities and social interactions (i.e., establish regular mealtimes with family members, arrange to meet a "buddy" at the skateboard park once per week). Over the next 4 months, his scores on the Beck Depression Inventory (Beck et al., 1979) declined from the mid-30s to the 5–15 range. However, he continued to experience periodic depressive episodes and anger outbursts, prompting a referral for a medication evaluation. He was prescribed fluoxetine. His response to the medication was carefully monitored by a psychiatrist, who was familiar with the treatment of autism. Though no single treatment has been demonstrated to be consistently effective in treating the symptoms of autism (Martin et al., 2000), Randy displayed further reduced depressive symptoms and less frequent anger outbursts with this treatment.

The therapy process itself raised several issues that required immediate

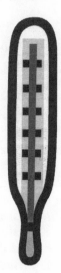

6. Boiling over!

5. Very angry

4. Moderately angry

3. Annoyed

2. A little angry

1. Not Angry

FIGURE 14.2. Randy's anger thermometer.

resolution. For example, the waiting room for clients was often quite noisy or the receptionist failed to immediately contact the therapist. Randy responded to both situations with anxiety and escalating hostility. Careful problem solving and planning led Randy to routinely bring material to read or a Game Boy to play, should he have to wait in the waiting room. He also devised a plan to reapproach the receptionist after 5 minutes of waiting and using a polite voice request to see the therapist again. These issues were addressed directly in therapy, as they were similar to issues Randy was having in the community. In this way, in therapy we could consider everyday obstacles and plan strategies to avoid or contend with such situations.

Six months after therapy was initiated, treatment moved to the next phase. In this second phase, greater emphasis was placed on establishing goals to promote Randy's independence and self-satisfaction. Many of the previous approaches (e.g., mood monitoring) continued, but additionally therapy focused on goal setting, identifying obstacles, and reviewing accomplishments. During this phase, visual supports continued to be important, as did homework assignments. For example, with the therapist's prompting, he examined his long-term life goals. With time, he acknowledged that, though he really wanted to pursue skateboarding, he wanted to have a job "in the meantime." This led to an exploration of his interests, which included computers, as well as the pros and cons of computer-related work. Using in-session time and homework assignments, he and the therapist developed a visual "career path" diagram, in which he drew footprints that incorporated the multiple steps (e.g., getting a degree, looking for jobs) that he needed to take to reach his goal of getting a job using computers (see Figure 14.3).

With the therapist's encouragement and role-playing exercises, Randy obtained additional information on what would be required to complete an associate's degree in computer science, then information on the specific requirements and schedule for each course. By writing these down on a sheet of paper, he was better able to negotiate his schedule to his satisfaction, and he faced fewer upsetting scheduling surprises.

As Randy accomplished his goals (e.g., associate's degree), he colored in the footprints on his "career path" and, with the therapist's support, focused on the skills he had successfully developed to reach that step. Emphasis was placed on how these skills might be generalized or extended to reach the next goal. Randy learned and practiced skills within the therapeutic session, such as doing job searches, calling prospective employers, writing letters of interest for prospective jobs, and role playing for job interviews. Randy's search for a job was lengthy and he sustained several setbacks that necessitated a reevaluation for depression as well as work on anger management. Randy had always been easy to anger, had a history of acting out (i.e., yelling), and displayed low impulse control, particularly in situations without clear social rules or those that were simply aggravating. Such situations were not frequent; however, when they occurred they posed

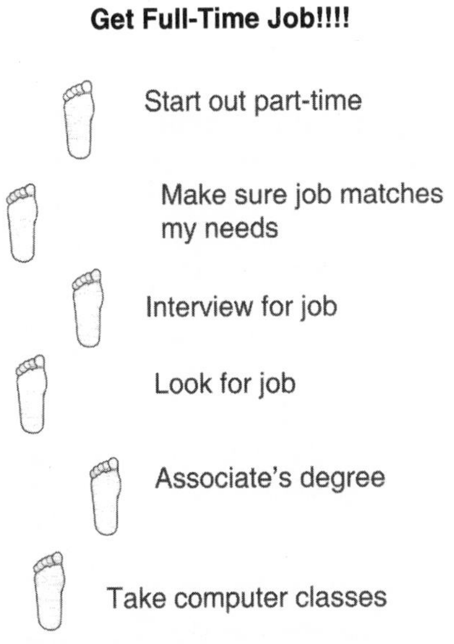

Get Full-Time Job!!!!

Start out part-time

Make sure job matches my needs

Interview for job

Look for job

Associate's degree

Take computer classes

FIGURE 14.3. Randy's career path diagram.

significant setbacks to his progress. Working with the therapist, Randy practiced a thought stopping technique that he was able to apply in situations in which he could identify becoming agitated. When this occurred, he kept a small stop sign in his wallet that would remind him to take several deep breaths, use rational self-talk, and consider his options and their consequences before he acted. Use of this technique required a great deal of practice and frequent reminders, but proved to be helpful in resolving several volatile situations.

His job search was particularly frustrating to him, as he had assumed that obtaining a position would be easy. After one problem-solving session, Randy spontaneously modified his "career path" chart to include finding a volunteer position that would provide him with job experience that he lacked. This proved to be a significant step. It was not only much easier to obtain a volunteer position than a paid position, but once he found a volunteer position he was able to practice the skills he needed to maintain a job. These skills included recognizing and responding appropriately to supervisors, working with others on the job, and handling corrective feedback. With Randy's consent, the therapist educated his supervisor about autism. This supervisor was much more amenable to providing supports once he understood the challenges Randy faced. This goal setting and training stage took approximately 9 months, and was marked by frequent setbacks in the context of overall progress.

After approximately 6 months in his volunteer position, Randy obtained gainful employment with a county office maintaining records on their computer network. This marked the transition into the third, and current, stage of therapy, which has focused on maintaining and extending the improvements he has made to date. Sessions have decreased to once every 2 weeks to once a month, with the understanding that more frequent involvement can occur as needed. His current supervisor is aware of his diagnosis and consults periodically with Randy's therapist. Both Randy's difficulties and his strengths have emerged at work. Randy is very dependable and punctual, and he completes his work with few or no errors. Though he has little contact with the public, he has had some difficulties with coworkers. These issues have been resolved through his supervisor and establishing clear rules for his behavior. For example, Randy has become frustrated when his work is interrupted and he is asked questions. He prefers to finish one task before starting on another. The therapist was able to address this issue during sessions using problem solving and role playing. Randy continues to work on goals at work. These include keeping himself appropriately occupied; at times Randy has been caught playing videogames while at work when he has completed all of his assigned work. His goals have now been revised to address his need to initiate appropriate activities at work—that is, to seek out work that needs to be done rather than rely on his routine activities. Randy and his supervisor periodically generate a list of tasks that need to be completed.

Randy has achieved his goal of obtaining gainful employment using the computer skills that he has developed. His overall level of functional adaptation has improved dramatically, indirectly illustrated by his "with treatment" typical weekday schedule in Figure 14.1. Currently, he does not exhibit or report significant ongoing depressive symptoms, but he continues to have difficulties from time to time in his coworker relationships. Defining acceptable behavior in a concrete manner and role playing in-session as well as outside of sessions is a constant requirement. Regular part-time employment has meant that Randy has had to make compromises in other aspects of his life, including the amount of time he spends on the Web and skateboarding. This has been a particular issue as he, his supervisor, and the therapist have gradually increased his hours and responsibilities. Concerns continue regarding his relative isolation from others and his tendency to prefer to participate in solitary activities, despite his expressed interest in building his social network. Moreover, he continues to function poorly in unplanned and fluid social situations. Finding the proper balance for Randy in the use of his time to interact with others as well as having time for himself remains a challenge, as is his ability to interact appropriately in difficult or unfamiliar situations.

Overall, cognitive-behavioral techniques and careful medication management have supported significant behavior change in Randy's case. In our experience, medication and cognitive-behavioral treatments are not incompatible, though careful consideration of the unique features of autism and of the specific client need to be kept in mind with both cases. At this point, the choice of whether to use psychotropic drugs, and the choice of agent and dosage, is a matter of clinical experience, rather than empirical knowledge (Martin et al., 2000). In Randy's case, a medication trial was indicated because, despite intensive CBT, he continued to display significant emotional disturbance that limited his quality of life and his adaptive functioning. The choice of agents was based upon the clinical experience of the prescribing psychiatrist, and upon Randy's past treatment history.

The cognitive-behavioral techniques used with Randy are common, but they were individualized to suit his strengths and weaknesses. Additionally, the techniques were useful across a range of circumstances and could be easily shaped to suit Randy's unique situations. At this point, Randy is feeling better about himself and what he has accomplished. Still, he displays core deficits in theory of mind, executive function, and central coherence, albeit with an increased coping repertoire. Problem situations arise to some degree on a regular basis, often bringing his autistic symptoms to the forefront (e.g., a conflict related to poor comprehension of a social situation). Moreover, his adaptive skills, especially in the social arena, remain well below those of similar intellectual and contextual background.

CONCLUSIONS

This case illustrated some of the challenges and techniques that may be used to build the adaptive functioning of adolescents and young adults with HFA/AS. It is important to note that the treatment was symptomatic, rather than curative. Despite significant positive behavior changes, the pervasive developmental disorder remained, raising ongoing adaptive challenges for the client and those working with him. This has necessitated a longer-term therapeutic relationship than is often seen with CBT. Moreover, as is typical in work with these clients, the therapist in this case study maintained a greater involvement with others in the client's natural environment than is typical of most CBT work. Though this work can be extremely challenging, it has been our clinical experience that, with therapist knowledge, patience, empathy, creativity, and realistic expectations, the payoff can be substantial in terms of greater client independence and overall adjustment.

REFERENCES

Albanese, A. L., San Miguel, S. K., & Koegel, R. L. (1995). Social support for families. In R. L. Koegel & L. K. Koegel (Eds.), *Teaching children with autism: Strategies for initiating positive interactions and improving learning opportunities* (pp. 95–104). Baltimore, MD: Paul Brookes.

American Psychiatric Association. (1994). *Diagnostic and statistical manual of mental disorders* (4th ed.). Washington, DC: Author.

Attwood, T. (1998). *Asperger's syndrome: A guide for parents and professionals.* Philadelphia: Jessica Kingsley.

Beck, A. T., Rush, A. J., Shaw, B. F., & Emery, G. (1979). *Cognitive therapy of depression.* New York: Guilford Press.

Bernard, M. E., & Joyce, M. R. (1993). Rational-emotive therapy with children and adolescents. In T. R. Kratochwill & R. J. Morris (Eds.), *Handbook of psychotherapy with children and adolescents* (pp. 221–246). Boston: Allyn & Bacon.

Charman, T. (1999). Autism resources and information on the internet or world wide web. *Autism, 3*(1), 97–100.

Cutler, B. C., & Kozloff, M. A. (1987). Living with autism: Effects on families and family needs. In D. J. Cohen, A. M. Donnellan, & R. Paul (Eds.), *Handbook of autism and pervasive developmental disorders* (pp. 513–527). New York: Wiley.

Ehlers, S., Gillberg, C., & Wing, L. (1999). A screening questionnaire for Asperger syndrome and other high-functioning autism spectrum disorders in school age children. *Journal of autism and developmental disorders, 29*(2), 129–141.

Eliasoph, E., & Donnellan, A. M. (1995). A group therapy program for individuals identified as autistic who are without speech and use facilitated communication. *International Journal of Group Psychotherapy, 45*(4), 549–560.

Faherty, C. (2000). *Asperger's: What does it mean to me?* Arlington, TX: Future Horizons.

Filipek, P. A. (1999). Neuroimaging in the developmental disorders: The state of the science. *Journal of Child Psychology and Psychiatry, 40*(1), 113–128.

Filipek, P. A., Accardo, P. J., Baranek, G. T., Cook, E. H., Dawson, G., Gordon, B., Gravel, J. S., Johnson, C. P., Kallen, R. J., Levy, S. E., Minshew, N. J., Prizant, B. M., Rapin, I., Rogers, S. J., Stone, W. L., Teplin, S., Tuchman, R. F., & Volkmar, F. R. (1999). The screening and diagnosis of autistic spectrum disorders. *Journal of Autism and Developmental Disorders, 29*(6), 439–484.

Ford, A. (1987). Sex education for individuals with autism: Structuring information and opportunities. In D. J. Cohen, A. M. Donnellan, & R. Paul (Eds.), *Handbook of autism and pervasive developmental disorders* (pp. 430–439). New York: Wiley.

Frith, U. (1989). Autism and "theory of mind. " In C. Gillberg (Ed.), *Diagnosis and treatment of autism* (pp. 33–52). New York: Plenum Press.

Fullerton, A., & Coyne, P. (1999). Developing skills and concepts for self-determination in young adults with autism. *Focus on autism and other developmental disabilities, 14*(1), 42–52, 63.

Gillberg, C. (1998). Asperger syndrome and high functioning autism. *British Journal of Psychiatry, 172*, 200–209.

Gillberg, C., & Schaumann, H. (1989). Autism: Specific problems of adolescence. In C. Gillberg (Ed.), *Diagnosis and treatment of autism* (pp. 375–382). New York: Plenum Press.

Grandin, T. (1995). *Thinking in pictures.* New York: Vintage.

Gray, C. A. (1998). Social stories and comic strip conversations with students with Asperger syndrome and high-functioning autism. In E. Schopler, G. B. Mesibov, & L. J. Kunce (Eds.), *Asperger syndrome or high-functioning autism?* (pp. 167–198). New York: Plenum Press.

Greene, R. W. (1998). *The explosive child.* New York: HarperCollins.

Heflin, L. J., & Simpson, R. L. (1998). Interventions for children and youth with autism: Prudent choices in a world of exaggerated claims and empty promises. *Focus on Autism and Other Developmental Disabilities, 13*(4), 194–211.

Howlin, P. (1999). *Children with autism and Asperger syndrome: A guide for practitioners and carers.* New York: Wiley.

Howlin, P., Baron-Cohen, S., & Hadwin. (1999). *Teaching children with autism to mind-read: A practical guide for teachers and parents.* New York: Wiley.

Hurley-Geffner, C. M. (1995). Friendships between children with and without developmental disabilities. In R. L. Koegel & L. K. Koegel (Eds.), *Teaching children with autism: Strategies for initiating positive interactions and improving learning opportunities* (pp. 105–125). Baltimore, MD: Paul Brookes.

Hurren, J. (1994). The therapeutic use of play, recreation, and leisure for children with autism and developmental disorders. *Journal on Developmental Disabilities, 3*(1), 51–62.

Jordan, R., & Powell, S. (1996). Encouraging flexibility in adults with autism. In H. Morgan (Ed.), *Adults with autism: A guide to theory and practice* (pp. 74–88). New York: Cambridge University Press.

Kendall, P. C. (1993). Cognitive-behavioral therapies with youth: Guiding theory, current status, and emerging developments. *Journal of Consulting and Clinical Psychology, 61*, 235–247.

Kendall, P. C., Marrs, A. L., & Chu, B. C. (1998). Cognitive-behavioral therapy. In T. Ollendick (Ed.), *Comprehensive clinical psychology: Children and adolescents. Clinical formulation and treatment* (pp. 131–147). New York: Elsevier.

Kendall, P. C., Panichelli-Mindel, S. M., & Gerow, M. A. (1995). Cognitive-behavioral therapy with children and adolescents. In H. P. J. G. van Bilsen, P. C. Kendall, & J. H. Slavenburg (Eds.), *Behavioral approaches for children and adolescents* (pp. 1–18). New York: Plenum Press.

Kimball, W., Nelson, W. M., & Politano, P. M. (1993). The role of developmental variables in cognitive-behavioral inteventions with children. In A. J. Finch, W. M. Nelson, E. S. Ott (Eds.), *Cognitive-behavioral procedures with children and adolescents* (pp. 25–66). Boston: Allyn & Bacon.

Klin, A., Sparrow, S. S., Marans, W. D., Carter, A., & Volkmar, F. R. (2000). Assessment issues in children and adolescents with Asperger syndrome. In A. Klin, F. R. Volkmar, & S. S. Sparrow (Eds.), *Asperger syndrome* (pp. 309–339). New York: Guilford Press.

Klin, A., & Volkmar, F. R. (2000). Treatment and intervention guidelines for individuals with Asperger syndrome. In A. Klin, F. R. Volkmar, & S. S. Sparrow (Eds.), *Asperger syndrome* (pp. 340–366). New York: Guilford Press.

Klin, A., Volkmar, F. R., & Sparrow, S. S. (Eds.). (2000). *Asperger syndrome.* New York: Guilford Press.

Koegel, R. L., & Koegel, L. K. (1995). *Teaching children with autism: Strategies for initiating positive interactions and improving learning opportunities.* Baltimore, MD: Paul Brookes.

Koegel, R. L., Koegel, L. K., & McNerney, E. K. (2001). Pivotal areas in intervention for autism. *Journal of Clinical Child Psychology, 30*, 19–32.

Koegel, R. L., Koegel, L. K., & Parks, D. R. (1995). "Teach the individual" model of generalization: Autonomy through self-management. In R. L. Koegel & L. K. Koegel (Eds.), *Teaching children with autism: Strategies for initiating positive interactions and improving learning opportunities* (pp. 67–77). Baltimore, MD: Paul Brookes.

Kunce, L., & Mesibov, G. B. (1998). Educational approaches to high-functioning autism and Asperger syndrome. In E. Schopler, G. B. Mesibov, & L. J. Kunce (Eds.), *Asperger syndrome or high-functioning autism?* (pp. 227–261). New York: Plenum Press.

Lord, C. (1995). Facilitating social inclusion: Examples from peer intervention programs. In E. Schopler & G. B. Mesibov (Eds.), *Learning and cognition in autism* (221–240). New York: Plenum Press.

Lord, C., Risi, S., Lambrecht, L., Cook, E. H., Leventhal, B. L., DiLavore, P. C., Pickles, A,, & Rutter, M. (2000). The autism diagnostic observation schedule-generic: A standard measure of social and communication deficits associated with the spectrum of autism. *Journal of Autism and Developmental Disorders, 30*, 205–223.

Lord, C., Rutter, M., DiLavore, P. C., & Risi, S. (1999). *Autism Diagnostic Observation Schedule.* Los Angeles: Western Psychological Services.

Lord, C., & Rutter, M. (1994). Autism and pervasive developmental disorders. In M.

Rutter, E. Taylor, & L. Hersov (Eds.), *Child and adolescent psychiatry* (3rd ed., pp. 569–593). Oxford, UK: Blackwell Science.

Lord, C., Rutter, M., & Le Couteur, A. (1994). Autism Diagnostic Interview—Revised: A revised version of a diagnostic interview for caregivers of individuals with possible pervasive developmental disorders. *Journal of Autism and Developmental Disorders, 24*(5), 659–685.

Martin, A., Patzer, D. K., & Volkmar, F. R. (2000). Psychpharmacological treatment of higher-functioning pervasive developmental disorders. In A. Klin, F. R. Volkmar, & S. S. Sparrow (Eds.), *Asperger syndrome* (pp. 210–228). New York: Guilford Press.

Matthews, A. (1996). Employment training and the development of a support model within employment for adults who experience Asperger syndrome and autism: The Gloucestershire group homes model. In H. Morgan (Ed.), *Adults with autism: A guide to theory and practice* (pp. 163–184). New York: Cambridge University Press.

Mesibov, G. B. (1992). Treatment issues with high-functioning adolescents and adults with autism. In E. Schopler & G. B. Mesibov (Eds.), *High functioning individuals with autism* (pp. 143–155). New York: Plenum Press.

Mesibov, G. B., Shea, V., & Adams, L. W. (2001). *Understanding Asperger syndrome and high functioning autism.* New York: Kluwer/Plenum.

Morgan, H. (1996). Appreciating the style of perception and learning as a basis for anticipating and responding to the challenging behaviour of adults with autism. In H. Morgan (Ed.), *Adults with autism: A guide to theory and practice* (pp. 231–248). New York: Cambridge University Press.

Myles, B. S., & Southwick, J. (1999). Asperger syndrome and difficult moments: Practical solutions for tantrums, rage and meltdown. Shawnee Mission, KS: Autism Asperger Publishing.

Ozonoff, S. (1998). Assessment and remediation of executive dysfunction in autism and Asperger syndrome. In E. Schopler, G. B. Mesibov, & L. J. Kunce (Eds.), *Asperger syndrome or high-functioning autism?* (pp. 263–289). New York: Plenum Press.

Ozonoff, S., & Griffith, E. M. (2000). Neuropsychological function and the external validity of Asperger syndrome. In A. Klin, F. R. Volkmar, & S. S. Sparrow (Eds.), *Asperger syndrome* (pp. 72–96). New York: Guilford Press.

Quinn, C., Swaggart, B. L., & Myles, B. S. (1994). Implementing cognitive behavior management programs for persons with autism: Guidelines for practitioners. *Focus on Autistic Behaviors, 9*(4), 1–13.

Robbins, T. W. (1997). Integrating the neurobiological and neuropsychological dimensions of autism. In J. Russel (Ed.), *Autism as an executive disorder* (pp. 21–53). New York: Oxford University Press.

Ronen, T. (1998). Linking developmental and emotional elements into child and family cognitive-behavioural therapy. In P. Graham (Ed.), *Cognitive-behaviour therapy for children and families* (pp. 1–17). New York: Cambridge University Press.

Schopler, E. (1989). Principles for directing both educational treatment and research. In C. Gillberg (Ed.), *Diagnosis and treatment of autism* (pp. 167–183). New York: Plenum Press.

Schopler, E., Mesibov, G. B., & Kunce, L. J. (Eds.). (1998). *Asperger syndrome or high functioning autism?* New York: Plenum Press.

Schopler, E., Reichler, R., & Rochen-Renner, B. (1988). *The Childhood Autism Rating Scale (CARS)*. Los Angeles: Western Psychological Services.

Schreibman, L. (1994). Autism. In L. W. Craighead, W. E. Craighead, A. E. Kazdin, & M. J. Mahoney (Eds.), *Cognitive and behavioral interventions: An empirical approach to mental health problems* (pp. 335–358). Boston: Allyn & Bacon.

Smith, T. (1993). Autism. In T. R. Giles (Ed.), *Handbook of effective psychotherapy* (pp. 107–133). New York: Plenum Press.

Sparrow, S. S., Balla, D. A., & Cicchetti, D. V. (1984). *Vineland Adaptive Behavior Scales*. Circle Pines, MN: American Guidance Service.

Stahmer, A. C. (1999). Using pivotal response training to facilitate appropriate play in children with autistic spectrum disorders. *Child Language Teaching and Therapy, 15*, 29–40.

Stoddart, K. P. (1998). The treatment of high-functioning pervasive developmental disorder and Asperger's disorder: Defining the social work role. *Focus on Autism and Other Developmental Disabilities, 13*(1), 45–52.

Tantam, D. (2000). Adolescence and adulthood of individuals with Asperger syndrome. In A. Klin, F. R. Volkmar, & S. S. Sparrow (Eds.), *Asperger syndrome* (pp. 367–399). New York: Guilford Press.

Tsai, L. Y. (1999). Recent neurobiological research in autism. In D. B. Zager (Ed.), *Autism: Identification, education, and treatment* (pp. 63–95). Mahwah, NJ: Erlbaum.

Twachtman, J. L. (1996). Improving the human condition through communication training in autism. In J. R. Cautela & W. Ishaq (Eds.), *Contemporary issues in behavior therapy: Improving the human condition* (pp. 207–231). New York: Plenum Press.

Twachtman-Cullen, D. (1998). Language and communication in high-functioning autism and Asperger syndrome. In E. Schopler, G. B. Mesibov, & L. J. Kunce (Eds.), *Asperger syndrome or high-functioning autism?* (pp. 199–225). New York: Plenum Press.

Volkmar, F. R., Klin, A., Schultz, D. J., & Cohen, D. J. (1998). "Nonautistic" pervasive developmental disorders. In C. E. Coffey & R. A. Brumback (Eds.), *Textbook of pediatric neuropsychiatry* (pp. 429–447). Washington, DC: American Psychiatric Press.

Wing, L. (1989). Autistic adults. In C. Gillberg (Ed.), *Diagnosis and treatment of autism* (pp. 419–432). New York: Plenum Press.

World Health Organization (1992). *The ICD-10 classification of mental and behavioural disorders: Clinical descriptions and guidelines*. Geneva: Author.

SUGGESTED READINGS

Heflin, L. J., & Simpson, R. L. (1998). Interventions for children and youth with autism: Prudent choices in a world of exaggerated claims and empty promises. *Focus on Autism and Other Developmental Disabilities, 13*(4), 194–211.

Howlin, P. (1999). *Children with autism and Asperger syndrome: A guide for practitioners and carers*. New York: Wiley.

Klin, A., Volkmar, F. R., & Sparrow, S. (Eds.). (2000). *Asperger syndrome*. New York: Guilford Press.

Koegel, R. L., & Koegel, L. K. (1995). *Teaching children with autism: Strategies for initiating positive interactions and improving learning opportunities*. Baltimore, MD: Paul Brookes.

Mesibov, G. B. (1992). Treatment issues with high-functioning adolescents and adults with autism. In E. Schopler & G. B. Mesibov (Eds.), *High functioning individuals with autism* (pp. 143–155). New York: Plenum Press.

Mesibov, G. B., Shea, V., & Adams, L. W. (2001). *Understanding Asperger syndrome and high functioning autism*. New York: Kluwer/Plenum.

Schopler, E., Mesibov, G. B., & Kunce, L. J. (Eds.). (1998). *Asperger syndrome or high functioning autism?* New York: Plenum Press.

Siegel, B. (1996). *The world of the autistic child: Understanding and treating autistic spectrum disorders*. New York: Oxford University Press.

Zager, D. B. (1999). *Autism: Identification, education, and treatment*. Mahwah, NJ: Erlbaum.

15

The Quadripartite Model Revisited

Promoting Positive Mental Health in Children and Adolescents

DAVID L. DuBOIS
ROBERT D. FELNER
ERIKA M. LOCKERD
GILBERT R. PARRA
CRISTY LOPEZ

In the first edition of this casebook, we described a quadripartite model for understanding and enhancing the social competence of children and adolescents (DuBois & Felner, 1996). The framework's underlying assumptions and general approach were rooted in a broader movement in the field toward greater consideration of positive mental health and adaptation, shifting away from a predominant focus on disorder and psychopathology. In the ensuing years this movement has, if anything, intensified. Building on earlier arguments for an increased emphasis on promoting positive mental health, investigators have proposed for further study such concepts as psychological wellness (Cowen, 2000), healthy youth development (Larson, 2000), and resilience in the form of positive adaptive outcomes for youth exposed to heightened levels of stress (Luthar, Cicchetti, & Becker, 2000; Wyman, Sandler, Wolchik, & Nelson, 2000). There also has been substantial interest in the promotion of positive mental health as an applied aim within both clinical and preventive interventions for children and adolescents (Cicchetti, Rappaport, Sandler, & Weissberg, 2000; Durlak, 1997).

Is positive mental health a relevant concept for cognitive therapy with children and adolescents? We argue that it is for several reasons. Cognitive-behavioral therapies, for the most part, have been concerned with achieving symptom reduction, yet it is critically important also to promote competencies and a sense of well-being in children and adolescents receiving treatment, thus moving beyond the mere absence of indications of disorder. In doing so, positive resources may be instilled in youth that facilitate progress during treatment as well as long-term maintenance of gains. From a consumer perspective, both youth and their parents also may respond more favorably when treatment recognizes and seeks to promote strengths, as opposed to focusing solely on deficit reduction. Cognitive-behavioral therapists working with youth, furthermore, already attend to a range of concerns that are amenable to a focus on positive mental health. These include, for example, aims of strengthening social skills, fostering accuracy in perceptions of self and others, improving mood and feelings of self-worth (i.e., self-esteem), increasing mastery beliefs and optimism about the future, and so on.

Efforts to promote positive mental health among youth, however, ideally should be informed by a comprehensive and well-delineated conceptual framework. The existing literature offers general principles and concepts that may be useful to consider in this regard. Lacking, however, is a more refined framework that offers enough detail to be of practical use for guiding the assessment and treatment of individual youth. The quadripartite model offers a promising starting point for this type of effort, given both its demonstrated utility for clinical application (DuBois & Felner, 1996; see also Felner, Lease, & Phillips, 1990) and the prominent role already afforded social competence in conceptualizations of positive mental health and functioning (Durlak, 2000). Nevertheless, social competence should not be equated with positive mental health; social competence rather may be best viewed as "a necessary component of, but . . . not equivalent to positive mental health" (Felner et al., 1990, p. 260). Empirically validated taxonomies of the essential components of positive mental health are in their relative infancy (Dinges, 1994). Available theoretical perspectives do converge, however, in pointing to indicators of psychological competence/well-being as constituting, along with social competence, a critical and distinct dimension of positive mental health during development (see Durlak, 2000; Goleman, 1997; Ryff & Singer, 1998). A twofold emphasis on psychological and social dimensions of positive mental health, furthermore, is analogous to the well-supported distinction between internalizing (or emotional) and externalizing (or behavioral) dimensions of mental health problems among youth (Achenbach, 1990; Mash & Dozois, 1996).

In the present chapter, we describe a revised version of the quadripartite model that incorporates psychological competence/well-being as a distinct dimension of positive mental health (see Figure 15.1). In doing so, we argue that the same four core areas hypothesized to constitute the internal structure of social competence apply equally to psychological competence and well-being. This quadripartite structure includes cognitive, behavioral, emotional, and motivational domains of influence. We posit that, as with social competence, it is essential to view the characteristics of the psychological dimension of positive mental health in relation to features of the youth's environmental context (i.e., person–environment transactions). The utility of the expanded model for clinical assessment and treatment is then illustrated with a case example. Finally, directions for further elaboration of the proposed framework and its application to clinical interventions with youth are discussed.

THE REVISED QUADRIPARTITE MODEL

Overview

The revised quadripartite model includes both psychological competence/well-being and social competence as distinct dimensions of positive mental health. Social competence refers to the degree to which youth demonstrate the capacities required for effective interpersonal functioning (Compas, 1993). Psychological competence or well-being, by comparison, refers to the extent to which the internal, and hence more subjective experiences that youth have of themselves and their lives are favorable and thus likely to facilitate their overall adaptation (Perry & Jessor, 1985). Certain constructs, such as social self-concept, clearly have relevance to both proposed components of positive mental health. Yet, consistent with their relative independence, there is also a potential for observed levels of social and psychological functioning to diverge significantly from one another. A youth could, for example, exhibit strong social competence (e.g., favorable relationships with peers and adults) but at the same time fail to demonstrate psychological signs of positive mental health (e.g., feelings of personal efficacy or life satisfaction). Conversely, prominent markers of adaptive social functioning (e.g., effective skills for interpersonal problem solving) may be lacking for a child or adolescent who nevertheless has relatively high levels of psychological competence/well-being (e.g., positive feelings of self-worth based on success in areas other than social relations).

Social competence and psychological competence/well-being are each expected to make unique contributions, in turn, to overall positive mental health (see Figure 15.1). This assumption notwithstanding, it is presumed that the implications of each dimension for positive mental health are most usefully considered in context of the characteristics and processes associated with the other. To illustrate, even if certain indicators of psychological well-being or competence are evident for a given youth, such as high self-esteem or a sense of mastery, these may not contribute to positive mental health if they are sustained by noxious social behaviors (e.g., aggression) or, relatedly, occur in the absence of meaningful interpersonal ties altogether. The two dimensions also are assumed to have the potential to influence each other reciprocally over the course of development (cf. DuBois &

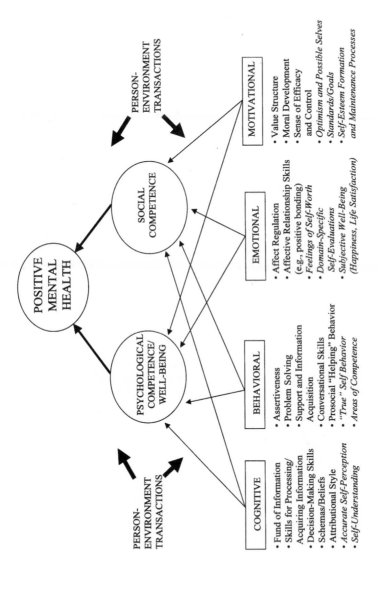

FIGURE 15.1. The revised quadripartite model of positive mental health (components added with specific relevance to psychological competence/well-being in *italics*).

405

Felner, 1996). Thus, gains in social competence for a given youth may contribute to enhanced psychological functioning, and vice versa.

As shown in Figure 15.1, each proposed dimension of positive mental health is shaped by the relative presence or absence of a wide range of skills/capacities within the four core areas of the model (i.e., cognitive, behavioral, emotional, and motivational). Mental health outcomes are assumed, furthermore, to be influenced primarily by the interaction of attributes within and across the core areas, rather than by any given element or core area in isolation (DuBois & Felner, 1996). As an example, even a youth who possesses a strong set of *cognitive* abilities for achieving social competence or psychological well-being would not necessarily be expected to be able to do so without accompanying *behavioral* skills for acting on such understandings, *emotional* capacities to regulate responses under situations of heightened arousal, and, of course, the *motivation* to initiate and direct efforts in these areas toward adaptive ends. Many of the specific skills and abilities within each of the core areas described previously as bearing on social competence (DuBois & Felner, 1996) also have relevance to psychological well-being or competence. Effective skills for decision making and problem solving, for example, although frequently emphasized as critical to social competence, may be additionally important for shaping the behavior and adaptive efforts of youth in directions that benefit key aspects of their psychological well-being (e.g., life satisfaction). The revised model also incorporates other abilities and personal qualities (highlighted in italics in Figure 15.1) that are not included in the original model but are important to consider because of their specific relevance to the psychological dimension of positive mental health. These elements include, for example, feelings of self-worth within the emotional domain and accurate self-perception and self-understanding within the cognitive realm.

A final key feature of the model is an emphasis on the importance of attending to contextual factors in efforts to assess or promote positive mental health. Socially competent functioning thus is conceptualized as "dependent not only on the sets of skills and abilities acquired by the youth, but also on *the degree to which these capacities are well suited or "matched" to the characteristics of the social environments in which they are employed*" (DuBois & Felner, 1996, p. 136, emphasis added). Accordingly, it is not enough to simply know the absolute level of skills within the four areas of the model. Rather, attention also must be given to their adaptive value within the youth's immediate contexts of development as well as the potential that exists within these settings for relevant capacities to be utilized to full advantage. In the present chapter, we extend this concept to include the importance of considering the "degree of fit" between psychological processes involved with mental health and the adaptive demands and opportunities that characterize the youth's environment.

The following sections describe aspects of the revised quadripartite model that seem especially relevant for assessing and promoting psychological competence/well-being as a distinct dimension of positive mental health. In doing so, we highlight several conceptual issues that are raised by distinguishing separate psychological and social dimensions of mental health for children and adolescents.

Components of Psychological Competence/Well-Being

As noted, the skills and qualities that serve as the foundation for psychological competence or well-being may include factors emphasized in discussions of social competence as well as additional characteristics with more distinctive relevance to psychological functioning. The following sections illustrate both possibilities with respect to each core area of the model. Neither the specific elements considered nor the somewhat broader sets of skills and qualities listed in Figure 15.1 are intended, however, to be comprehensive in nature.

Cognitive Domain

Within the cognitive domain, the availability of an adequate fund of culturally-relevant knowledge is necessary for competent social functioning, but also may have significant implications for psychological competence/well-being. In the short term, adverse psychological effects of deficits in this area (e.g., poor academic achievement) may be attenuated by a variety of compensatory factors. Many youth, for example, derive a sense of self-worth and well-being from alternative sources of gratification in their lives, such as peer relations or success in sports (Harter, 1999). Accordingly, levels of academic achievement among school-age children and adolescents typically predict only a relatively small proportion of the variation in their overall reported levels of self-esteem (DuBois & Tevendale, 1999). However, it should not be overlooked that, in the long term, academic knowledge deficiencies greatly increase the likelihood of outcomes such as school dropout and unemployment that have well-documented negative consequences for psychological well-being during later adolescence and adulthood (Dooley & Prause, 1997).

The capacities for accurate self-perception and self-understanding illustrate skill elements in the cognitive domain with direct implications for psychological functioning as a dimension of positive mental health (see Figure 15.1). Accurate self-assessment (Goleman, 1997) and intrapersonal understanding (Gardner, 1993) are distinct facets of personal competence or intelligence that are important for healthy functioning throughout the life span. The adverse implications of unrealistically negative beliefs about the self for psychological well-being are well recognized (Durlak, 2000). Recent research, however, also highlights a potential for self-perceptions that are biased in a *positive* or favorable direction to present significant liabilities for mental health (Bandmaster, Bushman, & Campbell, 2000; Colvin & Block, 1994; Harter, 1998). For youth, inflated self-perceptions may contribute to conflict and disagreements with others (e.g., parents), hypersensitivity in response to negative events and interpersonal feedback owing to the greater fragility of the self-concept (i.e., defensiveness), and difficulties stemming from limited self-understanding, such as poor decision making and problem solving (Harter, 1998). With specific relevance to psychological well-being, the pressure of living up to an inflated self-image itself also may take a significant toll directly on the emotional health of children and adolescents (Colvin & Block, 1994).

Complicating matters somewhat is a competing body of theory and research that points to potential desirable effects of inflated self-views (Taylor & Brown, 1999). Positive bias in self-perceptions, according to this literature, may enhance mood and facilitate more effective social and cognitive functioning. One suggestion has been that there is an "optimal margin of illusion" for views of the self, beyond which more extreme distortions become maladaptive (Bandmaster, 1989). Similar considerations may apply to other cognitive elements included in the revised model, such as the capacity to maintain a healthy but realistic sense of optimism about the future (Seligman, 1998). At present, these issues are far from resolved. Nevertheless, it does seem safe to conclude that the ability to maintain a reasonable degree of accuracy in perceptions of oneself and one's external life circumstances is indeed an important component of psychological competence and well-being for developing youth (Sandler, 2001).

At a more fundamental level, the cognitive capacities required for self-understanding and, hence, an appreciation of one's defining attributes as a person are important to healthy psychological functioning as well. Particularly for adolescents, these skills may be essential for the formation of a coherent and satisfying sense of identity (Erikson, 1968). Even those youth who feel that they know themselves, however, may not act in accordance with their true selves or "real me" when in the presence of others such as parents, teachers, or peers (Harter, 1999). Adolescents who tend to avoid engaging in true self behavior have been found in several studies to exhibit signs of poorer psychological adjustment (Harter, 1999). Such considerations illustrate the value of taking into account potential interactions across domains of the quadripartite model, in this case cognitive and behavioral. It is to the behavioral domain that our discussion now turns.

Behavioral Domain

Behavioral skills, in addition to their central, defining role in social competence, have implications for the psychological well-being of children and adolescents. Supportive relationships with significant others such as parents, peers, and teachers serve as building blocks for several key components of psychological health during development. These include an overall sense of self-worth (Harter, 1998), beliefs in personal control and self-efficacy (Flammer, 1995), and feelings of life satisfaction (Unger & Wandersman, 1988). As a result, the wide range of behavioral skills that have been viewed as instrumental underpinnings for social competence (e.g., prosocial "helping" behavior) also clearly are relevant to the psychological competence and well-being of developing youth.

It is important to note, however, that youth can demonstrate behavioral competence or ability in other areas that do not necessarily have a salient interpersonal component. Consider, for example, the capacity to problem solve effectively and show adaptive persistence when approaching tasks in various domains (e.g., school). These types of skills can be expected to contribute to the development of a strong internalized sense of self-efficacy and locus of control (Bandura, 1997), as well as positive feelings of self-worth (Rosenberg, 1979; White, 1960).

Specialized or unique areas of talent or aptitude also can make significant contributions to psychological aspects of positive mental health. By taking note of these at an early age and then fostering them, important aspects of well-being such as self-esteem and a sense of efficacy may be enhanced (Gardner, 1993). In accordance with this possibility, research has linked specialized areas of talent (e.g., music) among children and adolescents both to higher overall self-esteem (Vispoel, 1993) and to greater life course resilience and positive functioning (Werner, 1995).

A further specialized set of behavioral skills relevant to positive mental health are those pertaining to "environmental mastery" (Ryff, 1995; see also Compas, 1993). These include the capacity to make effective use of surrounding opportunities, to choose or create contexts suitable to personal needs and values, and to become involved in personally meaningful activities in one's environment. Individual youth, of course, may be limited in the "degrees of freedom" that their life circumstances afford them to exercise skills for environmental mastery. To the extent that such skills do contribute significantly to social and psychological components of positive mental health, however, this clearly would be consistent with the emphasis placed on the importance of person–environment transactions within the quadripartite model.

Emotional Domain

Affect regulation and other emotion-focused skills were included in the original version of the model in accordance with research linking such abilities directly to social competence. The inherently internalized quality of these capacities highlights their potential to contribute to the psychological competence and well-being of developing youth as well (Durlak, 2000).

This is illustrated by findings of recent research focusing on self-esteem stability (Kernis, 2002). Youth who demonstrate a high level of self-esteem stability are able to maintain consistency in their feelings about themselves across differing contexts and situations. This type of affective regulation has been linked to several indicators of psychological competence and well-being, including higher "baseline" or trait levels of self-esteem, positive mood, and intrinsic motivation for achievement and learning (Kernis, 2002).

Self-esteem, as reflected in overall feelings of self-worth, is itself illustrative of a core element of emotional functioning that may directly undergird the psychological functioning of youth, thereby contributing to positive mental health (Durlak, 2000). A major trend during the past decade has been increased attention to the multidimensional structure of self-esteem for children and adolescents (Harter, 1998). This research has revealed reliable differences in the evaluations that youth make about themselves with respect to specific domains in their lives such as school work, family, peer relations, physical appearance, athletic ability, and so on (Harter, 1998). Distinct facets or domains of self-evaluation emerge as early as the preschool years (Marsh & Hattie, 1996) and become increasingly numerous and differentiated with age (Harter, 1998). These differing dimensions of self-evaluation, in turn, have been found to each make unique contributions to youths' overall feelings of self-worth (also referred to as global self-esteem; Harter, 1999). Some areas of self-esteem, however, may assume greater importance than others at any given stage of development. Among young adolescents, for example, body-image and peer relations dimensions of self-evaluation are especially strong influences on feelings of self-worth (DuBois, Tevendale, Burk-Braxton, Swenson, & Hardesty, 2000).

Subjective well-being, as reflected in tendencies toward happiness and life satisfaction (Myers & Diener, 1995), is another important factor in the emotional domain contributing to the psychological mental health of children and adolescents. Components of subjective well-being (e.g., life satisfaction) for developing youth appear to follow a multidimensional, domain-specific structure similar to that noted previously for self-esteem (Huebner, 1994; Huebner, Gilman, & Laughlin, 1999). Available findings also suggest that factors contributing to subjective well-being constitute a distinct aspect of psychological mental health for children and adolescents (Huebner et al., 1999). A youth with high self-esteem and other indicators of psychological health (e.g., self-understanding), for example, may experience limited happiness and life satisfaction if environmental circumstances are inadequate to meet his or her needs. The manner in which multiple elements within and across domains may need to be taken into account to derive a full understanding of psychological well-being or competence continues to be useful to keep in mind as the discussion now broadens to include motivational concerns.

Motivational Domain

Motivational and expectancy sets, the final core area of the model, are important in shaping the "performance" aspects of social competence (DuBois & Felner, 1996). However, consistent with their internalized nature, they also may have significant implications for adaptive psychological functioning. Personal efficacy and control beliefs, frequently emphasized as core indicators of positive mental health for children and adolescents (Durlak, 2000), are illustrative in this regard. In accordance with their relevance to psychological well-being, youth reporting relatively strong perceptions of internal control and self-efficacy tend to score higher on measures of self-esteem (Tashakkori, 1992), positive mood (Treasure, Monson, & Lox, 1996), and life satisfaction (Huebner, 1991). As with other elements discussed (e.g., self-esteem), however, efficacy and control beliefs are likely to vary depending on the specific types of tasks or domains of activity involved (Bandura, 1997). Feelings of efficacy or control focused on certain domains (e.g., school work), furthermore, may have a significant influence on psychological well-being despite having few, if any, consequences for social competence.

Additional motivational components relevant to psychological functioning are indicated in Figure 15.1. These include a sense of optimism or hope (i.e., positive beliefs about the likelihood of future life outcomes; Scheier & Carver, 1985) as well as the closely related concept of possible selves (i.e., ideas youth have of personal roles and identities they could assume in the future; Markus & Nurius, 1986). A teenager, for example, might hold favorable expectations of finishing school (optimism/hope), while also envisioning herself as successful in adult roles such as a desired career path (possible selves). These future-oriented aspects of psychological functioning have been differentiated empirically from more contemporaneous indicators of well-being (e.g., self-esteem; Carvajal, Clair, Nash, & Evans, 1998; Markus & Nurius, 1986). Optimism and hope combined with self-esteem in research with adolescents, however, to form a single, higher-order factor or construct (Carvajal et al., 1998). This suggests the value of considering present- and future-oriented psychological elements in conjunction with one another.

The standards and goals that youth establish for themselves also are an important concern. When youth adopt highly demanding personal standards in areas such as physical appearance or school work (i.e., perfectionistic tendencies), this may interfere with key ingredients of positive psychological functioning such as feelings of self-worth (Harter, 1999). It is equally apparent, however, that an absence of age-appropriate goals and aspirations can contribute to failure experiences that are detrimental to psychological health (Bandura, 1986). Taking both of these considerations into account, youth who strive for challenging but realistic goals are most likely to enjoy healthy psychological functioning (Higgins, 1991).

A final set of motivational processes may lead youth to actively seek to enhance key aspects of their psychological well-being. Motivational strivings for feelings of self-worth (i.e., self-esteem motive) are illustrative in this regard (Harter, 1999). Normative sources of self-esteem during development include competence-building and success experiences, in conjunction with positive relationships with others (Harter, 1999). Obtaining self-esteem from these sources can be inherently reinforcing for youth and thus encourage them to make further efforts in these directions, thereby fostering sustained feelings of self-worth as well as other aspects of healthy psychological functioning (e.g., self-efficacy beliefs). Children and adolescents also exhibit varying degrees of reliance on self-protective and self-enhancing strategies as a means of responding to threats to their self-esteem (Kaplan, 1986; Rosenberg, 1979). These motivational strategies, too, may prove adaptive for psychological well-being, such as when youth are able to discount the importance of areas in which they experience less success (Harter, 1999). Unfortunately, though, in some instances such processes may instead serve over time to undermine positive mental health (Colvin & Block, 1994). Consider, for example, a youth who because of self-protective tendencies (e.g., defensiveness) fails to develop a capacity for accurate appraisal of personal strengths and limitations. As another example, some youth may begin to associate with deviant peers in an attempt to achieve a sense of being accepted and validated by others (Kaplan, 1986). It is not difficult to imagine either type of tendency having consequences that ultimately detract from both feelings of self-worth and other aspects of psychological well-being.

Person–Environment Transactions

Paralleling their significance for social competence (DuBois & Felner, 1996), person–environment transactions also are important in considering the adaptive implications of processes that relate to psychological aspects of positive mental health. According to one recently proposed model (DuBois, Bull, Sherman, & Roberts, 1998), for example, the consequences of self-esteem for adjustment are directly dependent on the adequacy of fit between the processes involved in supporting feelings of self-worth and the features of the youth's environment. Favorable outcomes are predicted when processes relied on by youth in attempting to meet their needs for self-esteem are congruent with the views, expectations, and values of significant others in their lives (e.g., parents) as well as the adaptive demands and norms that they encounter both in primary settings of development (e.g., school) and the larger society. In the absence of such congruence, adjustment may be compromised through several mechanisms. Some youth, for example, may experience interpersonal difficulties stemming from discrepancies between their own self-concepts and how they are perceived by others, such as parents or peers. For others, problems may stem from seeking to protect their sense of worth by devaluing success in key areas such as school. Of further note, the environments of some youth may fail to recognize and support specific areas in which they demonstrate competence (e.g., music), thus blocking avenues for deriving self-esteem in a developmentally appropriate manner (DuBois et al., 1998).

In addition to making it more difficult for youth to maintain strong feelings of self-worth, these types of environmental incongruence may interfere with aspects of their psychological well-being such as sense of mastery, life satisfaction, and optimism or hope for a positive future. Conversely, in other instances, there may be a good fit between self-esteem processes of youth and the same environmental dimensions. For example, others may share an appreciation of the youth's strengths or talents and actively support the youth's involvement in activities that nurture these areas of competence. Such congruence could be instrumental in promoting the youth's self-esteem and in strengthening a broad range of other key aspects of psychological functioning.

Achieving some degree of independence from environmental expectations or demands, however, may be equally important for the psychological well-being of developing youth. Of particular note, youth must have sufficient opportunities to derive feelings of worth on the basis of their own interests and values. When this occurs, a genuine or "true" (i.e., healthy) sense of self may develop, as opposed to one that is based primarily on conforming to externally imposed criteria (Deci & Ryan, 1995). In support of this perspective, "constructive" forms of deviance from conventional norms and expectations have been found to be associated with favorable adjustment among adolescents (Chassin, Presson, & Sherman, 1989). Such considerations underscore the value of conceptualizing psychological aspects of positive mental health within a contextual framework.

Psychological and Social Dimensions of Positive Mental Health

Relation of Psychological Well-Being to Social Competence

As we have seen, psychological competence/well-being may be influenced by many of the same elements within the core areas of the quadripartite model that are instrumental in providing a foundation for social competence. As a result, the model predicts that youth often will exhibit quite similar levels of psychological and social functioning. It also is assumed, however, that the two dimensions of positive mental health can diverge substantially for any given youth. Objective social competencies, for example, typically are reflected to only a partial extent on corresponding psychological measures such as social self-concept (Byrne & Shavelson, 1996) and social self-efficacy beliefs (Connolly, 1989). This may occur for a variety of reasons, including an inability of youth to accurately appraise or fully appreciate such strengths themselves. Psychological health also can be influenced by a wide range of experiences that have little, if any, direct relevance for effective social functioning. As noted, these include personal competencies in areas such as schoolwork and extracurricular activities. When the values and motivations of youth are directed toward such domains more than their interpersonal relationships, divergence between psychological and social dimensions of positive mental health may be especially likely to occur. Likewise, outside influences may affect one dimension of functioning more than the other. In the resilience literature, for example, it has been found that when youth demonstrate social competence in the context of high levels of stress, they still may fare relatively poorly on measures of psychological functioning (Luthar et al., 2000).

The model further assumes that psychological and social dimensions of positive mental health may influence each other reciprocally during the course of development. Consider, for example, that youth with low self-esteem or sense of self-efficacy may not attempt adaptive interpersonal behaviors that are nonetheless in their skill repertoires, thereby diminishing social competence (DuBois & Felner, 1996). The latter social tendencies could, in turn, interfere with aspects of psychological functioning such as feelings of happiness or life satisfaction. Available research provides support for both of these possible directions (e.g., Smokowski, 1999). In formulating approaches to promoting the positive mental health of children and adolescents, it thus may be critically important to consider the implications of current levels of each of the two proposed dimensions, as well as possible modifications in each, in the context of their likely implications for one another.

Relation of Psychological Well-Being and Social Competence to Positive Mental Health

As shown in Figure 15.1, psychological well-being and social competence each are posited to contribute uniquely to a superordinate construct of positive mental health. One implication of this feature of the model is that the most favorable levels of overall adaptation should be evident for youth who exhibit high levels of both psychological and social functioning. A psychological *and* social foundation for positive mental health also may promote other aspects of healthy functioning (e.g., school performance) and, furthermore, protect against the onset of mental disorder.

Finally, it is important to consider interactions between psychological and social dimensions of functioning that may contribute to positive mental health for youth. It is possible, for example, that strengths on one dimension may serve to protect or insulate youth against negative consequences for mental health associated with weaknesses on the other. Gains that accrue in both psychological and social facets of mental health, furthermore, may combine synergistically to facilitate more positive outcomes than would be expected on the basis of either in isolation. Improvements in social functioning, for example, may provide a more realistic foundation for beliefs in efficacy and self-worth, thus increasing their adaptive value. In a corresponding manner, growth in indicators of psychological well-being may facilitate improvements in interpersonal behaviors important to social competence. These scenarios highlight how consideration of both psychological and social dimensions of mental health may facilitate more holistic case conceptualization and treatment planning in clinical work with children and adolescents. With this in mind, we now apply the model to an illustrative case of a youth referred for treatment.

CASE EXAMPLE

Robert, an 11-year-old boy in the sixth grade, was referred for outpatient therapy by his family's primary care physician in a health maintenance organization. At the time of referral, Robert was living with his mother, a paralegal assistant, and his father, a skilled construction worker, along with three younger siblings. He was attending a K–6 elementary school, one of five "feeder" schools for a larger junior high school that he was scheduled to enter the following year.

Initial Assessment

Sources of information for the initial assessment included interviews with Robert, his parents, and his classroom teacher; several standardized, paper-and-pencil assessment measures; and behavioral observation at school. Robert's developmental and family history were largely unremarkable, although 3 years previously he had seen a counselor at school for help with his "social behavior." At the time of referral, both Robert's parents and his teacher expressed concerns regarding the quality of his relationships with peers. Their ratings on the Achenbach Checklist (Achenbach, 1991) placed him in the "clinical" (i.e., problem) range on the Social Problems subscale of this instrument. Robert indicated awareness of these difficulties as well, noting that he "needed to do better" at getting along with others his age. Of particular concern to his parents and teacher was Robert's inability to control his temper in interactions with peers. His difficulties in this area were reported to be a source of frequent altercations, many of which escalated into physical fights. It was noted, furthermore, that teasing often served as a "trigger" for Robert's anger, much of it focusing on aspects of his physical appearance (e.g., being called "Dumbo" in reference to the relatively large size of his ears). Scores on standardized measures, such as the Self-Control Rating Scale (Kendall & Braswell, 1993), confirmed that Robert lacked developmentally appropriate skills for both self-control and affect regulation.

Robert's interactions with peers at school were the predominant source of concern. Difficulties there had resulted in numerous disciplinary incidents and led to a "negative set" in the views and expectations of others toward him in that setting. His teacher, with whom Robert had frequent disagreements, described him as an "excellent manipulator." When observed at school, furthermore, it was clear that Robert was not well accepted by his classmates. He sat by himself at lunch, for example, and was unable to find a group to play with at recess. His reports and those of his teacher suggested that this type of isolation and estrangement from peers had become typical of his experiences at school.

Robert's self-esteem was another area of concern raised by his parents. When administered the Self-Esteem Questionnaire (SEQ; DuBois, Felner, Brand, Phillips, & Lease, 1996), Robert reported favorable overall feelings of worth (i.e., global self-esteem; see Figure 15.2). A mixed picture was evident, however, with respect to more circumscribed areas of self-esteem assessed on the measure. Particularly noteworthy, given presenting concerns, was his low score on the Peer Relations scale. His self-evaluations in this area were predominantly negative and well below norms for his age group (DuBois et al., 1996). Deficits in self-esteem also were evident for two other domains relevant to peer relations—Body Image and Sports/Athletics (see Figure 15.2).

No less noteworthy, however, are strengths that Robert exhibited in several areas. He was performing well above average academically (as assessed by standardized tests of achievement) and, according to his parents and teacher, was "creative" and a "quick learner" with strong verbal skills. Robert's intellectual curiosity was apparent in his keen interest in a wide range of topics outside of school, some of which were unusual for his age (e.g., astronomy). Strengths in intrapersonal aspects of intelligence, furthermore, were suggested by Robert's awareness of his current adaptive difficulties and his insight into relevant contributing factors (e.g., difficulties with temper control). It also will be recalled that he expressed motivation to get along better with peers. As evidence of a general orientation toward self-improvement, he was observed on the SEQ to write-in comments such as "I want to do better" even for domains in which he currently was doing relatively well (e.g., school). Finally, Robert's parents noted that he displayed a wide variety of prosocial behaviors at home (e.g., caring for younger siblings) as well as a capacity for independence and handling responsibility (e.g., paper route).

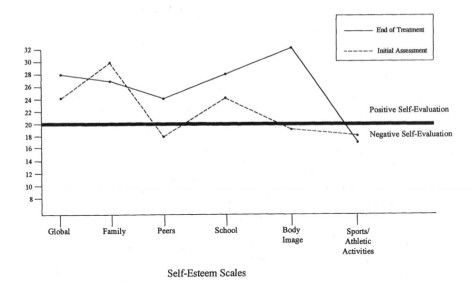

FIGURE 15.2. Robert's scores on the Self-Esteem Questionnaire at the time of initial assessment and end of treatment.

Diagnosis and Conceptualization

Diagnostically, Robert was found to meet several of the criteria in the fourth edition of the *Diagnostic and Statistical Manual of Mental Disorders* (DSM-IV; American Psychiatric Association, 1994) for attention-deficit/hyperactivity disorder (AD/HD), specifically the predominantly hyperactive–impulsive subtype of this disorder. Ratings by his classroom teacher on the ACTeRS rating scale (Ulmann, Sleator, & Sprague, 1984) were elevated on the Hyperactivity dimension of this measure, for example, based on his reported tendency to "overreact" and be "impulsive (act or talk without thinking)." These impressions were confirmed by direct observation of Robert's behavior at school and also were consistent with information shared by his parents. In several respects, however, Robert was far from a "classic" example of a youth with attention-deficit/hyperactivity disorder. Symptoms of inattentiveness were mostly absent, for example, and those relating to the hyperactivity–impulsivity dimension of the disorder were restricted primarily to impulsivity. These latter tendencies, at least those noted to be problematic, also were limited primarily to situations of high negative emotional arousal and a single setting (i.e., school).

Ratings of different informants on the Achenbach Checklist indicated clinical or "borderline" (i.e., subclinical) levels of both internalizing and externalizing problems, with specific elevations in the areas of social withdrawal, anxious/depressive symptomatology, and aggressive behavior. More detailed assessment revealed, however, that Robert failed to meet criteria definitively for a specific DSM-IV disorder within either the emotional or behavioral domains. Illustratively, notwithstanding reported feelings of sadness and other indications of a possible mood disturbance (e.g., social withdrawal), these were not severe or pervasive enough to warrant a diagnosis such as major depressive disorder or dysthymic disorder. Despite Robert's aggressive behavior at times toward peers, the absence of involvement in delinquent or other relatively more serious forms of misbehavior similarly precluded a diagnosis of conduct disorder.

A deficit- or disorder-based conceptualization thus had limited utility as a basis for understanding and guiding approaches to intervention with Robert. An alternative conceptualization based on a positive mental health perspective, however, was more promising. From the standpoint of the revised quadripartite model, the following issues were especially salient:

Cognitive

- Lack of utilization of problem-solving/decision-making skills, especially under conditions of emotional arousal
- Above average intellectual functioning
- Accurate self-perception/self-understanding (e.g., "I have trouble with losing my temper")

Behavioral

- Areas of competence that help to maintain self-esteem/sense of efficacy (e.g., academic achievement, outside interests and responsibilities)
- Well-developed repertoire of behaviors for positive social interaction (e.g., prosocial helping), although limited primarily to relations with adults at present
- Limited opportunities for rewarding utilization of desirable peer behaviors in current school environment due both to social withdrawal and negative expectations "set" of classmates

Emotional

- Difficulties with affect regulation (e.g., responses to peer teasing)
- Positive overall feelings of self-worth, but negative self-esteem for peer relations and related domains (e.g., body image)
- Social difficulties at school (e.g., rejection/lack of acceptance from classmates) elicit negative emotions on a regular basis, thus detracting from overall happiness and life satisfaction

Motivational

- Goal-oriented (i.e., aspirations for improvement in peer relations and other domains); high standards may be associated with some "perfectionistic" tendencies
- Self-esteem processes (e.g., realistic assessment of strengths and weaknesses, strivings for self-improvement in valued areas) represent good "fit" with environmental norms and demands; tendencies toward assertion and independence as emerging bases for self-identity, however, may prove problematic for interactions with adult authority figures (e.g., arguments with teachers)
- Sense of efficacy or personal control for improving social relations at school likely limited by "reputation effect" (e.g., classmates and teacher interpreting even well-intentioned actions in an unfavorable light)

As is evident from this list, Robert had levels of skills or resources that were somewhat "low" in absolute terms in each of the four core areas of the model. These areas of relative difficulty or weakness, furthermore, included factors likely to influence both social competence and psychological well-being. Robert's difficulties with affect regulation, for example, and a compounding lack of utilization of cognitive problem-solving/decision-making skills when experiencing emotional arousal, were major factors interacting to limit his current level of social competence. His tendencies toward negative self-evaluation in selected domains (e.g., peer relations), combined with the lack of a strong sense of efficacy or control over these areas, likewise represented significant threats to Robert's psychological well-being. These influences relating to psychological and social dimensions of Robert's mental health were conceptualized as interrelated, rather than distinct or independent sets of processes. Accordingly, limitations in Robert's social competence were viewed as having a negative effect on his psychological functioning and, in a reciprocal manner, his psychological areas of weakness (e.g., low peer efficacy beliefs) were seen as limiting the effectiveness of his social functioning.

Two further points of understanding, derived from the revised quadripartite model, also are important in considering Robert's presenting problems. First, areas of strength within each core domain of the model were evident to at least the same extent as those representing areas of weakness or liability. These assets were relevant to both social competence (e.g., prosocial behaviors) and psychological well-being (e.g., overall feelings of self-worth) as dimensions of positive mental health. Cumulatively, these strengths offered possible insight into Robert's relative immunity from a fully developed psychiatric syndrome or disorder (e.g., depression). Importantly, they also represented valuable personal resources that might be able to be mined for productive purposes within treatment. A second notewor-thy issue is the prominent role of person–environment transactions in Rob-ert's presenting problems. The most salient presenting concern, for exam-ple, was the negative relationship that existed between Robert and others in the school setting. Furthermore, even if not initially the source of his adap-tive difficulties, the expectation "sets" held by classmates and his teacher in this setting clearly had evolved to function as adverse forces in their own right.

Course of Treatment

Based on the preceding conceptualization, a decision was made to pursue treatment from the perspective of promoting positive mental health as op-posed to a more traditional approach focused on remediation of deficits or disorder. Application of a conventional, deficit-reduction model was viewed as likely to be of limited utility in comparison to one emphasizing positive mental health for at least two reasons. First, most available treat-ment protocols developed from a deficit-reduction perspective focus on the remediation of particular DSM-IV disorders. As noted, Robert's difficulties did not fall neatly into one of these categories. Some basis existed to con-sider using strategies focused on amelioration of Robert's AD/HD-related symptomatology. His parents, however, expressed a strong desire to not pursue any of the pharmacological approaches commonly used in treat-ment of this disorder (e.g., Ritalin). The difficulties he exhibited with im-pulse control and anger management suggested that he might alternatively be a good candidate for training in cognitive-behavioral decision-making skills (see Pardini & Lochman, Chapter 3, this volume). Still, given the na-ture and situational specificity of Robert's difficulties in these areas (i.e., circumstances eliciting emotional arousal when at school, particularly in relations with peers), it was concluded that this type of protocol would need to be integrated with other treatment components. These were derived from the quadripartite model and included efforts directed toward (1) enhanc-ing skills for affect regulation and (2) providing more neutral, nonschool settings in which to utilize newly acquired skills.

A second consideration that argued against using a deficit-oriented ap-proach to treatment is that doing so would not have been conducive to the use of strategies oriented toward promoting positive mental health. This latter aim seemed important to integrate into any treatment plan that was developed for Robert. It will be recalled in this regard that the presenting concerns of his parents focused on promotion of competencies (i.e., im-proving self-esteem, increasing positive relations with peers) rather than a desire to have particular "deficits" or signs of disorder addressed. Robert too seemed most interested in working toward goals of this nature. Accord-ingly, a positive mental health orientation was desirable from the standpoint of both good "consumerism" (i.e., respecting the priorities and interests of clients) and fostering client motivation in the change process (Compas, 1993). It was hoped, furthermore, that by promoting positive mental health in targeted areas, the diffuse yet noteworthy indications of behavioral maladaptation and emotional distress that Robert exhibited could be ameliorated. Importantly, Robert's existing areas of strength were regarded as a valuable resource that could be "exploited" to advantage in treatment (i.e., used as leverage for efforts to remediate his areas of relative weakness).

Promotion of Social Competence

The initial focus in treatment was on strengthening Robert's skills for interpersonal problem solving and impulse control. The training incorporated efforts to increase Robert's capacity to implement the skills under "real world" conditions of negative emotional arousal (i.e., anger management). These goals were pursued early in treatment because it was expected that the success of other intervention strategies would be dependent on Robert acquiring greater ability to handle interpersonal stressors effectively, especially those involving peers. Utilizing a standard protocol (Kendall & Braswell, 1993), Robert was taught a series of generic "Stop and Think" steps for social problem solving and impulse control. Capitalizing on his above average cognitive abilities, it was not difficult for him to master application of the procedures to relatively neutral or positive social situations. As scenarios were introduced that better approximated the specific circumstances involved in eliciting his problematic interactions with peers, however, his performance deteriorated markedly. He often experienced difficulty enacting desired behaviors due to high levels of emotional arousal. It also was not uncommon for him to decline to select appropriate solutions altogether because of skepticism regarding their effectiveness in producing desired outcomes.

Several strategies proved useful in combating these obstacles. These included training in labeling and discriminating differing feeling states to enhance Robert's capacities for coping with affective arousal, as well as instruction and practice in rational responding to dysfunctional cognitions to reduce the intensity of the negative emotions that he experienced in stressful social situations. Difficulties often can be encountered when attempting to implement cognitively oriented interventions of this nature with preadolescent youth. Robert nonetheless responded well, perhaps reflecting his relatively advanced cognitive abilities and capacity for introspection. Of additional benefit was a decision to increase the "ecological validity" of in-session practice exercises by having Robert bring in a friend from his neighborhood with whom he could try out his newly forming skills. The enhanced sense of efficacy that Robert experienced as a result of success in these role plays was pivotal in setting the stage for efforts to have him utilize the skills effectively in settings outside of therapy.

To facilitate the generalization process, Robert's parents and teacher were instructed in procedures for "dialoging" (i.e., guiding him through the necessary steps of skill implementation when applicable and providing reinforcement for these efforts; Shure & Spivak, 1988). To encourage compliance with this key phase of treatment and provide a basis for internalization of enhanced feelings of efficacy and esteem, Robert was asked to self-monitor his social problem-solving behavior. He also received encouragement for doing so through the use of a structured reward system. Following the introduction of these intervention components, significant reductions were observed in the frequency and intensity of Robert's conflicts with peers. Notably lacking, however, were indications of positive growth and enjoyment in his peer relationships. This was particularly noticeable with respect to classmates at school. Despite substantially fewer overt negative interactions, these relationships still clearly did not constitute a source of pleasure or support for him. The reasons for this did not appear to be simply a lack of necessary efforts on Robert's part. Rather, it was apparent that a negative expectations set toward him continued to be operating in the school setting and was thus interfering with his ability to form satisfying relationships with peers in that context.

To address this concern, a concerted effort was made to increase Robert's positive involvement with peers in nonschool settings. He was enrolled in a weekend activity program of the local department of parks and recreation, for example, thus affording opportunities for participation in a variety of structured activities with peers outside of school. Emphasis also was placed on promoting greater informal interaction with peers in his neighborhood. It is noteworthy in this regard that Robert's family had moved early in the process of treatment; accordingly, any negative reputation effects that his behavior in the prior neighborhood might have established were, in effect, circumvented. These nonschool settings proved to be venues in which Robert was able to establish notably more satisfying and rewarding relationships with peers. He enjoyed regular positive interactions with his teammates on a youth bowling team, for example, despite the competitive nature of the activity. He also developed a close friendship with a youth from his neighborhood, thus providing him with a significant source of peer social support.

Enhancement of Psychological Well-Being/Competence

Improvements in Robert's peer relationships also were expected to enhance his sense of psychological well-being and competence. It will be recalled, for example, that his reported profile of self-esteem included "localized" deficits in several peer-oriented areas. Self-evaluations in these domains, furthermore, are among the strongest predictors of overall feelings of self-worth for young adolescents such as Robert (Harter, 1999).

At the same time, there also was a rationale to include interventions that focused directly on esteem-enhancement. Given the problematic nature of Robert's situation at school, for example, it was not clear that either peers or adults there would be a sufficient source of "naturally occurring" reinforcement for any changes he was able to demonstrate in his behavior. Of further note was Robert's tendency toward some degree of perfectionism in evaluating his performance in different domains. This suggested that he might find it difficult to give himself sufficient "credit" for desirable progress toward treatment goals (e.g., anger management).

One strategy for addressing these concerns was to provide Robert with training in self-reinforcement (Meichenbaum, 1992). This included giving him a notebook to keep a daily log of his prosocial behaviors, thus encouraging his internalization of positive efforts in this area. The log proved to be a highly successful intervention, with Robert maintaining it on a consistent basis throughout treatment. Robert's log entries were detailed and insightful, reflecting his strengths for introspection and verbal expressiveness. They therefore served not only as an effective basis for self-reinforcement, but also as a useful tool for exploring different social situations he encountered outside of therapy.

To increase environmental support for Robert's positive behaviors, a school–home note program was established (Braswell, Bloomquist, & Pederson, 1991). These notes, initially provided on a daily basis, proved effective as an additional tool for esteem-enhancement. Illustratively, in one session, Robert proudly greeted the therapist to show him the set of "perfect" notes that he had earned. His teacher initially had expressed some reluctance regarding this aspect of treatment because of the time and effort involved (and, perhaps as well, some skepticism regarding its potential effectiveness given her views of Robert). She followed through reliably, however, in several instances including her own words of praise. These responses signaled a shift toward a more favorable relationship between her and Robert, thus providing a further basis for improved feelings about himself and his experiences at school.

Fading and Termination

The preceding aspects of treatment were implemented during nine weekly sessions that extended to the end of the school year. In view of the positive indications of progress, a decision was made at this time to move toward termination via a systematic fading process. One session was planned for immediately prior to the time of Robert's transition to his new school the next fall, while two others were to take place once the school year had begun. Research indicates that the transition from elementary to junior high school is a stressful experience for many youth (Eccles, Midgley, Wigfield, & Buchanan, 1993). Those who lack optimal levels of support from peers are at particularly high risk for experiencing increased psychological symptoms during the transition (Hirsch & DuBois, 1991). Providing therapeutic support during the move to the new school thus was viewed as necessary for ensuring maintenance of the gains that had accrued in treatment. The transition also represented an important "window of opportunity" for further progress to occur as a result of a more favorable pattern of transaction established between Robert and those in his new school environment. Insofar as he would have the chance to start "fresh" with a largely new peer group and different set of teachers, the negative expectations set that had limited his opportunities for positive adaptation within his previous school would no longer be a significant factor. A desire to "exploit" this situation served as an additional impetus for focusing remaining therapy sessions on the acute phase of adjustment to the new school.

Robert's subsequent transition to junior high school was successful, both socially and academically. Robert and his parents reported, for example, that he had made several new friends and acquaintances and was involved in a variety of extracurricular activities (e.g., intramural basketball, science club). Robert's principal similarly conveyed that he was regarded by his teachers as a highly capable and "energetic" student whose "free thinking" manner tended to set him apart from his classmates. A readministration of the Self-Esteem Questionnaire during this phase of treatment (approximately 10 months after initial assessment) revealed improvements in several areas, including peer relations and overall self-esteem (see Figure 15.2). Based on the converging indicators of healthy social and psychological functioning, treatment was terminated according to plan.

Long-Term Follow-Up

Extended follow-up was able to occur over several years as a result of informal updates received from Robert and his parents. Robert continued to exhibit positive social and academic adjustment throughout this period. He was successful in graduating from high school a year early, for example, while still nonetheless maintaining an active and rewarding social life with peers. Psychologically, he exuded a strong sense of self-confidence, goal-directedness, and optimism regarding the future. Issues did continue to arise, however, that were relevant to those addressed in treatment. Illustratively, following a nationally publicized incident of school violence, Robert and several friends decided to protest what they felt was unfair critical attention being given to the reported dress of the perpetrators (i.e., black "long coats"). They did so by wearing the very same attire to school themselves the next day. When confronted by the school's principal, Robert reported that he avoided having the incident escalate by remaining calm, "remembering my 'stop and think' steps," and realizing that it would be more appropriate to pursue other forms of protest. Following high school, Robert enlisted in a branch of the armed services. At last report, at age 20, he was adjusting well and had recently completed the initial stages of a competitive officer training program.

DISCUSSION

Since publication of the first edition of this book, there has been growing scholarly and applied interest in positive mental health and its implications for developmental outcomes of youth. This trend notwithstanding, available treatment protocols for children and adolescents have remained focused predominantly on the goals of deficit-reduction and alleviation of symptoms of disorder. At present, several important issues still are in need of clarification concerning the merits of promoting positive mental health in interventions with youth. These include the benefits that gains in positive mental health should be regarded as offering in their own right, their value in treatment approaches focused on remediation of symptoms of disorder, and, furthermore, the capacity for existing client strengths to provide leverage for addressing presenting problems in other areas. A second key set of concerns pertain to the internal structure and dynamics of positive mental health. These include the status of psychological well-being and social competence as distinct but overlapping and potentially interacting dimensions of positive mental health as well as their relations, in turn, to more circumscribed skills and abilities in differing domains. A final constellation of noteworthy issues involve the role of person–environment transactions. These include their implications for assessment and case conceptualization as well as the design of effective interventions when adopting a positive mental health perspective.

Several aspects of the case example indicate the importance of attending to the preceding sets of concerns in clinical work with children and adolescents. Prior literature advocating promotion of mental health (e.g., Dinges, 1994) has emphasized the long-term benefits for overall well-being and adjustment that may accrue when pursuing this aim within interventions. Robert's trajectory of adjustment following treatment, characterized by a well-rounded pattern of psychological, social, educational, and occupational functioning extending several years into early adulthood, is consistent with this perspective. A related benefit of adopting a focus on promotion of positive mental health is that youth and their parents may view treatment goals as more desirable and thus be more willing to work toward them. It will be recalled that Robert's parents presented with concerns regarding his self-esteem and the suboptimal status of his peer relationships; Robert too clearly was motivated to work toward treatment goals in these areas. By contrast, approaches focused on deficit-reduction or remediation of disorder (e.g., AD/HD) had limited applicability. This was evident not only from a pure assessment standpoint, but also because such approaches would have been largely irrelevant or, in some instances (e.g., medication), in direct opposition to client preferences.

Different aspects of the case also point toward ways in which positive mental health may function to protect against the emergence of disorder. The gains that accrued in indicators of positive mental health (e.g., self-esteem) during the course of treatment are illustrative in this regard. These may have helped to ensure that the subclinical threshold levels of symptomatology that Robert exhibited in various areas (e.g., depression) did not evolve into more serious difficulties that met full criteria for disorder. Progress also was facilitated by strengths that Robert demonstrated upon entering therapy. His capacity to accurately identify personal limitations, for example, coupled with goal-oriented motivation for self-improvement, clearly was important to the success of many aspects of treatment.

The profile of skills and other qualities that Robert exhibited across the core domains of the quadripartite model are consistent with viewing psychological well-being and social competence as distinct, yet interrelated dimensions of positive mental health for developing youth. Areas of limitation, for example, included subsets of concerns that could be distinguished according to whether they pertained primarily to traditional conceptualizations of social competence (e.g., anger management difficulties) or psychological well-being (e.g., low self-esteem). Robert's relatively demanding personal standards, furthermore, appear to have led to some divergence between his internalized self-evaluations of his functioning in differing areas and what was suggested to be the case on the basis of more objective indicators, such as those typically used in assessing social competence (Compas, 1993).

Treatment efforts focused on improving both psychological well-being and social competence. Notably, gains in each area appeared to facilitate positive change on the other dimension. Robert's expanding skill base for effective interactions with peers enhanced his feelings of being accepted and validated by others his own age, a key foundation for healthy self-esteem during development (Harter, 1999). In a reciprocal manner, Robert's growing sense of efficacy in this part of his life served to increase his objective level of social competence insofar as it promoted confidence and persistence in handling challenging situations with peers (Bandura, 1997).

Several aspects of the case report also illustrate the significance of attending to person–environment transactions within clinical interventions to promote the positive mental health of children and adolescents. These include Robert's move to a new school during the latter stages of treatment.

This setting change provided a valuable opportunity for him to apply his newly acquired skills within a more receptive environment. Interestingly, his family's move to a new neighborhood also may have been beneficial for similar reasons. When such fortuitous shifts in environmental contexts do not occur "naturally" in treatment, it may be useful to consider the need for planned intervention components directed toward such goals. Strategies that may prove beneficial in this regard clearly are not limited to shifts to entirely new settings (e.g., different school). It often may be more feasible to focus efforts on improving transactions within the contexts where difficulties are occurring (e.g., school-based consultation).

A related issue raised by the case example is the optimal balance to strive for between the competing concerns of helping youth fit in with but also not overconform to environmental demands. To a large extent, Robert's sense of self-worth at the time of referral was tied to both existing areas of success (e.g., high achievement in school) and aspirations for self-improvement (e.g., control temper) that were congruent with the value systems and adaptive demands of his surrounding environment. This facilitated attainment of desired outcomes in treatment in several respects. Robert already was highly motivated to put effort into reaching relevant goals (e.g., improved peer relations). In addition, many of the skills and capacities he demonstrated (e.g., engaging in prosocial behavior) could be relied on to advantage in the design of intervention strategies. At the same time, whereas Robert's tendencies toward self-assertion and independence generally can be regarded as strengths, they also clearly had the potential to generate unfavorable consequences depending on the norms and expectations that existed in different contexts (e.g., the protest incident during high school). Complicating matters of interpretation to some degree is Robert's surprising decision, in view of his nonconformist and individualistic tendencies, to enter the armed services. The favorable early indications of his adjustment to this environment, however, suggest that it can be beneficial for youth to seek out or be directed toward settings that complement (and hence possibly "keep in check"), rather than directly mirror, the most salient tendencies in their psychological make-up.

Future Directions

There are several promising directions for further elaborating the quadripartite model as a framework for promoting the positive mental health of children and adolescents. It would be valuable, for example, to have more data that bear directly on the basic structure of positive mental health. This includes the proposed status of social competence and psychological well-being as overlapping yet distinct dimensions of positive mental health for youth. Such a view allows for the possibility that many youth may exhibit similar degrees of favorable functioning on both dimensions. It also allows, however, for divergent patterns in which youth exhibit healthy adaptation on one dimension (e.g., social competence), but not the other (e.g., psychological well-being). Systematic investigation of these possibilities, in conjunction with identifying factors that contribute to differing patterns, will be needed to inform strategies for promoting positive mental health at various stages of development. The specific skills and attributes that constitute the fundamental bases for social competence and psychological well-being within each of the differing core domains of the model also merit investigation. Increased understanding in this area is necessary to ensure that approaches for assessing positive mental health are suitably broad and comprehensive, thereby facilitating identification of appropriate targets of intervention and accurate measurement of progress and outcomes in treatment.

Research is also needed to clarify the relation of positive mental health to traditionally recognized indicators of mental disorder for children and adolescents (e.g., DSM-IV diagnoses). Several pertinent issues in this regard already have been noted (e.g., role of positive mental health in protecting against onset of disorder). Additionally, it could be useful to explore the viability of incorporating both negative and positive dimensions of mental health within a more unified conceptual framework (Durlak, 2000). Efforts directed toward this goal could help to elucidate more encompassing, higher-order patterns in the psychosocial adjustment of developing youth, thereby helping to avoid limitations associated with a predominant focus on either positive mental health or disorder. Finally, in pursuing greater understanding of the role of person–environment transactions in relation to positive mental health, it seems crucial that cultural differences be taken into account (Ogbu, 1995). Cultural considerations should be examined not only with respect to the backgrounds of individual youth (e.g., race), but also the salient characteristics of the contexts to which they are adapting (e.g., urban vs. rural settings).

A further frontier that needs to be addressed is the relation between existing models of cognitive-behavioral therapy that have been used primarily to treat disorders and newly emerging approaches that focus on enhancing positive mental health. They may be found to differ in their relative appropriateness and effectiveness, for example, depending on considerations such as type of presenting concern, client preferences, and goals of treatment. As we have emphasized in this chapter, however, there are many important areas of overlap between cognitive-behavioral therapies and the underlying assumptions, techniques, and objectives of an orientation that focuses on mental health promotion. Accordingly, it may well be that an integrative approach yields the most favorable results. Controlled clinical trials could be used to address these questions, but are in their relative infancy in the adult literature (e.g., Fava, 1999) and to our knowledge have not yet been undertaken with children or adolescents.

Conclusion

In recent years, issues relating to positive mental health have begun to receive greater attention. This trend offers the promise of more effectively meeting the needs of youth both as clients in therapy and as participants in community-based programs that seek to promote health or prevent disorder. Such efforts offer a basis for deepened appreciation of developmental and ecological influences on the mental health outcomes of children and adolescents. Effective approaches to promotion of positive mental health thus may enhance sensitivity to individual differences among youth as well as the interplay of such differences with their surrounding environmental circumstances. The revised quadripartite model described in this chapter, although requiring additional investigation, is a promising framework for realizing this aim.

REFERENCES

Achenbach, T. M. (1990). Conceptualization of developmental psychopathology. In M. Lewis & S. M. Miller (Eds.), *Handbook of developmental psychopathology* (pp. 3–14). New York: Plenum Press.

Achenbach, T. M. (1991). *Integrative guide for the 1991 CBCL/4–18, YSR, and TRF Profiles*. Burlington: University of Vermont, Department of Psychiatry.

American Psychiatric Association. (1994). *Diagnostic and statistical manual of mental disorders* (4th ed.). Washington, DC: Author.

Bandura, A. (1986). *Social foundations of thought and action: A social cognitive theory*. Englewood Cliffs, NJ: Prentice-Hall.

Bandura, A. (1997). *Self-efficacy: The exercise of control*. New York: Freeman.

Bandmaster, R. F. (1989). The optimal margin of illusion. *Journal of Social and Clinical Psychology, 8,* 176–189.

Bandmaster, R. F., Bushman, B. J., & Campbell, W. K. (2000). Self-esteem, narcissism, and aggression: Does violence result from low self-esteem or from threatened egotism? *Current Directions in Psychological Science, 9,* 26–29.

Braswell, L., Bloomquist, M., & Pederson, S. (1991). *ADHD: A guide to understanding and helping children with attention deficit hyperactivity disorder in school settings*. Minneapolis: University of Minnesota.

Byrne, B. M., & Shavelson, R. J. (1996). On the structure of social self-concept for pre-, early, and late adolescents: A test of the Shavelson, Hubner, and Stanton (1976) model. *Journal of Personality and Social Psychology, 70,* 599–613.

Carvajal, S. C., Clair, S. D., Nash, S. G., & Evans, R. I. (1998). Relating optimism, hope, and self-esteem to social influences in deterring substance use in adolescents. *Journal of Social and Clinical Psychology, 17,* 443–465.

Chassin, L., Presson, C. C., & Sherman, S. J. (1989). "Constructive" vs. "destructive" deviance in adolescent health-related behaviors. *Journal of Youth and Adolescence, 18,* 245–262.

Cicchetti, D., Rappaport, J., Sandler, I., & Weissberg, R. P. (Eds.). (2000). *The promotion of wellness in children and adolescents*. Washington, DC: CWLA Press.

Colvin, C. R., & Block, J. (1994). Do positive illusions foster mental health?: An examination of the Taylor and Brown formulation. *Psychological Bulletin, 116*, 3–20.

Compas, B. E. (1993). Promoting positive mental health during adolescence. In S. G. Millstein, A. C. Petersen, & E. O. Nightingale (Eds.), *Promoting the health of adolescents: New directions for the twenty-first century* (pp. 159–179). New York: Oxford University Press.

Connolly, J. (1989). Social self-efficacy in adolescence: Relations with self-concept, social adjustment, and mental health. *Canadian Journal of Behavioural Science, 21*, 258–269.

Cowen, E. L. (2000). Psychological wellness: Some hopes for the future. In D. Cicchetti, J. Rappaport, I. Sandler, & R. P. Weissberg (Eds.), *The promotion of wellness in children and adolescents* (pp. 477–503). Washington, DC: CWLA Press.

Deci, E., L., & Ryan, R. M. (1995). Human autonomy: The basis for true self-esteem. In M. H. Kernis (Ed.), *Efficacy, agency, and self-esteem* (pp. 31–46). New York: Plenum Press.

Dinges, N. G. (1994). *Mental health promotion.* (Commissioned paper for the Institute of Medicine, available through National Technical Information Service, Order No. PB94-121860)

Dooley, D., & Prause, J. (1997). School-leavers' self-esteem and unemployment: Turning point or a station on a trajectory? In I. H. Gotlib & B. Wheaton (Eds.), *Stress and adversity over the life course: Trajectories and turning points* (pp. 91–113). New York: Cambridge University Press.

DuBois, D. L., Bull, C. A., Sherman, M. D., & Roberts, M. (1998). Self-esteem and adjustment in early adolescence: A social-contextual perspective. *Journal of Youth and Adolescence, 27*, 557–583.

DuBois, D. L., & Felner, R. D. (1996). The quadripartite model of social competence: Theory and applications to clinical intervention. In M. Reinecke, F. M. Dattilio, & A. Freeman (Eds.), *Cognitive therapy: A casebook for clinical practice* (pp. 124–152). New York: Guilford Press.

DuBois, D. L., Felner, R. D., Brand, S., Phillips, R. S. C., & Lease, A. M. (1996). Early adolescent self-esteem: A developmental-ecological framework and assessment strategy. *Journal of Research on Adolescence, 6*, 543–579.

DuBois, D. L., & Tevendale, H. D. (1999). Self-esteem in childhood and adolescence: Vaccine or epiphenomenon? *Applied and Preventive Psychology, 8*, 103–117.

DuBois, D. L., Tevendale, H. D., Burk-Braxton, C., Swenson, L. P., & Hardesty, J. L. (2000). Self-system influences during early adolescence: Investigation of an integrative model. *Journal of Early Adolescence, 20*, 12–43.

Durlak, J. A. (1997). *Successful prevention programs for children and adolescents.* New York: Plenum Press.

Durlak, J. A. (2000). Health promotion as a strategy in primary prevention. In D. Cicchetti, J. Rappaport, I. Sandler, & R. P. Weissberg (Eds.), *The promotion of wellness in children and adolescents* (pp. 221–241). Washington, DC: CWLA Press.

Eccles, J. S., Midgley, C., Wigfield, A., & Buchanan, C. M. (1993). Development during adolescence: The impact of stage-environment fit on young adolescents' experiences in schools and in families. *American Psychologist, 48*, 90–101.

Erikson, E. (1968). *Identity, youth and crisis.* New York: Norton.

Fava, G. A. (1999). Well-being therapy: Conceptual and technical issues. *Psychotherapy and Psychosomatics, 68,* 171–179.

Felner, R. D., Lease, A. M., & Phillips, R. S. C. (1990). Social competence and the language of adequacy as a subject matter for psychology: A quadripartite trilevel framework. In T. P. Gullotta & G. R. Adams (Eds.), *Developing social competency in adolescence* (pp. 245–264). Newbury Park, CA: Sage.

Flammer, A. (1995). Developmental analysis of control beliefs. In A. Bandura (Ed.), *Self-efficacy in changing societies* (pp. 69–113). New York: Cambridge University Press.

Gardner, H. G. (1993). *Multiple intelligences: The theory in practice.* New York: Basic Books.

Goleman, D. (1997). *Emotional intelligence.* New York: Bantam Books.

Harter, S. (1998). The development of self-representations. In W. Damon (Series Ed.) & N. Eisenberg (Vol. Ed.), *Handbook of child psychology: Vol. 3. Social, emotional, and personality development* (5th ed., pp. 553–617). New York: Wiley.

Harter, S. (1999). *The construction of the self: A developmental perspective.* New York: Guilford Press.

Higgins, E. T. (1991). Development of self-regulatory and self-evaluative processes: Costs, benefits, and tradeoffs. In M. R. Gunnar & L. A. Sroufe, (Eds.), *Self processes and development: The Minnesota symposia on child psychology* (Vol. 23, pp. 125–165). Hillsdale, NJ: Lawrence Erlbaum.

Hirsch, B. J., & DuBois, D. L. (1991). Self-esteem in early adolescence: The identification and prediction of contrasting longitudinal trajectories. *Journal of Youth and Adolescence, 20,* 53–72.

Huebner, E. S. (1991). Correlates of life satisfaction in children. *School Psychology Quarterly, 6,* 103–111.

Huebner, E. S. (1994). Preliminary development and validation of a multidimensional life satisfaction scale for children. *Psychological Assessment, 6,* 149–158.

Huebner, E. S., Gilman, R., & Laughlin, J. E. (1999). A multimethod investigation of the multidimensionality of children's well-being reports: Discriminant validity of life satisfaction and self-esteem. *Social Indicators Research, 46,* 1–22.

Kaplan, H. B. (1986). *Social psychology of self-referent behavior.* New York: Plenum Press.

Kendall, P. C., & Braswell, L. (1993). *Cognitive-behavioral therapy for impulsive children* (2nd ed.). New York: Guilford Press.

Kernis, M. H. (2002). Self-esteem as a multifaceted construct. In T. M. Brinthaupt & R. P. Lipka (Eds.), *Understanding early adolescent self and identity: Applications and interventions* (pp. 57–88). Albany: State University of New York Press.

Larson, R. W. (2000). Toward a psychology of positive youth development. *American Psychologist, 55,* 170–183.

Luthar, S. S., Cicchetti, D., & Becker, B. (2000). The construct of resilience: A critical evaluation and guidelines for future work. *Child Development, 71,* 543–562.

Markus, H., & Nurius, P. (1986). Possible selves. *American Psychologist, 41,* 954–969.

Marsh, H. W., & Hattie, J. (1996). Theoretical perspectives on the structure of the self-concept. In B. A. Bracken (Ed.), *Handbook of self-concept* (pp. 38–90). New York: Wiley.

Mash, E. J., & Dozois, D. J. A. (1996). Child psychopathology: A developmental–systems perspective. In E. J. Mash & R. A. Barkley (Eds.), *Child psychopathology* (pp. 3–60). New York: Guilford Press.

Meichenbaum, D. (1992). Evolution of cognitive behavior therapy: Origins, tenets, and clinical examples. In J. K. Zeig (Ed.), *The evolution of psychotherapy: The second conference* (pp. 114–128). New York: Brunner/Mazel.

Myers, D. G., & Diener, E. (1995). Who is happy? *Psychological Science, 6,* 10–19.

Ogbu, J. U. (1995). Origins of human competence: A cultural–ecological perspective. In N. R. Goldberger & J. B. Veroff (Eds.), *The culture and psychology reader* (pp. 245–275). New York: New York University Press.

Perry, C. L., & Jessor, R. (1985). The concept of health promotion and the prevention of adolescent drug abuse. *Health Education Quarterly, 12,* 169–184.

Rosenberg, M. (1979). *Conceiving the self.* New York: Basic Books.

Ryff, C. D. (1995). Psychological well-being in adult life. *Current Directions in Psychological Science, 4,* 99–104.

Ryff, C. D., & Singer, B. (1998). The contours of positive human health. *Psychological Inquiry, 9,* 1–28.

Sandler, I. (2001). Quality and ecology of adversity as common mechanisms of risk and resilience. *American Journal of Community Psychology, 29,* 19–61.

Scheier, M. F., & Carver, C. S. (1985). Optimism, coping, and health: Assessment and implications of generalized outcome expectancies. *Health Psychology, 4,* 219–247.

Seligman, M. E. P. (1998). The prediction and prevention of depression. In D. K. Routh, R. J. DeRubeis, & J. Robert (Eds.), *The science of clinical psychology: Accomplishments and future directions* (pp. 201–214). Washington, DC: American Psychological Association.

Shure, M. B., & Spivak, G. (1988). Interpersonal cognitive problem-solving. In R. H. Price, E. L. Cowen, R. P. Lorion, & J. Ramos-McKay (Eds.), *Fourteen ounces of prevention: A casebook for practitioners* (pp. 68–82). Washington, DC: American Psychological Association.

Smokowski, P. R. (1999). Ecological risk and resilience: A mixed-method analysis of disadvantaged, minority youth. *Dissertation Abstracts International, 60(05),* 1769A.

Tashakkori, A. (1992). Gender, ethnicity, and the structure of self-esteem: An attitude theory approach. *Journal of Social Psychology, 133,* 479–488.

Taylor, S. E., & Brown, J. D. (1999). Illusion and well-being: A social psychological perspective on mental health. In R. F. Bandmaster (Ed.), *The self in social psychology* (pp. 43–68). Philadelphia, PA: Psychology Press.

Treasure, D. C., Monson, J., & Lox, C. L. (1996). Relationship between self-efficacy, wrestling performance, and affect prior to competition. *Sport Psychologist, 10,* 73–83.

Ulmann, R. K., Sleator, E. K., & Sprague, R. (1984). A new rating scale for diagnosis and monitoring of ADD children. *Psychopharmacology Bulletin, 20,* 160–164.

Unger, D. G., & Wandersman, L. P. (1988). The relation of family and partner support to the adjustment of adolescent mothers. *Child Development, 59,* 1056–1060.

Vispoel, W. P. (1993). The development and validation of the Arts Self–Perception

Inventory for adolescents. *Educational and Psychological Measurement, 53,* 1023–1033.

Werner, E. E. (1995). Resilience in development. *Current Directions in Psychological Science, 4,* 81–85.

White, R. W. (1960). Competence and the psychosexual stages of development. In M. R. Jones (Ed.), *Nebraska Symposium on Motivation* (Vol. 8, pp. 97–141). Lincoln: University of Nebraska Press.

Wyman, P. A., Sandler, I., Wolchik, S., & Nelson, K. (2000). Resilience as cumulative competence promotion and stress protection: Theory and intervention. In D. Cicchetti, J. Rappaport, I. Sandler, & R. P. Weissberg (Eds.), *The promotion of wellness in children and adolescents* (pp. 133–184). Washington, DC: CWLA Press.

SUGGESTED READINGS

Cicchetti, D., Rappaport, J., Sandler, I., & Weissberg, R. P. (2000). *The promotion of wellness in children and adolescents.* Washington, DC: CWLA Press.

Compas, B. E. (1993). Promoting positive mental health during adolescence. In S. G. Millstein, A. C. Petersen, & E. O. Nightingale (Eds.), *Promoting the health of adolescents: New directions for the twenty-first century* (pp. 159–179). New York: Oxford University Press.

DuBois, D. L., & Tevendale, H. D. (1999). Self-esteem in childhood and adolescence: Vaccine or epiphenomenon? *Applied and Preventive Psychology, 8,* 103–117.

Larson, R. (2000). Toward a psychology of positive youth development. *American Psychologist, 55,* 170–183.

Ogbu, J. U. (1995). Origins of human competence: A cultural–ecological perspective. In N. R. Goldberger & J. B. Veroff (Eds.), *The culture and psychology reader* (pp. 245–275). New York: New York University Press.

Ryan, R. M., & Deci, E. L. (2000). Self-determination theory and the facilitation of intrinsic motivation, social development, and well-being. *American Psychologist, 55,* 68–78.

16

Personality Disorders among Children and Adolescents

Is It an Unlikely Diagnosis?

ARTHUR FREEMAN
ANDREA RIGBY

The childhood shows the man, As morning shows the day.
—JOHN MILTON, *Paradise Regained* (1671)

Allison was a quiet, studious 11-year-old child who did well in school. She had few friends and seemed to avoid work and play groups in school and at home. In gym class or during free time, she would sit by herself and read. Teachers had always seen Allison as "shy," but since she had always done well in school, did not appear unhappy, and caused no trouble, they did not see that she had any problems that should bring her to the attention of the school guidance or psychology staff or that they should alert Allison's parents.

Mitchell was a generally compliant, obsessive–compulsive, hard working, success-driven and sometimes demanding 13-year-old. He always scored at the highest level on classroom or standardized tests. If his scores were less than 95%, Mitchell could be counted on to go to the teacher and argue, beg, or attempt to cajole to gain another few points for answers that he believed were "close" and that should be worth additional credit. He was seen by teachers as a superior student, and his parents were proud of his achievements and shared their pride with him on many occasions. He received awards and praise for his success.

Alice was a ten-year-old who was aggressive to other children. She would bully them and take physical advantage of smaller children. It was rumored by the other children that she had killed kittens by putting them into a paper bag and then stepping on them. Where the rumor started was unclear. She was an average student but was intimidating to the other children (and to some teachers) who saw her as "someday being dangerous."

Eddie was 6 years old. When he entered first grade he carried with him reports from preschool and kindergarten teachers of his explosive temper. When he was not given what he demanded, he would have tantrums that could involve throwing things, destruction of property, attacking other children, and self-injurious behavior. This last act involved scratching his arms while screaming. His arms were often marked by the scratches. Eddie's mother tried to keep his nails short to avoid too much damage. She also made sure that he wore shirts that covered his arms.

Do any of these children "qualify" for a diagnosis of personality disorder? Are these children with certain traits that may be precursors to later personality disorder, or can they be diagnosed during childhood as having a personality disorder? The most frequent response is that children cannot be diagnosed as having a personality disorder for a number of reasons. Some reasons are theoretical, some conceptual, and some "legal." The goal of this chapter is to examine the premise and the diagnosis of personality disorders in children and adolescents by raising and discussing the conceptual, theoretical, and "legal" issues. This is followed by a discussion of a cognitive-behavioral treatment model and a case example and recommendations for revisions of the diagnostic criteria. Finally, we offer future directions for study.

DIAGNOSING PERSONALITY DISORDER

The diagnosis of personality disorder offers a useful categorization that allows for communication among professionals. We must recognize at the outset, however, that the specific disorders set out in the most recent revision of the *Diagnostic and Statistical Manual of Mental Disorders* (DSM-IV-TR; American Psychiatric Association, 2000) are not engraved in stone, but are far more plastic. The present DSM is the latest iteration in a series of diagnostic manuals going back to 1952. In each of the DSMs the specific disorders, the definitions of those disorders, and the diagnostic criteria for the disorders have changed. In some cases the changes have been quite minimal, but in other cases disorders have disappeared and others have appeared. The first two versions (DSM-I [American Psychiatric Association,

1952] and DSM-II [American Psychiatric Association, 1968]) offered the clinician general statements about disorders, though with little guidance about applying the offered definitions. Few, if any, criteria were set out, and the clinician could virtually "mix and match" diagnostic terms as they saw fit. Starting with the third edition, DSM-III (American Psychiatric Association, 1980), criteria sets were delineated for each disorder. The implication was that each disorder could be identified by a set of specific diagnostic criteria, and that the clinician was to stay as close to the criteria as possible and avoid making up their own diagnoses. Moreover, the emphasis shifted from definitions that were theoretically (psychodynamically) based to criteria sets that were more behaviorally based. The arrangement of the personality disorders in DSM-III into clusters suggested that the specific disorders must be seen as continua with a significant relationship between each diagnosis within a cluster.

Several questions emerge. At what point, then, are the behaviors of children or adolescents seen and diagnosed as personality disordered? When do traits and styles of responding become diagnosed as pathology? At what point should (and does) the mental health community step in and attempt to challenge or to modify the noted behavior? Are there issues present that require the inclusion of the criminal justice system or the child protective systems into the treatment plan? At what point do troubled or troubling children get diagnosed as personality disordered?

The most frequent answer is that these children cannot be diagnosed as personality disordered according to DSM-IV-TR. The use of the personality disorder diagnosis is, to the thinking of some clinicians, somewhere between inappropriate and illegal. But is this true? Certainly, the following statement is the prototypical introduction in DSM-IV-TR (American Psychiatric Association, 2000) to all the criteria sets for the personality disorders. These involve "a pervasive pattern of [descriptive statements] beginning by early adulthood and present in a variety of contexts, as indicated by [a number] or more of the following [criteria listing]." Without any further reading, this repeated statement gives the impression that personality disorders are manifestations of behavior, affect, and cognition that arise and can only be diagnosed beginning in the early adult years. This has generally meant individuals above age 18 years. It is not, however, simply a case of an adolescent having a birthday and, upon reaching the age of majority, being rewarded with graduation from school, a new car, and the official designation of having a personality disorder. Rather, the term personality disorder implies an enduring pattern whose beginnings can, at the very least, be traced back to adolescence, and often to childhood. The one exception noted by DSM-IV-TR is the diagnosis of antisocial personality disorder where a history of conduct disorder in childhood and adolescence is required (p. 706). DSM-IV-TR states, "The features of a personality dis-

order usually become recognizable during adolescence or early adult life."
(American Psychiatric Association, 2000, p. 688)

DSM-IV-TR (American Psychiatric Association, 2000) offers six broad
criteria for identifying personality disorders. Although these are usually
used to understand adult behavior, with a little extension they equally apply to children and adolescents. According to DSM-IV-TR, the essential
features of a personality disorder are the following:

> An enduring pattern of inner experience and behavior that deviates mark-
> edly from the expectations of the individual's culture and is manifested in at
> least two of the following areas: cognition, affectivity, interpersonal func-
> tioning, or impulse control (Criterion A). This enduring pattern is inflexible
> and pervasive across a broad range of personal and social situations (Crite-
> rion B) and leads to clinically significant distress or impairment in social,
> occupational, or other important areas of function (Criterion C). The pat-
> tern is stable and of long duration, and its onset can be traced back at least
> to adolescence or early adulthood (Criterion D). The pattern is not better
> accounted for as a manifestation or consequence of another mental disor-
> der (Criterion E) and is not due to the direct physiological effects of a sub-
> stance (e.g., a drug of abuse, a medication, exposure to a toxin) or a general
> medical condition (e.g., head trauma) (Criterion F). (p. 686)

According to these criteria, all the children described at the beginning
of this chapter could be diagnosed as having a personality disorder. The
patterns described are exhibited in a wide range of social, school, and interpersonal contexts; they are not better accounted for by another disorder or
by some developmental stage; they are stable and have been in place for a
significant duration of the children's lives; and they are not the result of
some chemical or toxic reaction.

Clinicians are often left in a confusing position. Child psychologists,
child psychiatrists, classroom teachers, pediatricians, child care workers,
and clinicians working in acute treatment and residential settings regularly
see children and adolescents who meet criteria for personality disorders
(Beren, 1998; Bleiberg, 2001; Shapiro, 1997, Vela, Gottlieb, & Gottlieb,
1997). But can clinicians apply these "adult" diagnoses to this small but
visible group of children? What are the advantages and disadvantages of
using these diagnoses for children and adolescents? What are the placement, treatment, and political ramifications of using personality disorder
diagnoses for children and adolescents? Finally, does using these "adult"
diagnoses have the effect of creating a trashcan category that will be used
for the most troubling of children or adolescents?

Bearing these questions in mind, it is our contention that personality
disorders can be manifested and identified among youth prior to age 18.
These disorders can be diagnosed by having met the same criteria used for

adults. Rather than trying to find euphemistic terms, titles, or diagnoses, or seeing the identified patterns as clinical precursors to the adult disorders, we believe that the clinical reality of personality disorders in childhood must be appropriately assessed, diagnosed, and treated. As a starting point, we can point to DSM-IV-TR. Contrary to popular belief, DSM-IV-TR states:

> *Personality Disorder categories may be applied to children or adolescents in those relatively unusual instances in which the individual's particular maladaptive personality traits appear to be pervasive, persistent, and unlikely to be limited to a particular developmental stage or an episode of an Axis I disorder.* It should be recognized that the traits of a Personality Disorder that appear in childhood will often not persist unchanged into adult life. *To diagnose a Personality Disorder in an individual under age 18 years, the features must have been present for at least 1 year.* The one exception to this is Antisocial Personality Disorder, which cannot be diagnosed in individuals under age 18 years. (p. 687, emphasis added)

Probably the easiest markers for understanding and identifying personality disorders are when the behavior(s) are inflexible (i.e., the individual seems to have little choice in his or her response style), compulsive (i.e., the individual will almost always respond in the same idiosyncratic way, even after seeing and understanding that the behavioral choice may have negative consequences), maladaptive (i.e., the behavior may serve to get the individual into trouble), and the cause of significant functional impairment (i.e., the individual's adaptive function is limited or impaired) and subjective distress (i.e., the individual experiences marked and frequent discomfort).

PERSONALITY DISORDERS IN CHILDHOOD

Early identification and intervention can, ideally, be mounted for maximizing the value of therapy by addressing behaviors before they have become more powerfully and frequently reinforced and habituated. It would be far better, we think, to address the identified early borderline personality disorder with a 12-year-old child than when the same individual seeks therapy as a 25-year-old adult. The 13 years in which the problem is not treated, or is treated tangentially or as some euphemistic precursor to borderline personality disorder, will not serve the child well. It makes much better sense to treat the disorder as the disorder. Most simply, if it walks like a duck, looks like a duck, and quacks like a duck, it would be useful to first treat it as a duck. It makes sense for practitioners to treat adolescents with borderline personality disorder accordingly, because it is likely more treatable at age

12 than it will be at age 25, when personality style has become more firmly entrenched and habituated.

By definition, the diagnosis of personality disorder generally requires an evaluation of the individual's long-term patterns of functioning as described in DSM, where "the pattern is stable and of long duration." We can, however, view the stability over time as relative to the life span. The existence of behavioral pattern(s) in children and adolescents will be of shorter duration, but involve a substantially longer percentage of the individual's life. A persistence of symptoms for 4 years represents 10% of the life of a person 40 years old. For a 12-year-old, the same 4 years represents 33% of the child's life.

The behavioral characteristics used to define these disorders in adults must also be distinguished from characteristics that are part of normal and predictable developmental patterns for children. Also, behavioral patterns may emerge in response to specific situational stressors or more transient mental states (e.g., mood or anxiety disorder, substance intoxication). For example, the clinging and dependent behavior seen in a 3- or 4-year-old may be developmentally appropriate and should not then be used as a diagnostic sign of a dependent personality. We are not suggesting that every behavioral pattern seen in childhood is in full, or in part, a personality disorder. Nor are we positing that every pattern in childhood will persist into the adult years and eventually become a personality disorder.

DiGiuseppe (personal communication, August, 1992) has stated, "Children are not so much disturbed as disturbing to others." Behaviors may be seen by an objective observer as strange or unusual when those behaviors are judged by the standards of the larger community or group. The characteristics that may meet criteria for a personality disorder may not be considered problematic by the individual or his or her family, despite appearing to the objective observer as self-defeating, self-injurious, or self-punitive. The observed individual, or the members of that individual's family group or cultural subgroup, may be unperturbed, sanguine or non-observant regarding that same behavior. For the family or cultural subgroup, the behavior may be seen as acceptable and even laudable. Obviously, judgments about personality functioning must take into account the individual's ethnic, cultural, and social background. When a clinician is evaluating someone from a background different from his or her own, it is essential to obtain additional information from informants who are familiar with the child's sociocultural history, background, and experience.

Making the diagnostic process even more complex is the fact that there are circumstances in which the behavior that is diagnosed as personality disordered in an adult individual may have been quite functional and strongly reinforced during that individual's childhood or adolescence. The patterns that are later used to establish a diagnosis of personality disorder may, during the childhood years, have had value and purpose that began to wear away as the child moved into the adult years. A personality style may move to disorder or be exacerbated following the loss of significant supporting persons (e.g., a parent) or previously stabilizing social situations (e.g., changing schools, moving to a new home). It is not always the case that children with unusual behaviors go through school unnoticed. Olin et al. (1997) found that teacher ratings of adolescents subsequently diagnosed as schizotypal personality disorder found that there were observable analogues of the adult disorder in late childhood or early adolescence. Wolff and colleagues found that of 32 children identified as schizoid personality in childhood, three-quarters later met DSM criteria for schizotypal personality disorder (Wolff, Townshend, McGuire, & Weeks, 1991). In fact, some of these patterns may be apparent by the end of preschool, between ages 4 and 6 (National Advisory Mental Health Council, 1995).

For example, Neil was a 20-year-old man who sought treatment because of what he termed his "chronic depression." He labeled his problem "low self-esteem." His negative view of himself stemmed, he said, from his inability to be successful. This was in spite of having graduated from high school at age 16, college at age 20, and having a high paying job in the computer industry.

He described a pattern of "organization" and "neatness" that was consistent and pervasive since childhood He described his "playing" with toy cars as a child as involving lining the cars up along one wall and then moving them to be evenly lined up and spaced along another wall. He stated that his mother had always bragged that she could dress him in white clothes and have him play in the mud and come home clean. When he was a teenager, his mother proudly showed friends and neighbors her adolescent son's clothes closet where everything was hung up, hangers evenly spaced, with all clothes arranged by type and color and all facing the same way.

As a child, Neil was perfectionistic, totally school- and academics-focused, had few friends, and was poorly skilled socially. He received certificates of excellence, praise at home and at school, and the admiration or envy of other children. Then, as now, Neil had little reason to question his behavior or to change it. As the clinician obtained Neil's history, it seemed clear that the perfectionistic and demanding behavior had been a lifelong pattern. Neil had shown an obsessive–compulsive personality disorder since childhood or adolescence. Now he complained of being isolated ("I have trouble maintaining a relationship"), misunderstood ("What's wrong with wanting to do your very best?"), and baffled ("What am I doing wrong?"). He would like to feel better but without giving up his pattern. What he states in session after session is encapsulated in the words of Popeye the Sailor: "I y'am wot I y'am." Treatment for Neil would need to focus on the depression that motivates him for treatment but also on the basic schema that eventuated in his self-demanding, perfectionistic style. It involved demands that he could not meet, thereby always "failing" despite his objective successes. Similarly, the child who is diagnosed by teachers as having a conduct disorder and who resists authorities and terrorizes his peers may be seen by his parents or others in their culture as a "real boy," or a kid that "doesn't take shit from anyone." The question is whether the aggression is isolated, occasional, and episodic or meets DSM-IV-TR criteria and is part of a pervasive pattern. If it is not pervasive, the DSM category of child or adolescent antisocial behavior (V71.02) might be used.

ARGUMENTS AGAINST DIAGNOSING PERSONALITY DISORDERS IN CHILDHOOD

The argument can be made that children below the age of 18 cannot, by definition, have a personality disorder. This argument posits that in childhood the personality is still forming and that to label it as disordered gives the impression that the personality of the child is fully formed, fixed, and encased in stone. We respond to this argument by pointing out that the age of 18 as the entry point to adulthood is not typical of all cultures. In certain cultures the age at which children reach their majority may be as low as 13. It is at that point that the child may be married, begin bearing children, and have adult responsibilities

A second argument against diagnosing personality disorders in childhood is that personality is in a constant and rapid state of development throughout these years. To take a "snapshot" of behavior at any point in those years and use that picture to draw conclusions gives an inaccurate view of the individual. These patterns may (and probably will) change. Our response to this criticism is that all diagnoses are conditional and can and should be revised as the clinician obtains additional data.

A third argument against using personality disorder diagnoses for children and adolescents has to do with the diagnosis or label *personality disorders*. Simply stated, the diagnosis of personality disorder for a child may have the effect of causing therapists and teachers to quickly give up on the child without trying to help. In addition, the diagnosis of personality disorder will follow that child throughout his or her school years and may be used as an excuse for limiting or even withholding treatment. We would, in fact, agree with this argument inasmuch as diagnoses in a child's record will be viewed, for good or ill, throughout his or her school career and possibly beyond. We are, in fact, very concerned that the acceptance of our thesis of childhood personality disorders will result in malpractice among therapists, teachers, and institutions.

A fourth concern, and an extension of the previous point, is that the diagnosis of personality disorders will be applied inappropriately to socially or culturally different groups. It would then become an easy way for individual therapists, or entire systems and institutions, not to treat minority group children. Here again, we are very concerned that the personality disorder diagnosis will be too quickly and inappropriately applied. If, by virtue of a child's having a personality disorder, adults choose to "give up" on the child, we will have a very serious problem. In point of fact, these children need to be diagnosed so that they can receive the best and most appropriate care. If it becomes a "copout" for therapists, then it is more a problem of the mental health system than of the need for, or validity of, the diagnosis. The system is truly broken if it avoids treating those who clearly most need treatment.

ARGUMENTS FOR DIAGNOSING PERSONALITY DISORDERS IN CHILDHOOD AND ADOLESCENCE

It is generally agreed that personality pathology originates in childhood and adolescence. We believe that it makes sense to diagnose the problems at the earliest possible opportunity, not only for the sake of the individual, but also for the families. Early detection and intervention may limit pervasiveness and chronicity. Identification and prevention become essential ingredients in the treatment (Harrington, 2001).

Since most adults with personality disorders can identify childhood and adolescent manifestations of the disorder, the therapy for the child can include extensive parental involvement. This might serve to limit some of the damage that is consequent to impaired parenting. For example, victims of early childhood abuse are four times more likely to be diagnosed with a personality disorder by early adulthood (Johnson, Cohen, Brown, Smailes, & Bernstein, 1999; (Johnson et al., 2001; Johnson, Smailes, Cohen, Brown, & Bernstein, 2000). Had the patterns of behavior and the abuse been identified earlier, possibly intervention could have been implemented.

If necessary, child protective services can be brought into the case management, along with intensive home-based services as needed. The school can be involved as an agency that identifies children for treatment and can then participate in the treatment. There may be the need for agency intervention, and opportunities for postvention over the years.

BIOLOGICAL, PHYSIOLOGICAL, AND NEUROCHEMICAL PERSPECTIVES

Various theorists have pointed to neurological disturbances that may be implicated in the onset of personality disorders. The occurrence of childhood abuse (verbal, physical, or sexual) experienced by many patients with personality disorders may precipitate neurological changes. Teicher et al. suggested that childhood abuse agitates the limbic system in a way that produces impulsivity, aggression, affective instability, and dissociative states (Teicher, Ito, Glod, Schiffer, & Gelbard, 1994). Goleman (1995) posits that continual emotional distress can create deficits in a child's intellectual abilities and damage the ability to learn in such a way that, as the child develops, subsequent rational decision-making abilities are impaired.

Personality disorders seem to be heritable. DSM-IV-TR notes that borderline personality disorder is five times more common in first degree relatives than in the general population (American Psychiatric Association, 2000). Although these data suggest a genetic component, there is more evidence linking environmental factors to the development of personality disorders. We cannot, however, dismiss the possibility of a biogenetic substrate for personality disorder.

DEVELOPMENTAL PERSPECTIVES

One explanation for the emergence of personality disorders in childhood centers on the mother–child relationship as described by object-relations theorists. According to them, the child's intrapsychic structure develops through differentiation of self from object with interrelated maturation of ego defenses (Masterson, 2000). Mahler (as discussed in Kramer and Akhtar, 1994) described four stages of development: autistic, symbiotic, separation–individuation, and object constancy. Problems encountered by the child in the separation–individuation phase, in particular, are implicated in the etiology of borderline personality disorder, for example. Kohut (as discussed in Kramer and Akhtar, 1994) examined the distortions of "self-object" that he thought arose from narcissistic injury to the child at a particularly vulnerable moment or developmental stage. This injury was thought to lead to the formation of personality disorders.

Beck, Freeman, and associates (1990) have pointed out that certain behaviors observed in children, such as clinging, shyness, or rebelliousness, tend to persist throughout various developmental periods into adulthood, at which point they are given the personality disorder labels such as dependent, avoidant, and antisocial. There is evidence that certain relatively stable temperaments and behavioral patterns are present at birth. These innate tendencies may be reinforced by significant others during infancy, or modeled as appropriate and sought-after behaviors during early childhood. For example, the infant or toddler who clings and cries is much more likely to be singled out for attention by caregivers, which in turn reinforces the care-eliciting behavior. The difficulty arises when these patterns persist long after the developmental period in which they might be adaptive.

Kernberg, Weiner, and Bardenstein (2000) comment that enduring patterns of personality are increasingly being described in preschoolers. These include patterns of aggressive behavior, inflexible coping strategies, and insecure attachment. Adult manifestations of these patterns might be depression, drug use, and criminal behavior. The progression of childhood conduct disorder to antisocial personality disorder suggests that personality disorders have their origins in earlier developmental stages (Kasen et al., 1999). Impulsivity and empathy are both apparent in children as young as age 2, and deviations in both impulsivity and empathy are components of certain personality disorders. The presence of concrete operational thinking in middle childhood makes it possible to discern thought disorders and impaired reality testing in school-age children.

FAMILY SYSTEM PERSPECTIVES

Family environment is thought to be an important contributing factor in the development of personality disorders in childhood. Families in which the child's attachment to primary caregivers is disrupted through death, divorce, or severe parental pathology, or otherwise chaotic family environments, may elicit maladaptive personality patterns in the child.

Family and systemic factors contribute to the development of personality disorders in children by providing learning experiences that lead to the formation of maladaptive schemas that persist throughout the developmental phases. These factors include the following:

1. Parents' failure to teach frustration tolerance. Even well-intentioned parents may fail to provide optimal training for dealing with frustrating experiences early in the child's life. This would include the setting and maintaining of clear and consistent boundaries.
2. Inappropriate child rearing and ignorance regarding child management skills. Overly punitive or overly permissive parenting may initiate disturbances in the child's sense of boundaries and self-regulation.
3. Skewed parental value systems. The highly achieving, perfectionistic child may be pushed by parents to excel, and reinforced by the parents' own need to succeed. Parents' beliefs are reflected in their choice of socialization strategies for their children, which in turn determine whether a child exhibits socially appropriate or socially deviant behavior (Rubin, Mills, & Rose-Krasnor, 1989). Cultural factors also come into play (Harkness & Super, 2000).
4. Parental psychopathology. The relationship between parental psychopathology and childhood oppositional disorder is quite strong. Hanish and Tolan (2001) and Hanish, Tolan, and Guerra (1996) have suggested that a parent with antisocial personality disorder, through the use of modeling and reinforcement, may transmit the

idea to the child that it is acceptable to defy authority. As the child internalizes this belief, he or she begins to oppose the parent, and eventually other authority figures.

5. Severe and persistent psychosocial stressors in the child's life. This might include financial problems, displacement of the home, parental/marital discord, or stressors with the community. Hanish et al. (1996) found that marital discord is a predictor of childhood behavior problems, specifically noncompliant, disruptive behavior.

6. Parental neglect and rejection. Parental neglect and rejection may lead to the development of schemas that suggest to the child that he or she is disconnected from primary attachment figures, and lead to a more pervasive sense of isolation.

7. Difficult child temperament. Children who are difficult infants may elicit responses from caregivers that contribute to the formation of maladaptive schemas. The crying, whining child may experience harsh punishment and more rejection, as well as excessive attention from frequent attempts on the part of the parents to soothe the child themselves rather than foster an ability in the infant to self-soothe.

8. Frequent and severe boundary violations. These violations can occur on the part of both the child and the parent. For example, if the child is forced into a dependent role at the expense of normal development of autonomy because of a parent's own need for dependence, then the child will have difficulty with individuation. Children who are inclined to introversion may delay or inhibit natural steps toward autonomy, and an overly punitive parenting style may thwart the child's first steps toward a clearly defined self. Instances of physical and sexual abuse are clear and severe boundary violations that have been linked with the development of several personality disorders.

IMPACT OF THE PERSONALITY
DISORDER ON FUNCTIONING

As with adults, the disorder itself may have either a positive or negative impact on the child or adolescent's interpersonal relationships, intrapersonal experience, school, work, or family relationships. For some children and adolescents, the disorder may cause significant and severe discomfort and dysfunction. For others, the personality style is ego-syntonic and the distress is from others (family, peers, school). For still others, the disorder is, at this point, functional. As noted earlier, the compliant, dependent, obsessive–compulsive, hard working, success-driven/demanding child will succeed at school and be seen as a hard worker and superior student. The results of the personality disorder in this instance may serve to enhance a child's school performance. In most cases, the squeakiest wheel will get the notice and attention. The externalizing child will be noticed while the internalizing child can be more easily ignored.

COGNITIVE-BEHAVIORAL CONCEPTUALIZATION OF THE PERSONALITY-DISORDERED CHILD

The clinician must work to identify schemas that are driving the child's cognitions, affect, and behavior (Freeman, 1983; Freeman & Leaf, 1989; Freeman, Pretzer, Fleming & Simon, 2003). Since these schemas evolve through assimilation and accommodation, the clinician must assess the schemas that are being used to address life problems. The range of schemas can encompass personal, family, gender, cultural, age-group, and religious schemas, with varying degrees of power and credibility for the child. For example, religious schemas may have more credibility and power for the child in a devoutly religious family than for the child whose family has no religious affiliation. The more powerful the reinforcers for schemas, and the more frequently they are reinforced, the more likely strong bonds will exist between the child and schemas. It is important to determine how early in life schemas are acquired, for the earlier-acquired schemas are the most powerful. The clinician needs to be aware that schemas can be acquired through multifaceted, multisensory learning, through cognitive, behavioral, motor/kinesthetic, visual, olfactory, and gustatory modes, for example. This means that even infants have the capacity to acquire schemas, hence the ensuing difficulty in attempting to modify early entrenched but maladaptive schemas.

Behaviors and beliefs can also be the result of modeling. The child observes significant others and learns that certain patterns of behavior are reinforced. The nature of the behavior may be adaptive or maladaptive, depending on the level of pathology present in parents. The child also gains reinforcement for a particular pattern of behaviors. Family environment and genetic predisposition may interact in unique ways, resulting in the development of a child who manifests a pattern of behaviors.

ASSESSMENT AND DIAGNOSTIC PERSPECTIVES

The clinician who suspects that the behavior of a child or adolescent may warrant an Axis II personality disorder diagnosis must thoroughly assess the child's behaviors, affect, and cognition across a variety of situations, as well as obtaining a thorough family and developmental history. The assessment should include contact with or reports from the child's pediatrician and teachers in earlier grades. This is required to assess the chronicity of the problem and whether the behaviors are pervasive. Data can be collected through structured clinical interviews with the child and his or her parent(s), from teachers and other school personnel (administrators or counselors), and through psychological testing, behavioral observations at home and at school, repeated self-report measures when possible, symptom behavioral checklists, school behavior report forms, family history, and the clinician's interview impressions.

Essential to making the diagnosis is a thorough grounding in developmental norms and an understanding of what is normative for that child in that setting, at that time. For example, when one sees an adolescent who is contrary, argumentative, impulsive, anti-authority, and risk taking, one might easily label this youth as normal. The assessment questions include the following:

- Does the reported and/or observed behavior have a normal developmental explanation?
- Does the behavior change over time or setting? Is it cyclical, variable, and unpredictable, or is it constant, consistent, and predictable?
- Could the behavior be the result of discrepancies between the child's chronological age and his or her cognitive, emotional, social and/or behavioral ages?
- Does the child function similarly in different environments? For example, does the behavior relate to the child's placement at home or in school?
- Is the behavior culturally related?
- Who has made the referral, and why was it made at this point?
- Is there agreement between parents, or between parent(s) and teacher(s), on the cause, need, or purpose of the referral?
- What are the expectations that are being made of the clinician in responding to the referral? For example, how does the child's behavior compare or contrast with the behavior of other children in that family or socioeconomic and sociocultural setting?
- How does the child's behavior compare or contrast with the behavior of other children in that age or social group?
- What is the history of the child's behavior in terms of length of existence, duration when stimulated, and ability of the child to control, contain, or withdraw from the behavior?
- Does the child have insight into the behavioral cues that trigger the behavior or the consequence of the behavior?
- Does the child see the behavior as something that he or she is interested in modifying?
- What are the differing views of the child's behavior? Are the clinician's sources of data reliable?
- The parent report is important in terms of the child's behavior at

home. How does the child relate to siblings, neighborhood friends, clubs, sports, organizations, church activities, adult relatives, pets, and self-care (activities of daily life).

- Has there been recurrent physical, emotional, sexual, or verbal abuse? The parental view of discipline versus child abuse is a key element to be considered.
- Within societal norms, is the parental behavior inappropriately sexual or seductive? Is incest suspected?
- What is the parent's view of privacy for the child?
- Are the parents inappropriately, unreasonably, or unjustifiably interfering with the child's relationships with other children?
- Within societal norms, are the parents inappropriately involved with the child's personal hygiene beyond the child's necessity?

Based on Kernberg et al. (2000), we would identify a number of specific factors to be considered in the assessment.

- The clinician must evaluate the child's temperament, which is likely based on biogenetic factors that then constitute a "disposition" influencing the child's interactions with his or her world. This temperamental filter will affect the nature, style, frequency, "volume," and content of the child's approach to the world.
- The child's internal, persistent, and developing mental construction of selfhood (identity) would need to be assessed.
- Gender plays a role inasmuch as it carries with it both self- and other expectations that would be based in the culture. While certainly a component of identity, gender also carries with it significant societal norms and demands.
- It would be critical to be able to identify any neuropsychological deficits related to cognitive functioning, and important to identify any problems in the manner in which the child organizes, processes and recalls information.
- The child's level, content, range, and repertoire of affect need to assessed.
- What is the child's characteristic mode of coping with internal and external stressors in his or her life? How does the child respond initially and how do his or her attempts at coping increase or decrease as the stressors persist?
- The clinician must assess the child's environment, which includes his or her family system, school experience, and religious environment, as well as the stability of all the above. It will be important to assess the reactivity and reciprocal behavior of others within the systems.
- The child's motivation and attempts to meet intrinsic and extrinsic

needs are important. This will reflect the "why" of the child's actions. What is the goal of the child's drives and actions?

- The child's social facility and repertoire of social interaction skills will assist the child in relating to and coping with significant others within the environment.
- The child's actions can be best understood in light of his or her level of cognitive development and integration. The child at preoperational levels cannot be expected to process information in the same manner as the child at the level of concrete or formal operations.
- What are the most active and compelling schemas that the child uses to understand and organize the world?

Frequently, the euphemisms used to describe the child can be added to the diagnostic mix. The child may be isolated and withdrawn (the schizoid child), suspicious (paranoid child), irritable or sensitive (borderline child), self-focused (narcissistic child), aggressive (antisocial child), attention seeking (histrionic child), conscientious and careful (obsessive–compulsive child), needy (dependent child), shy (avoidant child), or stubborn though apparently agreeable (passive–aggressive child).

We would identify a number of factors which can (and often do) complicate the differential diagnosis of personality disorder in adolescents. First and foremost is the typical adolescent "neurosis." Adolescents are exploring new roles, shedding old ones, and confronting new challenges, all the while trying to maintain a semblance of safety and stability. This describes much of adolescent behavior. The parent or other authority often responds to their actions by stating, "You should know better." There are significant hormonal surges that serve to influence the adolescent's behavior, cognitive processing, and affect. Significant mood shifts are typical of the adolescent and are rooted in his or her physiology. These mood shifts are similar to those seen in individuals with bipolar illness, that is, rapid alternation and shift of mood.

Adolescence presents everyone with a Kafkaesque experience of metamorphosis. There are rapid (and often significant) changes in size, weight, height, and the development of secondary sex characteristics and, therefore, body shape. These changes are expected and seemingly taken in stride with far greater equanimity than would be the case if an adult experienced these same physical changes in the same brief period of time. There are rapid alterations of identity. The adolescent moves from child to adult. Hank Ketcham, the cartoonist responsible for "Dennis the Menace" had Dennis state, "How come when I have to go to the doctor I am a big boy, but when its time for bed, I am still a little boy?" The adolescent tries out many identities in terms of dress, attitude, social circle, and relationship with family members. This shifting of identity could be mistaken as meeting criteria of personality disorder.

Adolescents end up in conflicts with parents, school authorities, or the justice system. Adolescence is filled with rebellion alternating with dependence. The push–pull of the relationship with parents is encapsulated by the adolescent's wanting greater freedom while asking for financial or social support. This dichotomizing is also indicative of certain personality disorders.

The adolescent may rebel by joining an apparently neurotic or antisocial group. Parents are concerned that the adolescent is hanging out with the "wrong group." In fact, the adolescent may make a very normal and appropriate adjustment to the group in the way he or she acts, dresses, talks, and responds to authorities and parents. The problem will be that the child or adolescent is not so much troubled, as troubling to others.

The emergence of sexual behavior serves as another confounding variable. The onset of this new behavior has implications for the adolescents' interpersonal actions, responsibility for their safety, and adherence to parental demands and expectations. The dividing line between socially approved sexuality as demonstrated by dress and action, seems increasingly to be blurred. The adolescent icons seen on MTV or in advertisements for clothing, music, foods, or recreation are overtly sexual.

Finally, there is a normal body dysmorphia during adolescence that relates to how one's body appears to self or to others. A skin eruption at the time of a date or important school function may be viewed as more than a pimple. It may be perceived as a cause for cloistering oneself and not appearing in public.

ELEMENTS FOR EXPLAINING THE BEHAVIOR

A central part of the assessment and, later, treatment is an explication and possible challenging of the parent's and teacher's thoughts and beliefs about the child. For example, in the "evil child" hypothesis, the adult sees the child's general behavior and specific reactions as the result of some genetic flaw. This is often presented as "This is a bad [evil] child" or "There is something just wrong with this child." A second hypothesis is that the child is purposely and vindictively causing trouble or making life difficult for others. The parent's or teacher's reaction may be rooted in rigid and unyielding rules about what is good, proper, appropriate, or expected behavior at home or in the classroom—rules that the child challenges or violates. A third factor may concern distributions of power in the classroom or home and demands by the adults for the child's loyalty to family codes of conduct or school expectations. Fourth, the clinician must examine in detail the family schemas regarding parent–parent behavior, children's behavior, child–parent behavior, boundaries, the ability or motivation to change, family rules, dealing with and possibly responding to authorities, and the interest, ability, and motivation to communicate.

The parental responses can be both written and verbal and should be utilized to disclose the child's behavior at present and historically. Information should be obtained about fearful reactions, repetitive/obsessive ruminations, compulsive behaviors, avoidance behaviors, instances of abuse, and reports of trauma.

SCHOOL AND TEACHER INVOLVEMENT

Teacher reports can provide excellent information regarding the child's responses pertaining to academic functioning, communication style, and relationship with other children, as well as his or her reaction to and relationship with the adults at school. The clinician will need to determine if the referral results from the teacher's lack of knowledge regarding normal development and developmental expectations. Similarly, the teacher's expectations for the child's behavior and the interrelationship between the teacher's behavior and that of the child should be explored. Are there classroom stressors that factor into the referral question and create an environment that exacerbates the situation? Is the identified behavior related and limited to peer interactions? How does the child typically handle new learning situations? Does the child withdraw from potentially dangerous situations, or increase his or her aggressive behavior as a result of anxiety or threat?

THE CHILD'S VIEW

The child's report of self-esteem, self-concept, fears, and views of others is essential. Data collected through interviewing and through psychological testing are useful. Such measures include Murray's Thematic Apperception Test (TAT, Murray, 1943) and Bellak's Child Apperception Test (CAT; Bellak & Bellak, 1948). Both can give the clinician an excellent "snapshot" of the child's cognitive, emotional, and behavioral percepts. For example, James, a ten-year-old boy, was referred by his teacher because of "shyness." He did not engage in interactions with other children and was reluctant or even resistant to respond in class. His teacher reported that there had been times when he acted "like an ostrich with his head in the sand," and explained: "I ask him a question and there are times that he acts as if he hasn't even heard the question. Then, when the other children start to giggle at his silence, he sometime stutters an inaudible response. I usually just let it go or just call on someone else." James' parents saw little reason for psychological referral, testing, or possible therapy. They were able quite easily to excuse, reframe, or reinterpret his behavior; for example: "He is just a quiet kid. Why does he have to speak up all of the time?" "He is a good kid. Isn't that enough?" "If you were to know him really well you would see a kid with a great memory, high intelligence, and good manners." "Everyone in our family is fairly quiet." "Uncle Joe is the same way. It runs in our family." "He does very well in school. He make sure of that." (It was discovered that James had an older brother who was diagnosed with a conduct disorder.)

James responded to card 1 on the TAT (a picture of a child with a violin) with the following story:

THERAPIST: What is happening in the picture?

JAMES: This boy is looking at a violin in a store window. He would really like to play the violin but can't. He is afraid to ask his parents for permission to take violin lessons because they will expect him to play for them all of the time. He'll have to show them what he has learned and it won't be any fun.

THERAPIST: What led up to this picture?

JAMES: I don't know. Maybe he saw a movie about a violin player?

THERAPIST: Okay, what is going to happen afterwards?

JAMES: He won't do it. When he is supposed to go for lessons he will probably just stay home and play video games. (*Jokingly.*) Maybe there is a video game about violins. (*Laughs.*) If they make him play for them he'll sound terrible and everyone will laugh.

Other responses had similar themes of concern about being judged harshly by others, looking foolish, the need to avoid being seen as foolish, and isolation as being preferable to any other state of interaction. Clearly, treatment goals for James would have to focus on the parent–child interaction(s), the expectations of the family and the school, and James' view of himself.

Direct observation of James was especially helpful. Data obtained through direct observation in the classroom helped the clinician to determine a baseline of behaviors that provided useful information to compare with that given by his parents.

Did James' behavior meet the criteria for personality disorder? Was it pervasive? Yes. Was it persistent and stable for a relatively long time—exceeding one year? Yes. Was the behavior outside the normal developmental limits for the child? Yes. Could it be better explained (without forcing the issue) by using an Axis I diagnosis? No. Based on these factors, James met criteria for the diagnosis of avoidant personality disorder.

TREATMENT COST

What if treatment recommendations are refused, and treatment is not initiated? Is there a possibility or even a probability that the identified behavior will spontaneously remit? If there is a minimal environmental shift, will the behavior then remit? Basically, the clinician must assess the "treatment cost" to the child. For example, if the child and his or her family are referred to therapy, is it possible that things may get worse for them? Who in the family can be called upon and trusted to participate in the therapy? What supports can be offered or provided for the child and the family? Who will fund the supports? For what period of time? In what context?

SELECTING THE OPTIMAL FOCUS FOR TREATMENT

The decision to engage the child in some form of psychological treatment is one that is ideally made in conjunction with, and with input from, a number of sources. At this point, it may be tempting to consider the child as the sole focus for treatment. However, such a singular emphasis on the child negates the reality that other forces are having an impact on the child and influencing the referral problem. This problem may result from the parent's lack of knowledge regarding norms of development and behavior in children and adolescents. The child's behavior may relate to parental behavior and expectations or to the parent's skills at parenting. Assessment of parenting skills deficits would thus be part of the intervention. In these circumstances, parent education is an essential ingredient of the treatment.

Given that a child spends half of his or her waking hours in school, it will be essential to engage not only the parents or other caretakers in the treatment plan, but also the school. The child must be included in the treatment planning. The "problem" would need to be explained to the child, along with the need for some intervention and the goals of treatment. Trying to treat a child who may have no idea why treatment is indicated may be a lost cause. The child may have little or no motivation to change, and may be frightened and opposed to any changes in his or her behavior or world.

Depending on the age and level of cognitive development of the child, treatment would have to be modified. For example, the child's developmental stage may not be adequate for verbal–abstract therapy. The child's verbal skills and ability to generalize, an important factor in therapy, may be similarly limited. Most children would have great difficulty being able to sit still, listen, concentrate, focus, and integrate the diverse pieces that arise in typical psychotherapy. Even spending an extended amount of time alone with an adult might be viewed as somewhere between strange and frightening for the child. Session length may have to be limited based on the child's ability to attend for a prescribed length of time.

THE THERAPY PROCESS

Once therapy has been agreed to, the actual therapy session is a small part of what must be viewed as an integrated whole. On a regular basis, the clinician needs to review the occurrence of target behaviors since the last session (based on parent and/or teacher report). Goals of therapy include expanding the child's "emotional vocabulary" to describe positive and negative feelings, helping the child to identify and dispute dysfunctional ideas, teaching self-instructional techniques, teaching problem-solving skills, including consequential thinking and finding alternatives, and role playing specific skills. When possible, significant others can act as therapy assistants by reinforcing learned skills in the child's home and/or school environment. Continued monitoring by parents and school personnel is encouraged for the purpose of collecting data, as well as fostering a sense of involvement and efficacy in those closest to the child.

It is assumed that the clinician has made a decision concerning the use of therapy to treat the child, the parent(s), the family, or the family system. The judicious use of time is essential. The clinician will want to set the agenda to allow the child and his or her parents to be alert to the goals of the session. When possible, both the child and the parents can suggest agenda items for discussion. Parents and teachers may be involved in assisting the child with homework assignments given in session, or with additional reinforcement of skills learned in session. The amount of time that is allocated to child work, parent work, or family work will be dependent on the clinician's assessment of where the focus must be at any particular point in the treatment.

The clinician will ascertain the child's capacity to "uncover" or "process" experience based on the child's cognitive level and response to therapy. For example, the child who is at the concrete operations level of thinking may respond best to therapeutic interventions that provide a limited range of choices for behavior. The focus of therapy should be on the change process itself. The therapist must develop a working alliance with the child by an assessment of the child's ability and willingness to connect both cognitively and emotionally. The therapist will be aided by an understanding of the basics of neuropsychology, the effects of anxiety on performance, the impact of learning problems on adaptive functioning, and developmental psychology.

CASE EXAMPLE

Edward (Eddie) White, the child described at the beginning of this chapter, was a 6-year-old boy referred by his classroom teacher to the school psychologist and then to a clinical psychologist. The reason for the referral was that Eddie was constantly throwing tantrums in the classroom, hitting other children, and threatening the teacher by waving his fist and saying "You better give me what I want or I'll get you." He destroyed the work of other children, and the teacher noted that there were things missing from the classroom that could not be accounted for. She suspected Eddie of having taken them.

The school psychologist decided that the issue was broader than just school-related issues and referred Eddie and his parents to an outside clinician.

Eddie was an only child. His mother was 35 years old, had earned a master's degree in education, and had taught elementary school for 2 years. His father, age 40 years, had a doctoral degree in history and was an senior administrator at a small college.

When his parents first met with the school psychologist, they were reportedly reluctant to accept the referral. Though Dr. White was quiet, Mrs. White was angry and attacked the teacher, the school psychologist, the school, the school system, and education in general. She needed to be calmed down on several occasions by her husband. She made numerous threats to have everyone's credentials publicly examined, demanded to see specific documentation for every act of which her son was "accused," and called into question the ability of the teacher to deal with her son ("He is brighter than most other children"; "He come from a better family"; "We have significant contacts in the educational community"; "He is protecting himself from the lower element in your school"). If her son actually did what he was reported to have done, she said, it was because he had been provoked by other children.

The school psychologist then decided to remove this referral from the school. Mrs. White demanded to know what would happen if she refused the referral. She was told that her son would be placed in a special class for emotionally disturbed children, as the teacher could not deal with him in the context of a regular class setting. Dr. White tried to calm his wife by patting her arm. Her response was to begin shouting at her husband and demanding, "Are you on their side? No one is going to hurt my son."

When they first met with the clinical psychologist, Mrs. White was calm and tried to portray the entire issue as a mistake and a "misunderstanding." It appeared as if Dr. and Mrs. White had prepared for this interview. Dr. White sat quietly looking around the room while Mrs. White did almost all of the talking.

Eddie, she said, was brighter than these other children after all. Since he was smarter and educationally advanced, he needed advanced class placement with older children so that he would not be frustrated. Mrs. White then asked the psychologist to write a letter, based on the initial interview, justifying her position and supporting her view that Eddie should be advanced in grade as the solution for the problem. She pointed out that she had been teaching Eddie to read since he was 2, that she read with him every night, gave him vocabulary quizzes based on the reading, had him do math problems, and took him to museums. She raised the issue of home schooling: "If the school cannot deal with a superior child, then we will educate him at home."

The therapist recorded this information and then asked several questions that quickly raised Mrs. White's ire.

THERAPIST: What does Eddie do for fun?

MRS. WHITE: He spends time with me. We play games, watch TV, and read together.

THERAPIST: Does Eddie have any friends in the neighborhood?

MRS. WHITE: Why? Why should he play with those ruffians? They are low class and would not appreciate him.

THERAPIST: Are you concerned that he has no social contacts except you?

MRS. WHITE: He'll have plenty of time for that after I'm gone. For now he needs me.

The therapist then asked about her pregnancy and delivery, and Eddie's progression through developmental milestones. Mrs. White became very suspicious.

MRS. WHITE: Why are you asking these questions? Why is this necessary. You are being very intrusive. All you need to do is to write a stupid letter. Is asking questions that are none of your business the way that you are trying to justify the enormous fee you are extorting from us? (*At this point her husband tried to calm her. She gave him a withering look, he withdrew his hand, and she continued.*) This is a set up, isn't it? You and that moron in the school have already decided what you're going to do, haven't you? I will tell you now, and I swear to God, you will not hurt my child.

THERAPIST: I understand how upsetting all of this must be. I can well understand how upset you both must have been to be called in to school. I have reviewed the school records, and I agree—Eddie is incredibly smart and academically advanced. I would like to help you, as much as I can, deal with the school on these issues.

Mrs. White, Dr. White, I have no reason to hurt your child. I have no agenda other than to gather information and decide how I can help YOU. I am working for and with YOU. Any work that I do will be for your benefit and the benefit of your son. Now to do that I need all of the information that you can share with me. I need to be able to present a case to the school on your behalf and on behalf of Eddie.

(*At this point, Mrs. White shifted markedly. Her tone of voice, demeanor, and verbal content changed.*)

MRS. WHITE: Thank you. We knew that we could trust you. What do you need to know?

Mrs. White described the fact that she and her husband could not conceive for many years and that Eddie was the result of several years of fertility work. ("Those stupid doctors had no idea what they were doing.") Her pregnancy was high risk and very difficult. She spent the last 2 months of her pregnancy in bed, and the final 3 weeks in the hospital. Eddie was born by cesarean section, an event that upset Mrs. White because of the scar it left. At this point, the time for the initial interview ran out. Dr. and Mrs. White were informed that the psychologist would want to continue the information gathering with them, even before meeting with Eddie. Mrs. White seemed relieved.

During the second information-gathering session, Dr. White was unavailable, so Mrs. White came to the session with Eddie. She stated that they had never left him with a babysitter and were not about to start. (The first session was held during school hours so that Eddie was in school at the time.) Eddie could only be described as a physically beautiful child. He had smooth blond hair, blue eyes, and fair skin. He was well proportioned and of appropriate size for his age. When initially greeted by the therapist, Eddie first looked to his mother. When she nodded, he said, "Hello."

Mrs. White brought several books for Eddie to read, and, for the most part, Eddie sat quietly in the waiting room during the session. On five occasions he tapped on the office door to ask his mother a question. These questions were, "Will we have dinner this evening?", "Can we watch television later?", etc.

Mrs. White started the session by telling the therapist how pleased she was that she could trust him to help Eddie, and that she could tell from the therapist's manner that he was accomplished, experienced, and sensitive. Mrs. White then began speaking as if the session was her own and not an information and evaluation session for her child. When the therapist tried to focus her on Eddie, she would say, "This is important. This will let you know about Eddie." In almost every instance the information was about her, which was ultimately revealing of her behavior toward her son.

Mrs. White was an only child of an absent father who was in the military and an alcoholic mother who, from Mrs. White's description, was verbally, physically, and emotionally abusive. During Mrs. White's childhood, her mother would slap her and demand that she not cry. Her mother said this was to prepare her for the cruelty of the world. By adolescence, Mrs. White no longer cried when she was struck. At that point, her mother would slap her, demanding, "Don't you have any feelings?" Mrs. White was then asked if she ever hit Eddie. Her anger returned and she demanded, "Why are you asking? Are you trying to take him away from me?" She stated that she knew about abuse reporting and that she wanted to make it clear that she had NEVER struck him. She reported that she did use threats of abandonment, threats of his being isolated and alone without her, of a future where he would not be able to cope because she wasn't there to help, support, love, and care for him. To show him what it was like being alone, she had on two occasions taken him to a mall and told him to sit on a bench and wait for her. She then did not return for an hour. Eddie dutifully sat on the bench and, when asked by passersby if he was lost, responded, "No. My mom will be right back." She then returned, crying about how much she missed him. When he saw her, he became very upset and began crying and clinging to her. On occasions when she returned and he was not also crying, she became furious and would not speak to him for the rest of the day. After that he would beg, "Please, please never leave me."

Mrs. White's mother told her that she had caused great difficulty during her mother's pregnancy. Mrs. White commented that "I was a bad fetus. I hurt my mother even before I was born. Eddie did the same to me." She then revealed that one of the reasons for her high-risk pregnancy was that she was so sure she was going to lose the baby that she tried to hurry the loss along. She would punch herself in the abdomen, run up and down stairs, and exercise beyond what was recommended just to "get it over with."

Her childhood was filled with many double messages. Her mother refused to allow her to attend college, knowing that it would mean that Mrs. White would leave home. Her mother constantly told her that a job as a cashier at a market or convenience store, an early marriage, and a home in town near to the mother was ideal. Her mother repeatedly stated, "I can't lose you. You are all that I have." This did not stop her mother from the constant physical abuse. With difficulty, Mrs. White attended a local community college. She then "broke her mother's heart" and went to the state university. This required that she move about an hour away from home. She stayed at the university after earning her bachelor's degree and completed a master's degree in education. It was in graduate school that she met her husband.

Mrs. White reported that she had no friends throughout her childhood and that only when she went away to school did she make friends. She joined a sorority in college and chose to live in the sorority house. After her first year, no one in the sorority wanted to share a room with her. She stated that she could not get along with the other girls. They were, she said, of low breeding and not what she had expected.

Based on Mrs. White's revelations, and a following meeting with her husband, it was decided that the approach to dealing with Eddie's behavior would be a combination of meeting with Eddie for about 10 minutes each week and, in the remaining balance of time, meeting with Mrs. White to help her with child-rearing skills. Surprisingly, she agreed to the second part (her being in therapy) but not to the first part (Eddie's therapy). It turned out that her concern was twofold: first, that if the therapist spent time with Eddie, Eddie would bond with him and no longer need her, and, second, that she wanted the therapist for herself.

There was also a long-term problem with Eddie's eating, a constant concern for Mrs. White. She would not allow him to eat anything that she did not prepare. If a child in school had a birthday and the child's mother brought cookies or cupcakes for the children, Eddie was not allowed to eat them. Though it appeared that she was concerned about the quality of food, the issue was more that she did not want Eddie to see anyone else as being able to nourish him. She breast-fed Eddie until the pediatrician demanded that she start feeding Eddie solid food. She refused, stating, "I can give him all that he needs." When she fed him, she would expose her breast, place the spoon next to her nipple, and feed him so that Eddie would connect sustenance with her alone.

Mrs. White was asked about Eddie's self-injurious behavior. She described that Eddie, when frustrated or angry, would scratch at his forearms until he bled. Mrs. White stated that she did her best do avoid the problem by clipping his nails daily and having him wear long sleeve shirts to hide the marks. She did not want to give the teacher "an excuse" for picking on her son.

The conceptualization of the problem was as follows:

1. Eddie had never been taught frustration tolerance. He would explode whenever there were any demands made on him by anyone.
2. Mrs. White's own behavior modeled this low frustration tolerance.
3. Mrs. White's behavior supported her son's tantrum behavior.
4. Eddie was the product of questionable and inappropriate child-rearing.
5. Although an elementary school teacher, Mrs. White seemed to be either ignorant or unskilled in basic child management or behavioral management skills.

6. There was clear parental psychopathology.
7. Eddie lived with severe and significant psychosocial stressors, always fearing abandonment.
8. There was an ongoing question as to whether Mrs. White's behavior was abusive and required child protective services.
9. Mrs. White was alternately rejecting and demanding of Eddie's love.
10. There were frequent boundary violations regarding eating.

Mrs. White met criteria for borderline personality disorder. Eddie met five of the criteria for the same disorder: (1) frantic efforts to avoid real or imagined abandonment, (2) a pattern of intense and unstable interpersonal relationships, (3) impulsivity, (4) self-mutilating behavior, and (5) difficulty controlling his anger.

The treatment of Mrs. White and Eddie lasted for 4 years. The therapist targeted specific social problems in school and worked with Mrs. White to help Eddie act in a more adaptive manner. The content of the sessions included basic developmental information, specific child rearing techniques, and explanations of how Mrs. White's behavior was possibly encouraging Eddie's dysfunctional behavior. Dr. White was included in many of these sessions.

The therapist maintained constant contact with the school and the classroom teachers. Eddie was maintained in a regular classroom. With Mrs. White's help, Eddie was "allowed" to make friends. He also became active in a soccer league, of which she attended every game and became the kind of soccer parent that every referee and coach would hate.

Eddie's building a life outside of her control was upsetting to Mrs. White. She was helped to see this as important for Eddie, even though it triggered her own abandonment schema. Her schemas about "good mothering" were enlisted to allow her to grant him a degree of freedom.

After 4 years of treatment, Dr. White was selected for a dean's position at a distant school. The family moved, and a referral was given for Mrs. White and Eddie in their new city. She chose to not accept the referral, stating that she did not want Eddie to have the stigma of therapy and that she did not want to start another relationship with a therapist, as the ending of therapy was so painful to her.

RECOMMENDATIONS FOR DSM-V

We would make several recommendations to be included in DSM-V. The first is a more explicit statement regarding the possibility of using personality disorder diagnoses with children and adolescents. This should include both the indications and the contraindications for the diagnosis.

Second, we would recommend that the headings for the criteria sets be revised to state that the criteria listed in each set could have begun in childhood and/or adolescence rather than, as presently stated, in early adulthood.

Third, the DSM text should include some statements regarding the treatability of these disorders, so that clinicians will not be immediately discouraged or frightened away from attempting treatment.

Fourth, the text should include material that will help the clinician make the differential diagnosis between Axis I and Axis II diagnoses.

Fifth, there needs to be the obvious, though necessary, injunction that the clinician be well versed in developmental norms.

Sixth, the criteria sets should include any particular childhood or adolescent manifestations of a personality disorder when such a manifestation differs substantially from the adult manifestation.

DISCUSSION AND CONCLUSIONS

"Cognitive therapy with children, as in work with adults, is founded upon the assumption that behavior is adaptive, and that there is an interaction between the individual's thoughts, feelings, and behaviors" (Reinecke, Dattilio, & Freeman, 1996, p. 2). Cognitive-behavioral treatments are of benefit to children, because they can be modified and tailored to meet the specific needs of the child. Therapeutic interventions focus on concrete concepts such as misinterpretation of information, reality testing, adaptive responses along a continuum, and basic problem-solving skills, rather than emphasizing insight. Everyday problems at school or home are addressed with the goal of developing a wider and better repertoire of coping skills. Using this basic framework, various cognitive-behavioral interventions can be utilized, such as time-management skills training, assertiveness training, problem-solving training, relaxation training, social skills training, self-management training, behavior analysis skills training, activity scheduling, self-monitoring, and developing adaptive self-talk.

Cognitive-behavioral therapy with children emphasizes the effects of maladaptive or dysfunctional beliefs and attitudes on current behavior. The presumption is made that the child's reaction to an event is influenced by the meanings he or she attaches to the event (Reinecke et al., 1996). When a child's behavioral and emotional responses to an event are maladaptive, it may be because the child lacks more appropriate behavioral skills or that his or her beliefs or problem-solving capacities are in some way disturbed (the cognitive elements). With this framework in mind, cognitive-behavioral therapists attempt to enable children to acquire new behavioral skills and provide them with experiences that foster cognitive change.

There is a need for protocols and research on each of the personality disorders in children and adolescents. We must develop new and more effective diagnostic tools, and sharpen our experience with existing tools. We have to evaluate "best practices" for treatment. What works best, with whom, in what time frame, and under what circumstances? We must be able to evaluate what are the idealistic goals for treatment, and what are the more realistic goals. Finally, we have to be ready to pay the price in staff time, clinician effort, and economic cost to treat these children.

Choosing to ignore the reality of personality disorders among children and adolescents, to downplay the problem, or to search for euphemistic terms all downplay the severity and impact of these disorders. The sooner we accept their reality, the sooner we will focus our efforts on treatment and relieve the suffering of these children.

REFERENCES

American Psychiatric Association. (1952). *Diagnostic and statistical manual of mental disorders*. Washington, DC: Author.

American Psychiatric Association. (1968). *Diagnostic and statistical manual of mental disorders* (2nd ed.). Washington, DC: Author.

American Psychiatric Association. (1980). *Diagnostic and statistical manual of mental disorders* (3rd ed.). Washington, DC: Author.

American Psychiatric Association. (2000). *Diagnostic and statistical manual of mental disorders* (4th ed., text rev.). Washington, DC: Author.

Beck, A. T., Freeman, A., & Associates. (1990). *Cognitive therapy of personality disorders*. New York: Guilford Press.

Bellak, L., & Bellak, S. S. (1948). *Children's Apperception Test*. Larchmont, NY: CPS.

Beren, P. (1998). *Narcissistic disorders in children and adolescents*. Northvale, NJ: Aronson.

Bleiberg, E. (2001). *Treating personality disorders in children and adolescents: A relational approach*. New York: Guilford Press.

Freeman, A. (1983). Cognitive therapy: An overview. In A. Freeman (Ed.), *Cognitive therapy with couples and groups* (pp. 1–10). New York: Plenum Press.

Freeman, A., & Leaf, R. (1989). Cognitive therapy of personality disorders. In A. Freeman, K. M. Simon, L. Beutler, & H. Arkowitz, *Comprehensive handbook of cognitive therapy* (pp. 403–434). New York: Plenum Press.

Freeman, A., Pretzer, J., Fleming, B., & Simon, K. M. (2003). *Clinical applications of cognitive therapy* (2nd ed.). New York: Kluwer Academic.

Goleman, D. (1995). *Emotional intelligence*. New York: Bantam Books.

Hanish, L. D., & Tolan, P. H. (2001). Antisocial behaviors in children and adolescents: Expanding the cognitive model. In W. J. Lyddon & J. V. Jones, Jr. (Eds.), *Empirically supported cognitive therapies: Current and future applications* (pp. 182–199). Springer.

Hanish, L. D., Tolan, P. H., & Guerra, N. G. (1996). Treatment of oppositional defiant disorder. In M. A. Reinecke, F. M. Dattilio, & A. Freeman (Eds.), *Cognitive therapy with children and adolescents* (pp. 62–78). New York: Guilford Press.

Harkness, S., & Super, C. M. (2000). Culture and psychopathology. In A. J. Sameroff, M. Lewis, & S. M. Miller (Eds.), *Handbook of developmental psychopathology* (pp. 197–214). New York: Kluwer Academic/Plenum.

Harrington, R. C. (2001). Childhood depression and conduct disorder: Different routes to the same outcome? *Archives of General Psychiatry, 58*(3), 237–238.

Johnson, J. G., Cohen, P., Brown, J., Smailes, E. M., & Bernstein, D. P. (1999). Childhood maltreatment increases risk for personality disorders during early adulthood. *Archives of General Psychiatry, 56*(7), 600–606.

Johnson, J. G., Cohen, P., Smailes, E. M., Skodol, A. E., Brown, J., & Oldham, J. M. (2001). Childhood verbal abuse and risk for personality disorders during adolescence and early adulthood. *Comprehensive Psychiatry, 42*(1), 16–23.

Johnson, J. G., Smailes, E. M., Cohen, P., Brown, J., & Bernstein, D. P. (2000). Associations between four types of childhood neglect and personality disorder symptoms during adolescence and early adulthood. Findings of a community-based study. *Journal of Personality Disorders, 14*(2), 171–187.

Kasen, S., Cohen, P., Skodol, A. E., Johnson, J. G., Smailes, E. M., Brook, J. S. (1999). Childhood depression and adult personality disorder: Alternate pathways of continuity. *Archives of General Psychiatry, 58*(3), 231–236.

Kernberg, P., Weiner, A. S., & Bardenstein, K. K. (2000). *Personality disorders in childhood and adolescence.* Northvale, NJ: Aronson.

Kramer, S., & Akhtar, S. (Eds.) (1994). *Mahler and Kohut: Perspectives on development, psychopathology, and technique.* Northvale, NJ: Aronson.

Masterson, J. (2000). *The personality disorders: A new look at the developmental self and object relations approach.* Phoenix, AZ: Zeig, Tucker.

Murray, H. A. (1943). *Thematic Apperception Test.* Cambridge, MA: Harvard University Press.

National Advisory Mental Health Council. (1995). Basic behavioral science research for mental health: A national investment: Emotion and motivation. *American Psychologist, 50*(10), 838–845.

Olin, S. S., Raine, A., Cannon, T. D., Parnas, J., Schulsinger, F., & Mednick, S. A. (1997). Childhood precursors of schizotypal personality disorder. *Schizophrenia Bulletin, 23*(1), 93–103.

Reinecke, M. A., Dattilio, F. M., & Freeman, A. (Eds.). (1996). *Cognitive therapy with children and adolescents.* New York: Guilford Press.

Ronen, T. (1997). *Cognitive developmental therapy with children.* New York: Wiley.

Rubin, K. H., Mills, R. S. L., & Rose-Krasnor, L. (1989). Maternal beliefs and child's competence. In B. H. Schneider, G. Attili, J. Nadel, & R. P. Weissberg (Eds.), *Social competence in developmental perspective* (pp. 313–331). Boston: Kluwer Academic.

Shapiro, T. (1997). The borderline syndrome in children. In K. S. Robson (Ed.), *The borderline child* (pp. 11–30). Northvale, NJ: Aronson.

Teicher, M. H., Ito, Y., Glod, C. A., Schiffer, F., & Gelbard, H. (1994). Early abuse, limbic system dysfunction, and borderline personality disorder. In K. R. Silk (Ed.), *Biological and neurobiological studies of borderline personality disorder* (pp. 177–207). Washington, DC: American Psychiatric Association.

Vela, R., Gottlieb, H., & Gottlieb, E. (1997). Borderline syndromes in children: A critical review. In K. S. Robson (Ed.), *The borderline child* (pp. 31–48). Northvale, NJ: Aronson.

Wolff, S., Townshend, R., McGuire, R. J., & Weeks, D. J. (1991). Schizoid personality in childhood and adult life: II. Adult adjustment and the continuity with schizotypal personality disorder. *British Journal of Psychiatry, 159,* 620–629.

SUGGESTED READINGS

Beck, A. T., Freeman, A., Davis, D. D., & Associates. (1990). *Cognitive therapy of personality disorders.* New York: Guilford Press.

Freeman, A., Pretzer, J., Fleming, B., & Simon, K. M. (2003). *Clinical applications of cognitive therapy* (2nd ed.). New York: Kluwer Academic.

Millon, T., & Davis, R. D. (1996). *Disorders of personality: DSM-IV and beyond.* New York: Wiley.

Perris, C., & McGorry, P. D. (Eds.). (1998). *Cognitive psychotherapy of psychotic and personality disorders.* New York: Wiley.

Index